Quality Evaluation in Non-Invasive Cardiovascular Imaging

Peter L. Tilkemeier • Robert C. Hendel
Gary V. Heller • James A. Case
Editors

Quality Evaluation in Non-Invasive Cardiovascular Imaging

Springer

Editors

Peter L. Tilkemeier
Department of Medicine
Greenville Health System
Greenville
South Carolina
USA

Gary V. Heller
Department of Cardiovascular Medicine
Atlantic Healthcare System
Morristown
New Jersey
USA

Robert C. Hendel
Miller School of Medicine
University of Miami
Miami
Florida
USA

James A. Case
Cardiovascular Imaging Technologies
Kansas City
Missouri
USA

ISBN 978-3-319-28009-7 ISBN 978-3-319-28011-0 (eBook)
DOI 10.1007/978-3-319-28011-0

Library of Congress Control Number: 2016936780

Printed on acid-free paper

This Springer imprint is published by Springer Nature
The registered company is Springer International Publishing AG Switzerland

Foreword

Quality: A Degree of Excellence

Quality. What does that word even mean? *"The standard of something as measured against other things of a similar kind; the degree of excellence of something." Oxford Dictionaries.*

In diagnostic testing, we can define quality as high value that leads to better outcomes for the patient tested.

But this does not happen by chance.

We have all seen those images, and perhaps more frequently, those reports of images, which are of low quality. They do not accurately represent the true state of the cardiac anatomy or physiology of the patient and cannot trustworthily guide further testing or management. The experienced referring physician may become less trusting of results, and may learn to adapt by layering tests, changing test referral patterns, or perhaps moving to more invasive testing strategies which they believe to be more definitive. The latter may increase costs and risks but also removes the potential diagnostic and prognostic benefit of non-invasive imaging.

In the USA, there is a move from volume-based to value-based purchasing of healthcare services. This transformation will dictate that 90 % of payments from Medicare will be related to quality measures within a few years of this printing. This includes mandatory laboratory accreditation for non-invasive imaging (as of 2012) and implementation of appropriate use criteria in decision support prior to ordering advanced cardiac imaging (as of 2017) in order to receive payments under the Medicare physician fee schedule.

This book is dedicated to increasing the level of quality in imaging by equipping the adaptable reader with the specific tools needed to navigate this sea change. Each area of non-invasive imaging has its own deep dive into how to improve quality. Whether motivated by our Hippocratic duty, medical liability concerns, or garnering fair payment for imaging services rendered, we all must strive for the highest level of quality in imaging. We must set and maintain quality as that degree of excellence, communicating it and even perseverating on it until it is uniform, commonplace, and widespread.

Chicago, IL, USA Kim Allan Williams, MD

Preface

Quality management is a journey, not a destination.
~Thomas H. Berry, leader in quality management development

A common theme among multiple international societies and organizations involved in cardiac imaging has become apparent in recent years: quality, due to its impact on all phases of cardiac imaging. Quality in imaging clearly has importance in clinical practice, is essential for accreditation, and signifies a laboratory that places patient care first. Quality in cardiac imaging impacts directly on patient care and may affect outcomes in a variety of ways. How quality initiatives are implemented in hospitals, clinics, and imaging centers is unclear and guidance is needed for laboratory's medical and technical directors and hospital administrators with regard to the development of quality improvement programs. This book is designed to serve as an important resource describing the importance of quality in cardiovascular imaging and how best to optimize an imaging laboratory.

Quality Evaluation in Non-Invasive Cardiovascular Imaging is designed to help physicians, technologists/technicians, and administrators develop their own quality programs. Discussions of each of the major cardiac imaging modalities (including computed tomography, cardiac magnetic resonance imaging, positron emission tomography, single-photon emission computed tomography, and echocardiography) are provided in a structured format. The first section addresses important global perspectives of the importance of quality, its relationship to value in the evolving role of non-invasive cardiac imaging, and the important role that accreditation plays in assuring quality. The final section presents tools for the reader to develop a meaningful quality improvement program, assists in preparing for accreditation, and suggests benchmarks for reporting quality. The overarching emphasis on quality in this book is of vital importance as part of the quest to advance the role of non-invasive cardiovascular imaging as "gatekeeper" to more expensive testing procedures and interventions.

As editors, we felt it important to assemble a group of authors that shared our vision as well as clinical expertise in each of the imaging modalities. With the group of experts contributing to this handbook, we believe that this book will be a valuable resource for all individuals interested in establishing high quality cardiac imaging services. Each modality-specific section is constructed of chapters addressing clinical applications of the imaging modality, appropriate patient and protocol selection and important elements for meaningful quality control and improvement programs addressing the needs for physician and technologist certification as well as laboratory accreditation. We anticipate that this book will serve as an important resource for the quality improvement activities in cardiac imaging laboratories and provide a day-to-day reference addressing quality issues as they may arise.

We invite you to begin on your quality improvement project for non-invasive cardiac imaging services and that Quality Imaging: A Handbook for Non-Invasive Cardiology will serve as a valuable resource in guiding you through that journey.

Greenville, SC, USA Peter L. Tilkemeier
Morristown, NJ, USA Gary V. Heller
Miami, FL, USA Robert C. Hendel
Kansas City, MO, USA James A. Case

Contents

Contributors

James A. Case, PhD Technical Director, Cardiovascular Imaging Technologies, Kansas City, MO, USA

Marcus Y. Chen, MD Cardiovascular and Pulmonary Branch, National Heart, Lung, and Blood Institute, National Institutes of Health, Bethesda, MD, USA

Cesia Gallegos, MD Department of Medicine, University of Miami Miller School of Medicine, Miami, FL, USA

Abhijit Ghatak, MD, MRCP Southwest Heart PC, Las Cruces, NM, USA

Linda D. Gillam, MD, MPH Department of Cardiovascular Medicine, Morristown Medical Center, Morristown, NJ, USA

Gary V. Heller, MD, PhD Department of Cardiovascular Medicine, Morristown Medical Center, Atlantic Healthcare System, Gagnon Cardiovascular Institute, Morristown, NJ, USA

Research Section, Intersocietal Accreditation Commission, Ellicott City, MD, USA

Robert C. Hendel, MD, FACC, FAHA, FASNC Cardiovascular Division Chief (Interim), University of Miami Miller School of Medicine, Miami, FL, USA

Steve W. Leung, MD Division of Cardiovascular Medicine, Departments of Medicine and Radiology, University of Kentucky, Lexington, KY, USA

Ryan Longmore, DO Department of Cardiology, Saint Luke's Hospital, Kansas City, MO, USA

Amgad N. Makaryus, MD, FACC, FACP, FASE, FSCCT Department of Cardiology, NuHealth, Nassau University Medical Center, East Meadow, NY, USA

Patty Reames, ARRT, CNMT, NCT, FASNC Practice Manager, Ohio State University Heart and Vascular Center, Bellefontaine, OH, USA

Ibrahim M. Saeed, MD, FACC, FAAP Saint Luke's Mid America Heart Institute Cardiovascular, University of Missouri, Kansas City, MO, USA

Sofia Shames, MD Department of Cardiology, Columbia University Medical Center, New York, NY, USA

Joseph Soltys, PhD MR Physics, Cardiovascular Imaging Technologies, LLC, Kansas City, MO, USA

Peter L. Tilkemeier, MD, MMM. Department of Medicine, Greenville Health System, Greenville, SC, USA

Seth Uretsky, MD, FACC Cardiovascular Fellowship Program, Atlantic Health System, Gagnon Cardiovascular Center, Morristown, NJ, USA

Part I
Overview

Chapter 1
The Importance of Quality

Peter L. Tilkemeier

Abstract Quality has evolved over the last five decades to a robust process assessing all aspects of the patient's, caregiver's, physician's and health system's experience and outcome. The importance of quality and the role it plays as we shift from volume to value based health care delivery systems is paramount. The quality process can be affected by all of those involved as well as the culture of the organization. Culture change can be an important part of ensuring high-quality outcomes. As health systems move from volume to value, imaging changes from a revenue center to an expense. Ensuring the highest quality outcomes from imaging, not just technically excellent images, but information that changes the delivery of healthcare at the patient level and affects satisfaction and morbidity and mortality will be essential.

Keywords Quality • Health care outcomes • Quality improvement processes

The quality improvement movement and medicine can be traced to the early 1900s when the Flexner report identified the lack of standardized requirements for medical schools. This initial standardization lead to the closing of a significant number of the medical schools at the time. In the late 1960s and early 1970s the work of Donabedian described the components of quality in terms of people, preferences, systems and effectiveness and the now familiar assessment paradigm of structure, process and outcome [1]. From this came the development of the ubiquitous quality assessment and quality assurance activities leading into the total quality management initiatives initiated by Toyota in the late 1980s. More recently, quality initiatives have been more centered around national initiatives such as the National Center for Quality Assurance (NCQA) and quality improvement efforts from the Center for Medicare and Medicaid Services (CMS). The current discussion is now one of changing the entire payment model for medicine from one of quantity to quality. Unfortunately, defining quality remains elusive due to the many different definitions and perspectives. Quality can be defined in many different ways. The definitions range from that

P.L. Tilkemeier, MD, MMM
Department of Medicine, Greenville Health System, Greenville, SC, USA
e-mail: ptilkemeier@gmail.com

P.L. Tilkemeier et al. (eds.), *Quality Evaluation in Non-Invasive Cardiovascular Imaging*, DOI 10.1007/978-3-319-28011-0_1

of the dictionary definition: (1) how good or bad something is (2) a characteristic or feature that someone or something has (3) something that can be noticed as a part of a person or thing: a high level of value or excellence [2]. To an individual perspective of "I know it when I see it" or as described by Deming, the father of the quality movement: (1) Quality is defined by the satisfaction of the customer; (2) Quality is dynamic and ever changing; and (3) To maintain a quality reputation, successful organizations must constantly adapt to change [3]. Depending upon the perspective of the person assessing, the definition of quality can vary widely. From a single patient perspective it may be exactly how something will affect them. From a physician perspective, quality can be measured as the effect on a single patient, multiple patients, their practice, or the group/hospital at which they practice. From an insurer perspective, the definition may look towards larger populations of patients and their overall outcome relative to a benchmark measures. Additionally, insurers may be assessing quality based upon the value of the care delivery which takes into account the cost necessary to achieve the quality measures [4].

The current emphasis on quality is driven by the poor performance outcomes noted in healthcare. Royer noted four drivers of the transformational change necessary if quality is to be improved. These are: (1) the lack of consistency in coordination of services among providers; (2) the high cost of care where prices and charges are unrelated to actual cost; (3) increasing physician dissatisfaction as physicians practice patterns become more guideline and protocol driven, and; (4) the current misalignment of vision with a focus on illness rather than wellness and volume rather than value [5]. In addition to these four drivers of transformational change in quality, other forces that are engaged in the marketplace include the increasing complexity of healthcare services and their delivery, customers and their knowledge, opinions, experience and other priorities. Furthermore, when taking a broader perspective, the cost and consequences of over use and inappropriate use and preventable errors enter into the equation.

One of the most important factors in limiting overuse, inappropriate use and preventable errors is a highly informed and engaged customer. Customer quality has been proposed as the third leg of the quality improvement effort [6]. Historically the quality improvement efforts have been focused around technical quality and service quality as defined by Berwick [7]. Technical quality has been defined as what the customer receives relative to what is known to be effective regarding the clinical or disease specific aspects of care and relates primarily to the healthcare provider. Service quality refers to the non-health aspects of care and the environment in which the care is delivered. It has been proposed that customer quality relates to those characteristics that the customer needs to effect improvement in the healthcare process, decision making and action to improve the quality of care delivered and received [6]. This conceptual scheme involves the customer in the delivery and decision making regarding their individual care. The use of the word "customer" can sometimes be sensitive as it relates to patients, however, in this setting many times the customer is not the patient. The customer can be a family member, a caregiver or a wellness visit patient and thus encompasses a much broader population than the use of the word patient alone.

Obtaining the highest level of quality of care delivery will require high levels of technical and service quality as well as high levels of customer quality. In order to achieve the highest level of customer quality three main attributes are necessary. These include a well-informed patient regarding knowing: (1) what and why to do; (2) how to do it and (3) the desire to do it [6]. Coaching a customer regarding these three major attributes will move the customer from a dependent stance to one who is interdependent and interacting effectively with all aspects of the healthcare delivery system. This important change in the paradigm of healthcare delivery will be necessary if we are truly going to affect the quality of care delivered.

Just as important as the empowered patient is to quality, the culture in which the care is delivered is essential. The first step in the necessary culture change to promote quality is one that is patient centric. In this model, provider convenience is relegated to a lesser importance. The major change in the perspective of the organizational culture that must be achieved are creating a safe and just culture within the organizational structure. Creating a culture of safety requires everyone in the organization to be practicing in a mindful and consciousness based manner while striving for perfection. This culture of mindfulness encourages the organization to be constantly evaluating workflow processes for any indications of a failure or hazard that may grow into an adverse event. If an organization is to obtain the high quality that will be necessary for the successful transformation of healthcare, it will be necessary to strive for perfection. Given the high volume with which healthcare organizations are functioning today, a small percentage error, are although seemingly acceptable, can lead to completely unacceptable population outcomes. It will no longer be acceptable to be good enough. Those organizations that hesitate in the process of quality improvement will soon find themselves passed by others that continue to strive for perfection. Thus an organization that was high performing becomes good while others strive for perfection and greatness [8]. For organizations to be successful and achieve this high functioning status, it will be necessary for them also to develop a just culture, characterized by a non-blaming quality improvement process [9]. This non-blaming process allows staff to report potential areas for improvement with the understanding that punitive measures will not be a result and requires civility on the part of all [10].

Those organizations which will be able to perform at the highest levels of quality are those that will include all of the tools mentioned as part of their quality initiatives to ensure a highly reliable and safe environment (Fig. 1.1). In addition to the utilization of the previously mentioned tools, understanding the importance of process improvement tools such as DMAIC: define, measure, analyze, improve and control; and their implementation in all aspects of the organization will be necessary to ensure quality outcomes. As part of this analysis, it is important to ensure that there is a continual return on investment as an organization strives to obtain perfection with regard to its quality. Most importantly, the return on investment is more than just a financial measure. As the organization is investing leadership, personnel, patient's and family's time and well-being, and the organizations dollars, the return on investment is important to be measured in other outcomes. These can include performance measures regarding the organization's mission, vision and values as well as goals outlined in the strategic plan from a leadership perspective. Second, patient satisfaction, well-being

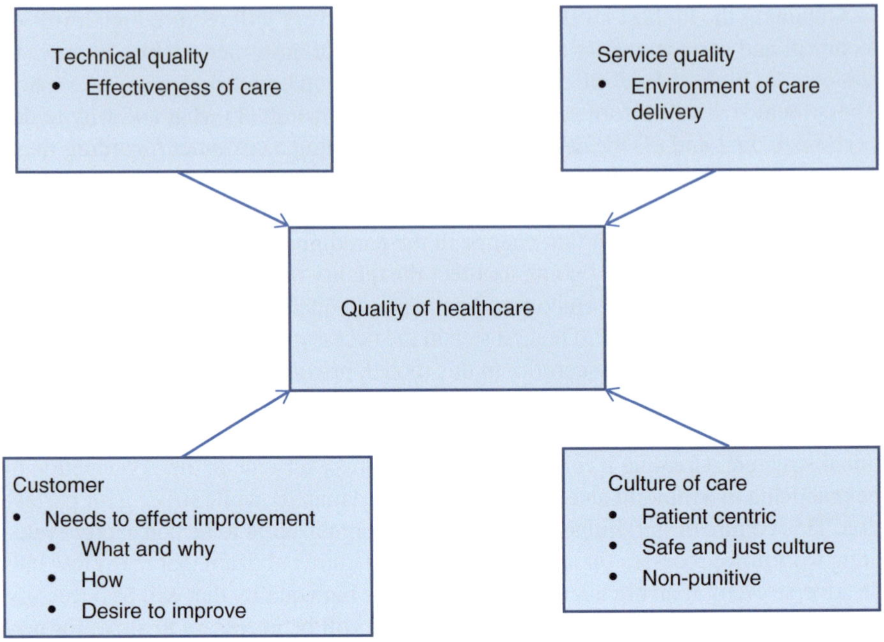

Fig. 1.1 Conceptual diagram outlining the four major components influencing quality in healthcare

and clinical outcomes from a patient and family perspective are important measures of success. Finally, financial outcomes given the financial resources that are invested in an effort to achieve the outcomes should be evaluated [10].

Therefore, quality is becoming central to everything that we will be doing in healthcare especially with regard to imaging. Developing tools and processes that allow us to continually improve, empowered patients and caregivers, and that have definable, measurable and comparable outcomes that allow assessment of organizational performance will be essential moving forward. If these are all done correctly patient, physician, insurer, regulatory agencies and large populations will all benefit [11]. The implications for imaging are significant. Quality of services delivered will become paramount, as imaging will become an expense rather than a revenue center as we move from volume to value. Determining the quality of an imaging study will no longer be determined only by the technical quality of the images but in terms of downstream care and health events such as functional status, quality of life, and reductions in morbidity and mortality [12].

References

1. Strite S, Stuart ME. Closing the quality and value gaps (part 3). Physician Exec. 2005;31(3):58–61.
2. http://www.merriam-webster.com/dictionary/quality. Accessed 1/3/15.

3. Deming WE. Out of the crisis. Cambridge, MA: Massachusetts Institute of Technology Center for Advanced Engineering Study; 1986.
4. Larson JS, Muller A. Managing the quality of health care. J Health Hum Serv Adm. 2002;25(3):280.
5. Royer TC. Adapting to the new healthcare market. Front Health Serv Manage. 2013;29(3):28–34.
6. Tabrizi JS, Wilson AJ, O'Rourke PK. Customer quality in health care. Letter to the editor. Patient Educ Couns. 2009;74(1):130–1. doi:10.1016/j.pec.2008.08.011. Epub 2008 Oct 1.
7. Kenagy J, Berwick D. Service quality in health care. J Am Med Assoc. 1999;281:661–5.
8. Cosgrove D, Fisher M, Gabow G, Gottleib G, Halvorson G, James B, Kaplan G, Perlin J, Petzel R, Steele G, Toussant J. A CEO checklist for high-value health care. Institute of Medicine (Internet). Published 5 Jun. Available from: www.iom.edu/~/media/Files/Perspectives-files/2012/Discussion-Papers/CEOHigh-ValueChecklist.pdf.
9. Marx D. Whack a mole: the prices we pay for expecting perfection. Plano: By Your Side Studios; 2009.
10. Blouin AS. High reliability: truly achieving healthcare quality and safety. Front Health Serv Manage. 2013;29(3):35–40.
11. Tooker J. The importance of measuring quality and performance in healthcare. Medscape Gen Med. 2005;7(2):49.
12. Lausing B. Patient-centered outcomes measuring quality and proving value in imaging. [Internet]. 2012 [cited 2015 Jan 10]. Available from: http://www.advisory.com/research/imaging-performance-partnership/the-reading-room/2012/11/patient-centered-outcomes-measuring-quality-and-proving-value-in-imaging.

Chapter 2
The Quality Cycle

Peter L. Tilkemeier

Abstract Due to the iterative pattern of quality improvement, numerous models have been developed that are referred to as quality cycles. Each model can offer unique advantages and disadvantages depending on the settings in which they are applied. The concept of cycles was foundational to the early quality efforts with the inception of the Plan-Do-Check-Act (PDCA) by Shewhart and Deming. Numerous variations based on this original model have been developed. As the sophistication of the processes that were being studied and improved increased, the models evolved into complex tools requiring special training and teams of individuals to implement and monitor. Each major quality cycle will be reviewed including the usual settings in which they can be most effective. Understanding these concepts allows evaluation and implementation of the methodology that is most likely to succeed in a particular setting.

Keywords Quality cycle • Plan-do-check-act • Lean • Six Sigma • Bridges to excellence • FMEA • Rapid cycle testing • Milestones • Breakthrough series model

The process of quality improvement is inherently iterative until a predetermined goal is reached. Following attainment of the goal, a monitoring process must be part of the plan to insure the process that was altered remains effective and maintains the desired outcome. As a result, models that have been developed to meet specific needs all rely on a cyclical process of evaluating the current state and describing an ideal future state; developing tools to implement the changes required; assessing the effectiveness of those tools and then repeating the process. This process has resulted in a number of quality cycle models being developed. A quality cycle model can range from a simple four step process to a much more complicated matrix methodology. It has evolved over the decades to meet the individual needs of the quality improvement process. As a result, it is important to know the various quality cycle models that are available and the strengths and weaknesses of each as it pertains to the quality improvement process that is being undertaken. Fourteen

P.L. Tilkemeier, MD, MMM
Department of Medicine, Greenville Health System, Greenville, SC, USA
e-mail: ptilkemeier@gmail.com

P.L. Tilkemeier et al. (eds.), *Quality Evaluation in Non-Invasive Cardiovascular Imaging*, DOI 10.1007/978-3-319-28011-0_2

quality cycle models will be described in this chapter describing their implementation, specific applications, scope, size and special features (Table 2.1), five will be considered in greater depth.

Table 2.1 Comparison of quality cycle models

Quality cycle	Project scope	Project size	Special features
PDCA/PDSA model	Variable – narrow to broad iterative	Small to large	Basis of other models
API model	Scalability regarding complexity of issues; used to develop new models or improve old models	Variable model dependent on team/project size	Three questions added to PDCA cycle
FOCUS-PDCA model	Maximize performance of pre-existing processes	Small to large	Developed by Hospital Corporation of America; variation of PDCA
FADE model	Problem focused	Small	Variation of PDCA
LEAN	Reduction of inefficiencies and waste adversely affecting performance	Usually large and multi-step serial processes	Numerous tools developed to facilitate. Need trained staff to facilitate improvement process
Six Sigma model	Reduce variation in currently functioning processes	Usually large and complex projects involving numerous teams	Reduces variability in process resulting in reduced waste and inventory and improved throughput
FMEA model	Predict future product failures due to prior failures; usually applied to new designs and processes	Usually utilized in multi-step cross departmental processes	Analysis based on severity, likelihood of occurrence and ability to detect future failure
5S model	Individual process improvement	Individual	Easily accomplished with training
Rapid cycle testing model	Decreasing time for implementation of improvements	Small to large, more effective in smaller populations	Developed by IHI, serial overlapping improvement process
Breakthrough series model	Collaboration among organizations to promote broad scope change	Large projects	Developed by IHI; barriers to success are required transparency among organizations that may be competitive
Milestones model	Assessment of process most likely to succeed;	Small to large	Serial process requiring completion of a step before proceeding to next step
Meyer model	Analysis of quality improvement and disconnect between data measurement and improvement	Aimed at physician change – small to large group	Numerous strategies included to promote change

(continued)

Table 2.1 (continued)

Quality cycle	Project scope	Project size	Special features
Al-Asaaf model	10 step model encompassing QA, QI, QC and total quality management	Large scale	Unifies all the major concepts of quality measurement and improvement
Bridges to excellence model	New process development to assure ability to apply Six Sigma improvement methodology following implementation	Small to large	Design of a process to allow implementation of Six Sigma improvement tools

PDCA Plan-D-Check-Act, *PDSA* Plan-Do-Study-Act, *API* Associates in Process Improvement, *FOCUS* Finding-Organizing-Clarification-Understanding-Selecting, *FADE* Focus-Analyze-Develop-Execute, *FMEA* failure mode effect analysis, *5S* sort, straighten, shine, standardized, sustain, *IHI* Institute for Healthcare Improvement, *QA* quality assurance, *QI* quality improvement, *QC* quality control

The concept of a quality improvement cycle was first published by Shewhart in the mid-1920s. Deming utilized this tool extensively and as such, he is often credited with its inception [1]. The Deming/Shewhart tool is especially useful in healthcare applications due to the inherent knowledge base of the healthcare delivery model as well as its values and disciplines by those who are implementing quality improvement [2]. In all of the quality improvement cycles, each step is dependent on the preceding step in that there must be significant coordination and balance between all of the steps to ensure an affective outcome [3]. This is reflected in the concept of "for a process to be improved it must be able to be measured" and the corollary argument of "do not measure things that you do not want to or cannot improve". It is also important to note and one of the difficulties with quality improvement processes is that they tend to be unique to the setting in which they are implemented. A successful quality improvement cycle implementation may require an entirely different set of tools to be successful in an institution with a different culture, mission, vision and values. This has made the generalizability of a particular quality improvement mechanism difficult and a reason for skepticism on the part of the practicing clinician when approached to participate in these activities. To better understand the unique characteristics of each quality cycle, the different models will be examined independently with regard to their strengths, weaknesses and usual implementation settings.

Plan-Do-Check-Act or Plan-Do-Study-Act (PDCA/PDSA)

The basis of all of the performance improvement models or quality cycles has some relation to the original quality improvement concept of Plan-Do-Check-Act or Plan-Do-Study-Act (PDCA/PDSA). The "planning" phase of this cycle includes defining an objective for the improvement project followed by inquiry into what the leaders think will happen during the process resulting in questions and projections. Having defined these two areas, a plan to carry out the cycle involving the necessary quality improvement team members, the goal of the project, a prospective timeline for major milestones in its accomplishment and the sites of implementation would need to be defined. The "doing" phase of the cycle is comprised of four major components: (1) Educating and training the staff who will be involved in the quality improvement process; (2) Developing a plan that allows implementation on a small scale or testing prior to broader implementation of the change; (3) Having implemented the small scale change, it is important to document any problems or unexpected observations that may occur during this phase of the change cycle; (4) Data generated from this small scale change project can begin to be analyzed using the quality control tools which are described in a later chapter. This completes the "doing" phase of the cycle. The third phase of the cycle entitled "Check/Study", includes an assessment and determination of the effect of the intervention with regards to the successful attainment of the goal or objective outlined in the planning phase. Detailed comparison of the results of the small scale change relative to predictions occurs during this phase. The lessons learned from the intervention are documented and shared with others as the team determines what changes are necessary for broad scale implementation. The final phase of the PDCA/PDSA cycle is "Act". During this phase organizational change is implemented depending upon the lessons learned during the prior three phases. Leadership will need to determine whether the plan can be implemented or if a second cycle is required to evaluate implementation of knowledge learned during the first cycle. Necessary changes to business processes will need to be implemented. Once implemented on a broad scale it is important to continue to evaluate the impact on quality improvement to identify any gaps in processes or performance of the initial intervention when more broadly applied within the organization. If further intervention is required due to the inability to obtain control of the process, the cycle can be restarted based upon the new knowledge obtained from the organization and implementation of the first cycle [4].

Associates in Process Improvement (API) Model

A variation on the PDCA cycle was the API improvement model. This model added three questions to the initiation and completion of the PDCA cycle. These questions were: what are we trying to accomplish, how do we know that the change results in improvement, and what change can we implement that will result in improvement? Focus on these three questions allowed scalability regarding the complexity of issues to be addressed through the improvement model. It additionally allowed variation based upon the size of the quality improvement team or whether this was to develop a new model or improve an old model of quality improvement [5].

"FOCUS"-PDCA Model

In the early 1990s, the Hospital Corporation of America formulated the next variation to the PDCA cycle. The key feature of this process was to maximize the performance of pre-existing processes. The preliminary steps leading up to the usual PDCA phase is the FOCUS acronym. In the focus acronym, "F" stands for finding a process that is in need of improvement. This includes defining the beginning and end of the process and determining who will benefit from the improvement. The "O" is for organizing a team of people knowledgeable regarding a process and should cross various levels of the organization. "C" is for clarification of current processes and the changes needed to achieve improvement. "U" is for understanding the potential for real causes of variation by measuring performance and whether or not the process to be improved is currently in a state of statistical process control. Finally, "S" is for selecting actions that are felt necessary to improve the process. Once these actions have been selected, the PDCA process can be implemented on those actions by the team that was identified [6, 7].

Focus Analyze Develop Execute (FADE) Model

The next variation on the PDCA improvement cycle is the FADE model developed by Organizational Dynamics. This was developed in early 2006. The methodology is more problem focused rather than systematic in its approach. The four phases are: Focus-choosing a problem and writing a statement to describe it; Analyze-learning more about the problem by gathering performance data; Develop-development of a solution and plan for implementing the solution; and Execute-implementing the plan and monitoring results with adjustments as necessary until success is documented [6].

LEAN Model

The LEAN model is specifically focused on reduction of inefficiencies which can adversely affect performance. This model originated in the Japanese automobile industry in the early 1990s. There is broad application of this methodology in healthcare in an effort to reduce waste within the healthcare system. Five principal areas of process improvement include value, value stream, flow, pull, and perfection. Value is defined as that which is important to the customers and ensures focus on their perspective, value stream insures all activities are necessary and valued to the process, flow implies the need for continuous processing throughout the value stream, pull signifies the drive for production due to demand and finally perfection is aimed at preventing defects and rework. There are eight

Table 2.2 Detailed steps in the LEAN process model

Step	Detail
1.	Definition of the performance problem from customer's perspective
2.	Examine current work procedures and diagram processes
3.	Gather improvement opportunities
4.	Identify root causes of the problem
5.	Develop proposed process diagram to address root causes
6.	Design an implementation plan for the change to include measures to determine success and a timeline

types of waste that were identified as part of the early LEAN work. These include unnecessary human movement, waiting for something needed to do your work, doing more than is necessary to meet requirements, poor quality work and rework to fix mistakes, excessive inventories resulting in resources that are waiting to be used, unnecessary movement of people, supplies and equipment in the process, products and services that customer's view as unnecessary to deliver the product and overproduction resulting in doing things that do not add value to the process.

The steps in a LEAN process include definition of the performance problem from the customers perspective as a first step (Table 2.2). Current work procedures are then examined and a diagram of the current process is created. This will help clarify the cause of the performance problem and provides the best information when described by those directly involved in the process. Improvement opportunities are gathered along with data to inform the team regarding the severity and frequency of the problem. As a result of the above, root causes of the problem can be identified and investigated. In response to the root causes that were identified, a proposed process diagram for a better way to do the work is evaluated and finally an implementation plan for the proposed new process is designed. This design includes measures to determine success as well as a completion timeline [6]. The LEAN process is very robust and designed to deal with complex system improvement throughout an organization. There is a broad spectrum of tools that are available to analyze and improve processes. There are numerous opportunities for specific training to acquire the skills necessary to fully utilize these tools as well as implement the Lean process in an organization.

Six Sigma Model

The Six Sigma model was developed in the 1980s and 1990s as a mechanism to reduce variation in business processes. It was initially implemented at Motorola and later refined by General Electric. It is quite popular in practice today with more than 20 % of recently surveyed physician executives utilizing this tool to improve healthcare performance. Reducing performance variability is the essence of a Six

Table 2.3 Detailed steps in the Six Sigma model

Step	Detail
1.	Defining the problem
2.	Measuring key aspects of current process
3.	Analyzing data from current process
4.	Implementing new processes
5.	Ensure control and improvement sustainability

Sigma quality improvement project. If successful, the defect rate should be less than 4 per 1 million opportunities. The five steps in a Six Sigma project include defining the problem, measuring key aspects of the process, data analysis, implementing improvements and finally ensuring control and sustainability of the improvement (Table 2.3). The process relies on three areas of emphasis which are: process variation control, an orientation towards results and the use of data to drive the process. Secondary effects of a uniform process derived from the implementation of Six Sigma are reduced waste, improved throughput and just in time inventory control [4, 6]. The Six Sigma process is very powerful in reducing variability and errors in processes. The process requires significant resources regarding data collection analysis and implementation of plans to correct error along with continuous reporting to ensure process change remains in place and there is no return to the prior practices.

Failure Mode Effect Analysis (FMEA) Model

Failure mode effect analysis is a mechanism to predict future product failure due to past failures [4]. This is usually reserved for evaluation of new designs and processes. The mechanism is primarily focused on the steps in a process that have the greatest potential for failure before that failure actually occurs. This results in a prioritization of failure modes based on severity, likelihood of recurrence and the ability to detect the potential for future failure. This is particularly helpful in the development of new processes within healthcare organizations given the multiple steps that could result in significant patient harm.

Five Steps (5S) Model

On an individual level there is a Japanese tool entitled 5S. The five steps allow a worker to implement change within their individual workplace to assure highest quality and productivity. The five steps are: sort, keeping only necessary items; straighten, arranging and identifying those items so that they can be easily retrieved; shine, keeping the workspace neat and clean; standardized, using best practice consistently; and sustained, maintaining current gains along with commitment to the process [4]. Implementation of the 5S model is at the individual level and fairly easily accomplished with minimal training. As this methodology is more individual, maintaining the process relies upon the individual's initiative to maintain improvement.

Rapid Cycle Testing Model

The Institute for Healthcare Improvement (IHI) has provided two mechanisms for quality improvement in the clinical setting. The first of these is rapid cycle testing or fast cycle time. This is a process designed to shorten the time for improvement from months to days for new process implementation while building significant staff engagement in the new process. It is important to note that rapid cycle improvement is not aimed at shorter development schedules or doubling the speed of current work as this will only increase the number of mistakes and limit the number of short-lived successes. For a rapid cycle time process to be successful, it is necessary for an organization to be redesigned into multifunctional teams with highly visible and measurable timelines and accountability to each other. This process also requires excellent communication skills between the teams. Additionally to be successful, rapid cycle improvement requires highest level leadership support as the process is very resource intensive. To be most effective, rapid cycle improvement requires overlap between implementation of the first change and evaluation, analysis and development of a second change in the cycle. The second cycle then is implemented while the third cycle starts the evaluation, analysis and development of the third change in the process. This is an iterative process until the goals are met for the process change project [4, 8]. Rapid cycle testing can be highly effective in an organization that needs to adapt quickly to changes in the surrounding environment with regard to its basic processes. The methodology garners support from large numbers of staff due to significant involvement at some stage in the process change. It does require excellent communication skills among the teams if it is to be successful.

Breakthrough Series Model

The second methodology that was derived from IHI is the breakthrough series model. The principal focus of this model is collaboration between large numbers of organizations working together over a defined period of time to improve a specific area of performance. Different models of change can be implemented in each of the organizations and then best practices are shared across those organizations including lessons learned and barriers to improvement. Leadership is provided by the IHI along with national experts. The use of this model results in implementation of widespread change affecting a larger population due to the broad collaborative nature of the team involved in developing the change. Barriers to success of this methodology include the need to openly share both successes and failures with other team members who may be in competitive markets, development of new communication models to share best practices across organizations, and the need for high level resources to accomplish and overcome these barriers [9]. The breakthrough series model affords the opportunity for collaboration across multiple organizations and thus affects change on a broader basis. Due to the need to build consensus regarding this change the process is not appropriate for those quality improvement initiatives that require more rapid implementation. Communication and sharing of information across organizations which are not used to this level of transparency can be a hindrance to its utilization.

Milestones Model

Also important in the clinical application of a quality cycle is the ability of an organization to evaluate its processes and measures to determine those which have the greatest opportunity for improvement. This is a more recent paradigm for evaluation developed by Lloyd and presented as seven milestones for an organization to be successful (Table 2.4). The seven milestones are: (1) Developing a measurement philosophy and involvement of measurement in the day-to-day functioning within the organization. A measurement of success in this milestone is that data is not being collected because you are told to but because someone wants to learn more about process variation within the organization. (2) Identifying the types and categories of concepts to be measured. This milestone ties the organizations strategic objectives to its quality improvement work. (3) Identifying specific measures for improvement. Specificity regarding the measure and ensuring appropriate data collection is an important part of this milestone. (4) Development of operational definitions of specific measures. It is important that an organization understands the definition to ensure consistent data collection and focus on a question for analytics. (5) The fifth step is to develop a data collection plan and gathering of the data. Many times the organization will fall into the predicament of utilizing current data because

Table 2.4 Detailed steps for the milestones for quality improvement model

Step	Detail
1.	Developing a measurement culture and incorporating into daily function
2.	Identify types and categories to be measured
3.	Identify specific measurements for improvement
4.	Develop operational definitions of the measures
5.	Develop and implement a data collection plan
6.	Data analytics using process control tools
7.	Develop and implement process improvement plans

it is easily available, however, not the most applicable to the question at hand. Specific data collection tools and resources to ensure adequate sampling and recording of the data is a necessary outcome from this step. This may require outside expertise to ensure consistency and reliability. (6) The sixth step in the process is data analytics including utilization of statistical process control methodology described in a later chapter and development of analytics for potential future processes. (7) The last step is the data collection necessary for the organization to develop plans regarding process improvement including implementation plans. This includes the investment in the resources for and the actual potential for execution of the process improvement [10]. The milestones model encourages an organization to address change in a serial manner. In order to progress to the next milestone, the requirements for all of the prior ones must be met. Although this can slow process, it insures success due to completion of each of the steps required to affect change.

Meyer Model

In a more specific model aimed at analyzing quality improvement and the disconnect between data measurement and improvement, Meyer proposes the following quality improvement cycle. The steps in the cycle include identification of an opportunity for improvement which leads to a plan for improvement followed by an intervention to the process. Outcomes from the intervention are then measured and compared to results that were available prior to the intervention or from other organizations. Based on the results from this comparison, further changes to the process are implemented and the cycle restarts with identification of new opportunities for improvement. As this cycle is principally based on physician change and quality improvement, Meyer additionally noted some representative strategies which could be applied. These included audit and feedback, use of regulations, focused incentives, behavioral interventions, the use of local opinion leaders and outreach visits to improve information, educational interventions including continuing medical education and self-instructed learning, and the use of information systems including reminder systems and computer decision support systems as mechanisms to affect improvement [3]. Many times a multifactorial approach with regard to application of the strategies is necessary for success.

Al-Assaf Model

In an effort to incorporate the concepts of quality assurance, quality improvement, quality control and total quality management, Al-Assaf developed a ten step quality management cycle. The first step is to plan for the process change, step 2 is standards setting, step 3 is communication of the standards, step 4 is monitoring the current process to insure it is in control, step 5 is to identify and prioritize opportunities for improvement, step 6 defines the opportunities for improvement, step 7 identifies the team to work on opportunities for improvement, step 8 analyzes and studies the opportunity for improvement with data gathering and analysis, step 9 is choosing and designing a solution to address the problem and step 10 is implementation of the solution. Step 10 can lead to further cycles that can start either at step 1, 2, 3 or 4 depending upon the solution and its implementation plan. This cycle applies all four quality activities. In the early steps of the process quality assurance is addressed, quality control is addressed in step 4 and quality improvement in steps 5 through 10. Total quality management is addressed throughout the entire cycle. This cycle follows all aspects of quality improvement in modern healthcare organizations [11].

Bridges to Excellence Model

The most recent model for quality improvement was derived by General Electric and is a variation on its previously described Six Sigma methodology. GE realized that if it was to utilize Six Sigma methodology to minimize defects, improve quality and reduce cost that it would be imperative to design processes that would be amenable to Six Sigma analysis. This new design methodology when applied in healthcare was entitled Bridges to Excellence. The process involves five steps. The first is initiation during which the need is defined including the scope, timeline and resources necessary for success. The second step is to define those measures which are critical to quality and define the customer's needs. Examples of this include well-defined performance measures that are within the provider's control, thresholds that are attainable and the provision of accurate and comprehensive data. The third step in the process is to define program specifications including high level design and evaluation of the design. The fourth step is to develop detailed designs, evaluation of those detailed designs and development and verification of a control plan regarding the process once implemented. Finally, is executing a pilot program and analysis of the results from this pilot with implementation in full scale production along with future vision for the product. Important key elements to success include ensuring that the rewards for excellence are as meaningful as possible, that the program's administratively simple and that the implementation of new processes would not be disruptive to current successful processes [12]. The Bridges to Excellence program is unique in that it is designed to build a process that is amenable to the application of other quality improvement processes, such as Six Sigma. This is a powerful tool and serves as recognition of the importance of ongoing quality improvement processes for organizational success.

In summary, the process of quality and the cyclical nature of its improvement mechanisms have been in place for almost a century. There has been significant evolution in the processes over that timeframe given the increasing complexity of the systems and which will work whether it be manufacturing or the delivery of healthcare. Cardiac imaging, as will be noted in Chap. 4, is a complex process which should benefit significantly from application of the quality cycle methodology.

As healthcare workers in the field of cardiac imaging, it is important to understand how each of these quality cycle tools can help to improve the quality within each of our facilities. Those that have had the greatest success in healthcare applications have been evaluated in greater depth and include: FOCUS-PDCA, LEAN, Six Sigma, FMEA and the Milestones models. Evaluation of the relative strength, weaknesses, and resources necessary for success and potential outcomes will ensure the ability to select the correct quality cycle improvement tool when addressing a specific problem.

References

1. Deming WE. Out of the crisis. 2nd ed. Cambridge, MA: MIT Center for Advanced Engineering Study; 1986.
2. Deming WE. The new economics for industry, education, government. Cambridge, MA: MIT Center for Advanced Engineering Study; 1993.
3. Meyer GS. Balancing the quality cycle: tackling the measurement-improvement gap in health care. Part I. Nutrition. 2001;17(2):172–4.
4. Warren K. Quality improvement: the foundation, processes, tools, and knowledge transfer techniques. In: Ransom ER, Joshi MS, Nash DB, Ransom SB, editors. The healthcare quality book: vision, strategy, and tools. 2nd ed. Chicago: Health Administration Press; 2008.
5. Langley G, Nolan K, Nolan T, Norman C, Provost L. The improvement guide: a practical approach to enhancing organizational performance. San Francisco: Jossey-Bass; 1996.
6. Spath PL. Introduction to healthcare quality management. 2nd ed. Chicago: Health Administration Press; 2013. p. 111–30. Chapter 5, Continuous improvement.
7. McLauglin CP, Kaluzny AD. Continuous quality improvement in healthcare: theory, implementation, and applications. 2nd ed. Gaithersburg: Aspen Publishers; 1999. p. 3–33. Chapter 1, Defining quality improvement: past, present, and future.
8. Choperena AM. Fast cycle time-driver of innovation and quality. Res Technol Manag. 1996;39(3):36–40.
9. Institute for Healthcare Improvement. Home page. [Internet]. 2015 [cited 10 Jan 2015]. Available from: http://www.ihi.org.
10. Lloyd RC. Milestones in the quality measurement journey. In: Ransom ER, Joshi MS, Nash DB, Ransom SB, editors. The healthcare quality book: vision, strategy, and tools. 2nd ed. Chicago: Health Administration Press; 2008.
11. Al-Assaf A. Organizational quality infrastructure: how does an organization staff quality? In: Ransom ER, Joshi MS, Nash DB, Ransom SB, editors. The healthcare quality book: vision, strategy, and tools. 2nd ed. Chicago: Health Administration Press; 2008.
12. De Brantes F. How purchasers select and pay for quality. In: Ransom ER, Joshi MS, Nash DB, Ransom SB, editors. The healthcare quality book: vision, strategy, and tools. 2nd ed. Chicago: Health Administration Press; 2008.

Chapter 3
The Quality/Cost/Value Relationship

Peter L. Tilkemeier

Abstract The cost of healthcare in the United States is growing at a rate that is non-sustainable given its percentage of the gross domestic product. This is in the setting of poor quality as defined by preventable mortality, access to care and equitable and efficient care delivery measured relative to other nations. Given the potential significant growth in individuals requiring healthcare, emphasis must be placed on the improvement in the value of care delivery. In order to improve the value, quality must be improved, or cost/or volume must be reduced in order to effect the value = quality/cost equation. The cost of quality theoretical model will be reviewed to understand how this has evolved as we move through the quality improvement era. Mechanisms to improve quality and cost including value stream analysis, value on investment and the use of interdisciplinary teams to improve the value of healthcare delivery will be examined.

Keywords Quality • Cost • Value • Interdisciplinary collaboration • Cost of quality modeling • Value analysis • Value on investment • Process improvement programs

There is uniform awareness that the cost of healthcare in the United States continues to grow more rapidly than the gross domestic product with a prediction in 2015 that the total healthcare spending will consume approximately 20 % of the gross domestic product [1]. Despite this significant level of spending, in 2009 the United States ranked 27 out of 34 Organization for Economic Co-operation and Development Nations in terms of life expectancy at birth [2]. This is not a tenable situation and suggests that unless intense efforts regarding changing the paradigm of healthcare delivery and reimbursement should be implemented. An important part of this paradigm change is the introduction of value into the equation. Value can be defined as the quality of the care received divided by the cost to deliver the care [3, 4]. Most recently the Agency for Healthcare Research and Quality and its 2007 report entitled National Health Care Quality noted three important aspects: (1) Healthcare quality continues to improve but at a slower rate; (2) Variation in healthcare quality delivery is diminishing but not for all measures; and (3) We have a long way to go to reach a target [5].

P.L. Tilkemeier, MD, MMM
Department of Medicine, Greenville Health System, Greenville, SC, USA
e-mail: ptilkemeier@gmail.com

P.L. Tilkemeier et al. (eds.), *Quality Evaluation in Non-Invasive Cardiovascular Imaging*, DOI 10.1007/978-3-319-28011-0_3

Defining quality can be difficult as we are moving towards more population-based decision-making. Additionally, standard outcome measures such as event free survival, control of the underlying condition, or other measures which would traditionally be used in a randomized phase III clinical trial are now potentially facilitated by the addition of health-related quality of life and comparative effectiveness research [6]. The benefit of these measures in the definition of the quality portion of the equation is important as many clinical decisions can or no longer will be based on randomized clinical trials. This may be due to the inherent biases among the trialists or the potential inability to randomize due to ethical concerns for certain trials. The ability to use large registry based populations in the comparative effectiveness analysis will facilitate the definition of quality in the equation.

There are two major approaches to improving the value of healthcare. The first would diminish the cost side of the equation while the second would improve the quality factor. Addressing the cost side of the equation from the provision of care perspective, the most important factors include the increasing prevalence of chronic disease in the population, the increasing size of the population at risk, increasing cost associated with technological advances and the impact of defensive medical practice. Examples of these include the greater than twofold increase in the prevalence of obesity in the US population as estimated by the Centers for Disease Control, a near threefold increase in 30 years in the prevalence of diabetes, and a very high prevalence of risk factors for coronary artery disease [7–9]. Improving technology has led to significant expansion of the cost side of the equation. Estimates have the increase in technology responsible for slightly more than 50 % of the rising healthcare spending in the last 50 years [10]. Most of these advanced technologies have been focused on the treatment of chronic conditions as opposed to the cure of acute problems. This further adds to the problem of increasing life expectancy and resulting longer care with high cost technology. The cost of defensive medicine continues to rise and will do so until appropriate reform is in place. Finally, the aging of the baby boomer generation with increasing life expectancy has led to the US Census Bureau projecting from 2010 to 2050 that the number of Americans over age 65 will double to 84 million and those over 85 increase to 18 million [11, 12]. With all of these simultaneous effects on the cost side of the equation, if we are to obtain any increase in value, there will need to be significant improvement with regard to quality or in the way in which we receive payment for these services.

Important mechanisms to address cost control are starting to be put into place today with greater sharing of data across healthcare systems to eliminate duplicative testing. Efforts at this have been unsuccessful in the past, perhaps because of attempting to initiate changes in a setting where cost savings was not of paramount importance. Other efforts underway to improve the cost side of the equation include care standardization and redesign, care coordination across multiple care settings and the use of decision support to predict those patients which are most likely to have negative outcomes allowing for reallocation of resources to address this increased risk. Additionally, this is happening in an environment of greater sharing of the cost of healthcare with the patients. The sharing of costs has produced greater patient engagement. This increased engagement has resulted in increasing healthy behaviors, improved adherence to disease management strategies and alignment of overall goals [13].

From the quality perspective, it will be important to address all potential quality measures. The measures that will be most important will depend upon the perspective of the person or organization performing the measurement. For example, the healthcare system or insurer will be most interested in the ability to change a population outcome. From a patient perspective, quality may be measured much differently. This could include the perceived quality of the care delivered, the achievement of a favorable outcome, such as control of blood pressure and do I feel better with the initiation of the therapy and finally, is it affordable. From the provider perspective, the quality definition will also vary. Factors included in this variability will potentially be tied to compensation, sense of ability to deliver high-quality care and satisfied patients, financial viability of the practice and ability to meet national standards and insurer goals. There are currently and will be a plethora of measures and measurement tools developed in an effort to define quality. It will be important to have these coordinated across specialties, health care delivery systems, and payors. Efforts by the National Committee on Quality Assurance to define the measures including numerator and denominator inclusion and exclusion characteristics will be key to this moving forward.

Theoretical Modeling

From a theoretical perspective, the cost of quality model was developed in the late 1980s to help understand the relationship between the cost of a unit of good product compared to the performance in quality [14]. As shown in Fig. 3.1, the model proposed that the lowest cost of production of a product was determined by the intersection of the costs of failure and the costs of achieving perfection. This was usually at a quality level of less than perfection secondary to the high cost of achieving perfection. With the introduction of the quality improvement initiatives initiated by Shewhart and Deming, the cost of perfection was lowered. This caused the curve to change from a U-shaped model (representing the increased cost associated with increased quality) to one more approximating a hockey stick (relatively flat costs once high quality is achieved). There is no greater cost in this model than not conforming to 100 % quality. This second model seems more appropriate to the delivery of healthcare today. The progression to "perfection" is demonstrated in Fig. 3.2. With increased emphasis on improvement in quality, the curve changes shape over time leading to the lowest cost being 100 % quality performance. This is a model in which we note the quality of care changing and achieving highest value through reduction in cost to achieve 100 % quality performance. This is important to consider as we look at both individual and population based health care delivery. Whether it is an individual patient's out-of-pocket expense or a healthcare system's total dollars spent, perfection is the lowest possible cost in today's system. This will, however, be difficult to achieve. Multiple efforts have been aimed at both cost and quality, but as demonstrated by this model, more importantly quality will be essential if we are to achieve highest value with delivery of care today.

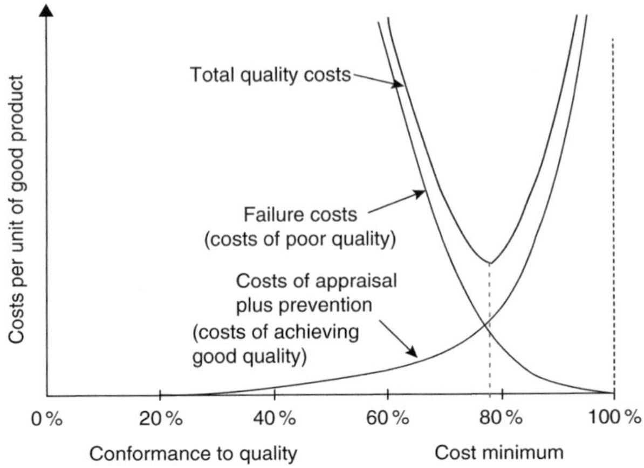

Fig. 3.1 The cost of quality. The cost minimum is achieved where the cost of failure and the cost of quality is lowest. This model assumes increasing cost to achieve 100 % quality and that less than 100 % quality is acceptable (From Freiesleben [22] published by Taylor & Francis Ltd. Reprinted by permission of Taylor & Francis Ltd.)

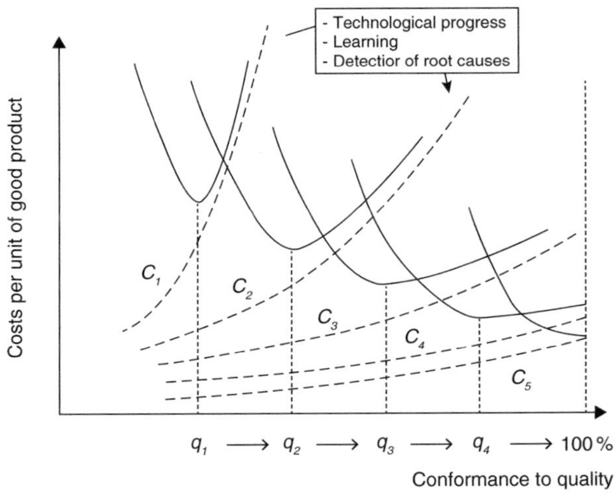

Fig. 3.2 The cost of quality. As systems evolve to a state of 100 % quality, the cost of achieving this declines as shown by the five different condition c1–c5. As the cost of less than 100 % quality is high, the goal is 100 % quality and this becomes the lowest cost point (From Freiesleben [22] published by Taylor & Francis Ltd. Reprinted by permission of Taylor & Francis Ltd.)

Mechanisms for Achieving Value

There are many examples of ways that value has been introduced into the quality of healthcare. These include value analysis programs and professionals, value on investment assessment of tools to improve quality and decrease cost, and process improvement programs. As value analysis has become an important part of the healthcare delivery system, educational and professional organizations have developed leading to the Association of Healthcare Value Analysis Professionals and their statement of purpose: “A value analysis professional is dedicated to clinicians and multidisciplinary teams to ensure optimal patient outcomes through clinical efficacy of healthcare products and services for the greatest financial value” [15]. Through the use of value analysis professionals in an organization the greatest effect is seen on the cost portion of the equation. The value analysis professional leads value analysis teams creating synergy between clinicians and supply chain providers. This ensures consistent decision making and support across the continuum of procurement. Furthermore, the value analysis professional will help organize supply utilization to ensure optimal use of scarce commodities. The use of evidence-based processes to assess and compare clinical value where available allows the greatest leverage to a decision that is fact based and objective and aligns with high-quality medical care. Utilization of resources to automate the value analysis process will be important for its ongoing success. Examples might include providing clinicians with the cost of a procedure based upon real time use of resources along with comparison to their peer groups within the organization [16, 17].

With regard to tools that assist with determining the value on investment, computerized physician ordering entry is an excellent example. The utilization of computerized physician order entry has been shown to significantly decrease medication errors as well as decrease the time spent in processing paper orders. An important part of an investment in new technology, like computerized physician order entry is to assure that the value statement that was proposed when this was being considered is actually met after implementation. Important baseline measures need to be identified and followed throughout the process to ensure that the organization is truly meeting its value on investment that was planned at inception of the project. Seldom does investment in technology allow reduction in staffing; better utilization of the staffing to improve quality and care delivery can be an expected outcome. Value on investment initiatives can improve both core and support processes through the utilization of key performance indicators such as access and revenue cycle, ordering in pharmacy, health information management, clinical documentation and information technology. These will potentially benefit the strategic areas of operational benefits; patient, physician and staff satisfaction; improvement in quality; and greater compliance with numerous regulatory bodies. Utilizing these core and support process measures, the system can measure value on investment and result in improved performance throughout the system. This could potentially replace the traditional return on investment as measured by financial performance alone [18].

Process improvement programs have been developed to help systems of care improve delivery of value in the healthcare setting. Whether it is on a large model driven basis or through individual projects within organizations, the importance of value to the organization cannot be stressed enough. A unifying theme across all of these initiatives is the importance of interdisciplinary collaboration. Development of an interdisciplinary team to improve a process is necessary in today's complex, matrix management healthcare delivery models. Representatives from all aspects of the patient care experience are essential if changes in care delivery to improve the value are to be successful. As one example, demonstrated by Britto-Rossi, the implementation of interdisciplinary teams can add significantly to both the cost and quality portions of the equation driving both in a favorable direction [19]. On a more theoretical basis, an eight step approach to a sustainable value proposition has been proposed. In recognition of the array of challenges that can occur in creating a sustainable value proposition the steps are relatively broad in scope. The eight steps include: (1) Establish an institutional vision; (2) Develop organizational structure; (3) Decide what to measure; (4) Collect the right data; (5) Analyze the relevant data; (6) Interpret the relevant data; (7) Create internal transparency; (8) Create external transparency (Fig. 3.3). Within each of these process steps, the author's identify models of implementation which will be more easy or difficult to achieve. Those that are more easily achieved include an internal focus with relatively available data and low-level analytics with small group implementation. Those that are more difficult include looking outside of the organization to establish broadly accepted measures, use large data and population based analysis leading to risk adjusted methods methodologies and system, region or network implementation [20]. A group of eleven large healthcare system CEOs have also developed a checklist of ten strategies aimed at improving quality and reducing cost leading to higher value performance. These are summarized in Table 3.1 and include: (1) A culture of continuous improvement; (2) Embedded safeguards; (3) Use of evidence protocols; (4) Ensuring high value is a governance priority; (5) Integrating care; (6) Internal transparency; (7) Information technology best practices are implemented; (8) Programmatic assessment of resource utilization; (9) Implementation of shared decision making; and (10) Targeted services. As a system of care moves through this eight step model or the ten strategies the value curve noted in Fig. 3.2 becomes more easily achiev-

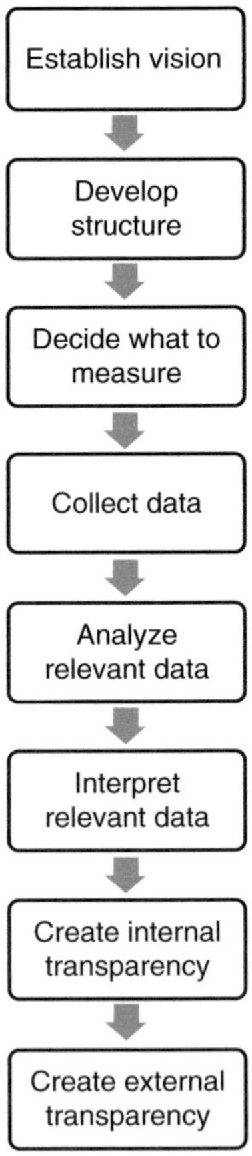

Fig. 3.3 Proposed eight step approach to a sustainable value proposition

Table 3.1 Checklist of ten strategies leading to higher value performance

	Strategy
1.	Culture of continuous improvement
2.	Embedded safeguards
3.	Use of evidence protocols
4.	Ensuring high value is a governance priority
5.	Integrating care
6.	Internal transparency
7.	Best practices in information technology
8.	Programmatic assessment of resource utilization
9.	Implementation of shred decision making
10.	Targeted services

able as the organization is delivering the highest possible quality at the lowest possible cost [21, 22]. Implementation of all or some of these initiatives, either partially or completely, will improve the ability of the organization to respond to the change from volume to value and maximize quality during the transition.

Summary

The relationship between quality, cost, volume and value is a complex one. There are numerous mechanisms proposed to evaluate each of the factors contributing to overall value. Some of these are more developed and readily implemented than are others. It is important for healthcare delivery systems to understand the absolute need to deliver value in today's world. These systems can be as small as the local practice office or as large as a multi-state clinically integrated network. Utilizing interdisciplinary approaches and value analysis methodology will be essential if society is successful in improving the value of health care delivered today.

References

1. Centers for Medicare and Medicaid Services. National health expenditure data. [Internet] 2008 [cited 2015 Feb 17]. Available from: http://www.cms.gov/Research-Statistics-Data-and-Systems/Statistics-Trends-and-Reports/NationalHealthExpendData/index.html?redirect=/NationalHealthExpendData/25_NHE_Fact_Sheet.asp#TopOfPage.
2. The World Bank. Health expenditure, total (% of GDP). [Internet] 2013 [cited 2015 Feb 16]. Available from: http://data.worldbank.org/indicator/SH.XPD.TOTL.ZS?order=wbapi_data_value_2011+wbapi_data_value+wbapi_data_value-last&sort=desc.
3. Healthcare Financial Management Association. Common definitions. [Internet] 2015 [cited 2015 Feb 17]. Available from: http://www.hfma.org/Content.aspx?id=24225.

4. Agency for Healthcare Research and Quality. National Healthcare Quality Report 2007. [Internet] 2007 [cited 2015 Feb 17]. Available from: http://archive.ahrq.gov/qual/nhqr07/nhqr07.pdf.
5. Healthcare Financial Management Association. The future of U.S. health care: value = quality/cost. (Industry Update). 2009 Buyer's Resource Guide. Healthc Financ Manage. 2008:22–5.
6. Konski A. Cost, quality, and value in healthcare: a new paradigm. Oncology (Williston Park). 2010;24(6):542–3.
7. Ogden CL, Carroll MD, Kit BK, Flegal KM. Prevalence of obesity in the United States, 2009–2010. NCHS Data Brief. 2012;82:1–8.
8. Centers for Disease Control and Prevention. Crude and age-adjusted percentage of civilian, noninstitutionalized adults with diagnosed diabetes, United States, 1980–2012. [Internet] 2013 [cited Feb 17]. Available from: http://www.cdc.gov/diabetes/statistics/prev/national/figage.htm.
9. Centers for Disease Control and Prevention. Division for heart disease and stroke prevention: data trends & maps. [Internet] 2015 [cited 2015 Feb 17]. Available from: http://nccd.cdc.gov/DHDSP_DTM/Default.aspx.
10. Congressional Budget Office. Technological change and the growth of health care spending. [Internet] 2008 [cited Feb 17]. Available from: http://www.cbo.gov/sites/default/files/cbofiles/ftpdocs/89xx/doc8947/01-31-techhealth.pdf.
11. US Census Bureau. Population: estimates and projections by age, sex, race/ethnicity. [Internet] 2012 [cited Feb 17]. Available from: https://www.census.gov/compendia/statab/cats/population/estimates_and_projections_by_age_sex_raceethnicity.html.
12. US Census Bureau. 2012 National population projections: summary tables. [Internet] 2012 [cited Feb 17]. Available from: https://www.census.gov/population/projections/data/national/2012/summarytables.html.
13. Gordon JE, Leiman JM, Deland EL, Pardes H. Delivering value: provider efforts to improve the quality and reduce the cost of health care. Annu Rev Med. 2014;65:447–58.
14. Plunkett JJ, Dale BG. Quality costs: a critique of some "economic cost of quality" models. Int J Prod Res. 1988;26(11):1713–26.
15. Association of Healthcare Value Analysis Professionals. Homepage. [Internet] 2015 [cited Feb 17]. Available from: http://www.ahvap.org.
16. Yokl RW, Tinker P. Having my say: leading practices in value analysis drive quality, cost effectiveness. [Internet]. 2014 [cited 2015 Feb 8]. Available from: http://www.hpnonline.com/inside/2014-06/1406-HMS-AHVAP.html.
17. Association for Healthcare Resource & Materials Management. White paper – cost, quality, and outcomes: the supply chain value equation. [Internet]. 2014 [cited 2015 Feb 8]. Available from: http://www.ahrmm.org/ahrmm/kc_documents/whitepapers_case_studies/2013_AHRMM_Executive_Thought_Leader_Forum.jsp.
18. Taylor R, Manzo J, Sinnett M. Quantifying value for physician order-entry systems: a balance of cost and quality. Healthc Financ Manage. 2002;56(7):44–8.
19. Brita-Rossi P, Adduci D, Kaufman J, Lipson SJ, Totte C, Wasserman K. Improving the process of care: the cost-quality value of interdisciplinary collaboration. J Nurs Care Qual. 1996;10(2):10–6.
20. Makadon HJ, Bharucha F, Gavin M, Oliveira J, Wietecha M. Value management: optimizing quality, service, and cost. J Healthc Qual. 2010;32(1):29–34.
21. Evans M. Higher-value performance: checklist's 10 strategies aimed at improving quality, cutting costs. Mod Healthc. 2012;42(24):8–9.
22. Freiesleben J. On the limited value of cost of quality models. Total Qual Manag Bus Excell. 2004;15(7):959–69.

Chapter 4
The Complexity of the Non-invasive Cardiac Imaging Process

Peter L. Tilkemeier

Abstract The noninvasive cardiac imaging clinical processes are complex secondary to the numerous providers and staff involved from initial patient evaluation through to test completion and communication of results. Factors which additionally impact the clinical processes include appropriate use criteria, utilization management, test selection, "cost" of the test, potential risk and communication of the results with implications for next diagnostic and/or therapeutic steps. The importance of guideline development and clinical implementation of decision support algorithms to simplify the process in the future will be necessary.

Keywords Multi-modality imaging • Appropriate use criteria • Clinical guidelines • Test substitution • Decision support algorithms • Physician communication • Physician education

Cardiac imaging is one of the most complex clinical processes that we have in medicine. It is a series of steps occurring in either a parallel or serial fashion resulting in a report to their referring physician/healthcare provider regarding a patient's condition (Fig. 4.1). The complexity of cardiac imaging is amplified by the multiple modalities presently available, the cost of the procedure, the potential risk to the patient, requirements for training of the staff performing the procedure, clear communication of the results and understanding of the impact of the results regarding the next step in providing care to the patient. Other confounding factors include the training and knowledge of the physician ordering the study to insure the test ordered is the most appropriate for answering the clinical question. Each of these steps will be examined separately to allow focus on their impact on the entire process.

P.L. Tilkemeier, MD, MMM
Department of Medicine, Greenville Health System, Greenville, SC, USA
e-mail: ptilkemeier@gmail.com

P.L. Tilkemeier et al. (eds.), *Quality Evaluation in Non-Invasive Cardiovascular Imaging*, DOI 10.1007/978-3-319-28011-0_4

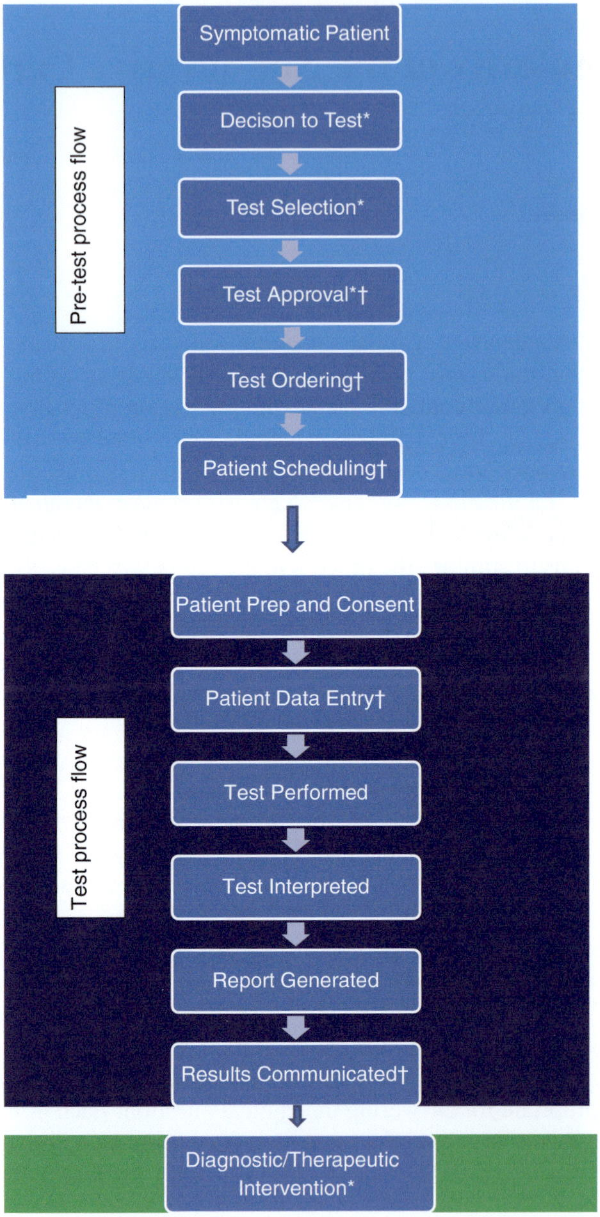

Fig. 4.1 Flow chart outlining the complexity of the non-invasive imaging process. * Step that could be influenced by decision support software; † step that could be facilitated by integrated data exchange, e.g. Integrating the Healthcare Enterprise

Test Selection

As will be addressed in each of the sections of this book, the multiple modalities of noninvasive cardiac imaging that are available today at times compete for the opportunity to diagnose certain conditions. For example, the diagnosis of coronary artery disease can be approached with an ECG stress test, stress echocardiogram, or stress myocardial perfusion imaging with either SPECT, PET, CT or MRI [1]. There are nuances to each of these modalities that may cause one to be preferred over another in the particular patient or patient population. In addition, the role of local expertise in the performance, interpretation and reporting of a particular modality must not be underemphasized. Thus, if there is local expertise in one type of procedure but not another, this test may be preferred. Additional factors that may impact test selection include the perceived cost of the test, difficulty ordering the test due to preauthorization, length of delay between ordering the test and the procedure being performed, perceived areas of expertise, or other factors. In order to be effective regarding selection of the right test for the right patient, there must be significant education of the ordering practitioner. The major areas of emphasis for each of the modalities are outlined in Table 4.1. As can be seen, there is significant overlap between the modalities with regard to their areas of diagnostic performance. As electronic health records and clinical decision support software continues to improve along with a better data driven understanding of the relative strength of each modality, the ability to choose the best test for the patient will become less problematic.

Cost and Risk

Procedural cost can be defined in many ways and thus can have varying impact regarding the complexity of the cardiac imaging process. One of the costs is the true financial cost of performing the test. Unfortunately, due to the high degree of variability in the insurance marketplace, this cost is only relatively understood. Certainly, an ECG stress test will be less expensive than the competing modalities

Table 4.1 Potential functionalities of each non-invasive cardiovascular imaging modality

	Functionality			
Modality	Perfusion	Function	Structural	Peripheral
CT	X	X	X	X
MRI	X	X	X	X
PET	X	X		
SPECT	X	X		
Echocardiogram	X	X	X	
Vascular ultrasound				X

for the initial cost of the test, however, the potential need for additive testing may not have been considered in the initial test selection. An example would be performing an exercise ECG stress test in a patient with poor physical capacity and a moderate pretest likelihood of disease. A test with the ability to perform pharmacologic stress with imaging will most certainly be needed in a high percentage of these patients. Therefore, the cost of the entire diagnostic evaluation has been raised by inappropriate test selection to start with. There are times that selecting a higher cost test initially may decrease the total cost of the diagnostic evaluation [2]. There is additionally variability in the cost of testing based on regional differences in cost and reimbursement. For example, the cost of a stress echocardiogram is higher in the Northeast than elsewhere in the United States.

The second cost that must be attributed to the test are the potential expense of downstream care depending on test selection. As was noted previously, improper test selection for particular patient can lead to the need for secondary testing to arrive at the correct diagnosis. Additionally, the selection of a test with mismatch between the sensitivity and specificity of the test and the incidence of disease in the population being tested can lead to either increased false positives or false negatives. Each of these results can have significant implications on the cost of future care. In the case of the false positive, additional testing is required to exclude the diagnosis, and in the case of false negatives, future care and or adverse outcomes may result due to false reassurances regarding the presence of disease. Third, the "cost" of the test with regard to future risk to the patient needs to be considered. For example, exposure to radiation as part of a nuclear based myocardial perfusion imaging study can have an impact on the future risk of developing cancer if used inappropriately. This cost, although poorly defined, should also be factored into the process [3].

The other potential risks to the patient that must be considered in addition to the potential for false positives, negatives and radiation exposure include the potential for contrast based reactions, test misinterpretation, or other errors in the process of image acquisition, such as patient misidentification, miscommunication regarding site and side (confusing left for right as an example), or other common procedural complications. It is imperative that the physician/healthcare provider ordering the test be knowledgeable regarding the potential risks and be able to discuss them with the patient, or facilitate discussion with someone who is knowledgeable regarding those risks, prior to the test being performed.

Training

The adequate training of the technical and professional staff involved in the performance of noninvasive cardiovascular imaging is essential to the diagnostic quality of the study. To facilitate this, multiple certification mechanisms have been developed for the technical and professional staff. These include board examinations, ongoing continuing education programs, and facility based accreditation programs. Technical staff must have the required classroom and practical training followed by an orientation program to understand equipment functionality and/or new settings for delivery of care. The same is true for the professional staff that oversees the function of the facility, participates in the interpretation and reporting of studies, and implements quality programs. Mechanisms for ongoing training of the technical and professional staff regarding new developments in the field are an essential element of a highly functioning and evolving facility to reflect the changes that could affect patient care. This should always be considered whenever new equipment or updates to existing equipment occur which can alter the current facility based processes. As a method to insure minimal standards for education and current knowledge, mechanisms are in place from a regulatory perspective regarding the requirements necessary for maintenance of licensure as well as maintenance of certification for both the technical and professional staff [4]. The professional accrediting societies are raising the standards for both those who perform the testing procedures as well as those who read the studies.

Communication

Communication is one of the most difficult aspects in any process today. Given the multiple mechanisms for communication and the sheer volume of information that is pushed to everyone on a daily basis, identifying the most effective mechanism for communication can be challenging. As can be identified in Fig. 4.1, there are multiple opportunities for poor communication to adversely affect the complex imaging process. Providing information to the ordering physician regarding the best test selection is the first of these. The ordering physician/healthcare provider may or may not have significant expertise regarding which test is preferred. Selection of the preferred test may be achieved through formal or informal consultation with a specialist in the field or with the physician in charge of the imaging modality. This may be facilitated through a decision support algorithm within the electronic health record. The broader implementation of electronic health records and the ability to access their content should improve the ability to communicate regarding preferred test selection and the results of the test. Mechanisms to facilitate this interoperability, such as Integrating the Healthcare Enterprise, will be essential to an effective communication system regarding test selection and results [5].

Furthermore, the imaging specialist responsible for interpretation of the test will need to assist in putting the test in the correct clinical context to ensure that appropriate next steps are implemented. The imaging specialist in consultation with the referring physician/healthcare provider can contribute valuable input regarding the need for additional testing, initiation of medications, or invasive therapeutic options. These decisions may additionally involve a consultant in the process in order to place the results, risks, patient factors and current literature in perspective regarding the next step in the care of the patient. Communicating the results clearly to all of the parties that are involved in the patient's care is necessary to ensure appropriate diagnostic testing or therapeutic intervention.

Appropriate Use Criteria and Pre-authorization

An important step in the imaging process is the application of appropriate use criteria and/or a preauthorization process for diagnostic imaging. There are many mechanisms for the implementation of either of these. Appropriate use criteria have been developed by the American College of Cardiology and the American College of Radiology and have been widely published for all of the diagnostic imaging modalities. The methodology for development of the criteria is well-established and quite rigorous [6]. Appropriate use criteria were developed initially on a modality basis. More recently they are being developed on a multimodality basis for a particular disease, such as congestive heart failure or ischemic heart disease [1, 7].

Appropriate use criteria have also been developed for therapeutic options. A significant portion of these include results from the noninvasive imaging studies. It is therefore essential that the results of the noninvasive imaging study include the matching criteria for those of the therapeutic appropriate use criteria [8]. The American College of Cardiology has developed a clinical tool for improving physician/healthcare provider education, which can be utilized as part of required physician training. The Formation of Optimal Cardiovascular Utilization Strategies (FOCUS) program is based upon the implementation of appropriate use criteria and modifying physician/healthcare provider behavior to reduce rarely appropriate studies in clinical practice [9]. Clinical trials regarding different mechanisms to change physician behavior have met with variable results and need further refinement if these programs are to be successful [10, 11].

The preauthorization process can be cumbersome in clinical implementation. Realizing the relatively high cost, volume and potential overutilization of noninvasive cardiac imaging, insurers have utilized preauthorization as a mechanism to control this. Whether it is using the ACC appropriate use criteria, a radiology benefits manager, or mechanism internal to the insurer, the process remains relatively similar although with different levels of impact on the practice. To effectively manage a preapproval process, many practices have had to add additional staff and physician/healthcare provider resources to acquire approval from the insurer prior to the study. Depending upon which studies require preauthorization, the potential for test shifting from a required study to one for which there is no requirement exists. This may result in sub-optimal test selection and the potential for increased cost secondary to this.

Next Steps

Given the complexity of the noninvasive imaging process for cardiovascular disease, our next steps must do anything and everything to simplify this. Development of guidelines regarding appropriate test selection in specific clinical settings that are broadly agreed upon will be essential. Development of tools that allow us to apply the clinical guidelines in practice, such as decision support, and integration of those tools into the electronic health record will also be essential to simplify the process. This implementation will also allow access to all providers at the point of care. The result of clinical decision support implementation at the point of care will be decreased variability among providers as well as improved test utilization in similar risk populations. Additional research comparing the effectiveness of the modalities for particular diagnoses will be necessary to inform the development of multimodality clinical guidelines for test utilization. Implementation and development of guidelines where they do not exist for clinical reporting along with mechanisms to allow structured, standardized reporting will also be essential.

References

1. Wolk MJ, Bailey SR, Doherty JU, Douglas PS, Hendel RC, Kramer CM, Min JK, Patel MR, Rosenbaum L, Shaw LJ, Stainback RF, Allen JM. ACCF/AHA/ASE/ASNC/HFSA/HRS/SCAI/SCCT/SCMR/STS 2013 multimodality appropriate use criteria for the detection and risk assessment of stable ischemic heart disease. J Am Coll Cardiol. 2014;63(4):380–406. doi:10.1016/j.jacc.2013.11.009.
2. Hachamovitch R, Berman DS, Shaw LJ, Kiat H, Cohen I, Cabico JA, Friedman J, Diamond GA. Incremental prognostic value of myocardial perfusion single photon emission computed tomography for the prediction of cardiac death differential stratification for risk of cardiac death and myocardial infarction. Circulation. 1998;97:535–43. doi:10.1161/01.CIR.97.6.535.
3. Einstein AJ, Berman D, Min JK, Hendel RC, Gerber TC, Carr J, Cerqueira MD, Cullom J, DeKemp R, Cullom J, DeKemp R, Dickert M, Dorbala S, Garcia EV, Gibbons RJ, Halliburton SS, Hausleiter J, Heller GV, Jerome S, Lesser JR, Fazel R, Raffe GL, Tilkemeier PL, Williams KA, Shaw LJ. Patient-centered imaging: shared decision making for cardiac imaging procedures with exposure to ionizing radiation. J Am Coll Cardiol. 2014. doi:10.1016/j.jacc.2013.10.092.
4. American Board of Internal Medicine. Maintenance of certification guide. [Internet] 2001–2015. [Cited 12/20/2014]. Available from: http://www.abim.org/maintenance-of-certification/.
5. Integrating the Healthcare Enterprise. [Internet]. 2003. [Cited 12/20/2014] Available from: http://www.ihe.net/.
6. Carr JJ, Hendel RC, White RD, Patel MR, Wolk MJ, Rettmann MA, Douglas PS, Rybicki FJ, Krmaer CM, Woodard PK, Shaw LJ, Yucel EK. 2013 appropriate utilization of cardiovascular imaging a methodology for the development of joint criteria for the appropriate utilization of cardiovascular imaging by the American College of Cardiology Foundation and American College of Radiology. J Am Coll Cardiol. 2013;61(21):2199–206. doi:10.1016/j.jacc.2013.02.010.
7. Patel MR, White RD, Abbara S, Bluemke DA, Herfkens RJ, Picard M, Shaw LJ, Silver M, Stillman AE, Udelson J. 2013 ACCF/ACR/ASE/ASNC/SCCT/SCMR appropriate utilization of cardiovascular imaging in heart failure a joint report of the American college of radiology appropriateness criteria committee and the American college of cardiology foundation appropriate use criteria task force. J Am Coll Cardiol. 2013;61(21):2207–31. doi:10.1016/j.jacc.2013.02.005.
8. Patel MR, Dehmer GJ, Hirshfeld JW, Smoth PK, Spertus JA. ACCF/SCAI/STS/AATS/AHA/ASNC/HFSA/SCCT 2012 appropriate use criteria for coronary revascularization focused update a report of the American College of Cardiology Foundation Appropriate Use Criteria Task Force, Society for Cardiovascular Angiography and Interventions, Society of Thoracic Surgeons, American Association for Thoracic Surgery, American Heart Association, American Society of Nuclear Cardiology, and the Society of Cardiovascular Computed Tomography. J Am Coll Cardiol. 2012;59(9):857–81. doi:10.1016/j.jacc.2011.12.001.

9. American College of Cardiology. Imaging in "FOCUS" [Internet] 2015. [Cited 12-20-2014] Available from: http://cardiosource.org/Science-And-Quality/Quality-Programs/Imaging-in-FOCUS.aspx?w_nav=Search&WT.oss=FOCUS&WT.oss_r=2844&.
10. Hendel RC, Cerqueira M, Douglas PS, Caruth KC, Allen JM, Jensen NC, Pan W, Brindis R, Wolk M. A multicenter assessment of the use of single-photon emission computed tomography myocardial perfusion imaging with appropriateness criteria. J Am Coll Cardiol. 2010;55(2):156–62. doi:10.1016/j.jacc.2009.11.004.
11. Saifi S, Taylor AH, Allen J, Hendel R. The use of a learning community and online evaluation of utilization of SPECT myocardial perfusion imaging. JACC Cardiovasc Imaging. 2013;6:823–9.

Chapter 5
Accreditation and International Perspectives

Peter L. Tilkemeier

Abstract Accreditation, whether from a United States or international perspective, is a multidimensional process with a goal of assuring and improving quality with regard to personnel qualifications, study performance, reporting of results and quality assurance programs. Depending upon the location of the facility, accreditation can be more likely to be performed by governmental agency compared to being overseen by a legislative process. Furthermore, the benefits of accreditation can vary from preferential access to resources to punitive actions regarding reimbursement. The European process tends to be one that is regulated and overseen directly by the government with preferential access to resources as opposed to the process in the United States which has been implemented by organizations meeting legislative standards with the potential for punitive action regarding reimbursement at the facility level. From both perspectives, the future vision is one of a continuous process built into the daily operations of the facility and following a continuous improvement algorithm.

Keywords Accreditation • Certification • Quality assurance • Accreditation organizations • Continuous quality improvement cycle

Accreditation

Accreditation is a multidimensional process with a goal of assuring and improving quality from all perspectives. This process varies according to setting of the accrediting organization. The different settings are determined by the accrediting body, philosophical approach to accreditation, such as mandated by government in an effort to improve quality, insurers in an effort to improve the value of a process to their clients, by the facilities themselves to gain a competitive advantage in the marketplace given competition from others and/or those that have been independently driven to assess and improve quality in their facility. Given these different motivating

P.L. Tilkemeier, MD, MMM
Department of Medicine, Greenville Health System, Greenville, SC, USA
e-mail: ptilkemeier@gmail.com

P.L. Tilkemeier et al. (eds.), *Quality Evaluation in Non-Invasive Cardiovascular Imaging*, DOI 10.1007/978-3-319-28011-0_5

factors, multiple driving forces for accreditation have evolved internationally. Within each model, the mechanisms for accreditation vary and each will be examined.

International Perspective

From an international perspective, there have been three major approaches. These have been different in the United Kingdom, Europe and the United States. The approach in the United Kingdom has been focused on the regulation of the provider with the assumption that this will result in assuring the quality of the study performed in the facilities which they are supervising. The focus thus far has been limited to echocardiography and cardiac computed tomography. This has recently been in evolution given changes in the evaluation of physicians in training. These changes have included the implementation of workplace-based assessments with senior physicians and insuring competency of those in training as opposed to experience based training requirement specific volumes which was supposed to translate into competency [1]. As the focus has changed more to competency-based training programs, the accreditation process has been able to change its focus from accreditation of individuals to accreditation of departments in which the training programs reside [2].

Departmental accreditation has provided the focus to be to inclusive of staff competency, equipment adequacy and standardized departmental processes in addition to implementing and assessing ongoing quality assurance programs. Through this process the British system has been able to identify centers of excellence and to utilize those centers to ensure high quality advanced imaging training feeding back into increased competency of the imaging facility staff. The continual quality assurance programs have also given the opportunity for more equitable distribution of resources across the system when resources have been scarce. Unfortunately, the current process remains in a period of transition for those individuals who have completed training prior to its implementation. The newly developed competency-based pathway is not available to them, hence the accreditation based pathway needs to remain in place for these individuals. Possible changes to this methodology may occur as accredited physicians will require revalidation of their competence and as methodologies are expanded into all imaging modalities [3].

The European Perspective

From a European perspective the accreditation pathway is completely voluntary and is modality specific. Accreditation was initiated in the field of echocardiography where the process initially started with individual accreditation. Initially begun as accreditation of individuals by the European Association of Echocardiography the process has now shifted to the facility level. It is important to note that this was and still remains a voluntary process in Europe. The accreditation process does not supersede and must harmonize with both national and local regulations for facility performance; however the accreditation model was designed to apply to all countries. It additionally includes both basic and advanced standards. One of the initial drivers for participation was felt to be access to capital dollars based upon the review by the accreditation body [4]. The accreditation process in Europe also is somewhat unique in that it is society-based as opposed to independent organization(s) providing the framework for accreditation. The echocardiography accreditation process realized early on that collaboration with other expert associations such as anesthesia for trans-esophageal echocardiography and pediatrics for congenital heart disease in the adult were important to their success with regard to accreditation in these advanced standards.

The accreditation standard for the European Association of Echocardiography has evolved over time with an updated version of the standards released in 2006 following a review of the first 3 years of voluntary accreditation. This review suggested that the process was working well and expanded the offering to an electronic format. Initial opportunities for improvement were focused around demographics of the facility [5]. Over time the European Association of Echocardiography expanded its focus to include all of cardiovascular imaging and in 2014 released the third update to the standards and processes for accreditation echocardiography facilities as the European Association of Cardiovascular Imaging (EACVI). The basic standards recommendations remain similar from the prior standards. There was increased emphasis on quality measures and process. It was thought that the benefit of accreditation fell into four major areas. The first is educational with four subareas: (1) preferential access to grants, (2) preferential participation in educational projects, (3) preferential access for fellowship and advanced imaging, and (4) preference for selection and participation in educational courses meetings. The second is a scientific perspective which should result in preference to participation in multicenter scientific projects. Third is the research perspective with accreditation by the EACVI potentially resulting in strong preference for research programs participation and fourth, from an economical perspective preference to be selected for clinical trials and sub studies that require clear quality control requirements and the potential for increased access to capital through objective assessment of facility needs [6]. When evaluated over time the accreditation process showed slow uptake in European countries however this has improved with greater recognition of the benefits of accreditation [7].

Following in the successful pattern of echocardiography, Cardiac magnetic resonance (CMR) imaging initially started with individual certification and progressed to facility accreditation. One of the challenges for the CMR process was the concept CMR is performed by both cardiology and/or radiology departments depending upon the local setting. This has added to the complexity of the issues. It was perceived that the driving force for voluntary CMR accreditation was the desire of trainees to receive their training in the accredited facilities. The accreditation process has utilized and leveraged the European cardiovascular magnetic resonance registry as a mechanism to ensure quality control with random audits of cases submitted to the registry.

In the initial document outlining requirements for individual accreditation, requirements were developed from the cardiovascular magnetic resonance working group of the European Society of Cardiology. A number of benefits of participation as well as recommendations for the future were developed. These benefits included: (1) Setting a European standard of practice for training of individuals in CMR; (2) Accreditation will afford demonstration of quality, and credibility for both study performance and training; (3) Accreditation was thought to be an advantage in negotiation with funding sources; (4) The ability to link to the European CMR registry allows the opportunity for quality control; (5) The accreditation process is not compulsory or regulatory with the regulatory standards defined by national laws and regulations, and (6) Realization that reciprocity with the accreditation process of the Society of Cardiovascular Magnetic Resonance imaging affords an opportunity for wider acceptance [7]. Their recommendations included the goal that a joint European mechanism be developed for training in cardiac imaging that is multimodality [8].

With regard to radionuclide myocardial perfusion imaging a different pathway has developed for monitoring the performance in Europe. The clinical audit tool was initiated by the European Commission in 1997 as the preferred mechanism for ensuring quality radionuclide use in the medical setting [9]. This process involves a systematic examination seeking to improve quality, patient care through the analysis of the usual structure, process and outcomes pathway of quality improvement. The European structure allows the clinical audit to be of various types and levels, either comprehensive, assessing the whole process, or partial focused audits assessing a critical part of the process. The use of this tool was reaffirmed in the European Commission 2009 update [10].

The clinical audit can be implemented in either an internal or external mechanism. This allows for a focused internal audit to assess a particular process or perhaps a larger external audit encompassing the entire department. It is distinctly different from the usual local or national regulatory inspections surrounding use of radioactive materials. Furthermore, the clinical audit can be performed either locally with on-site visitors or through a distant review with submission of data electronically. The audit process utilizes best practice statements and guidelines as a benchmark for comparison. One of the major difficulties with this approach is that there are many areas in which only expert opinion provides the basis for the benchmark.

Unfortunately, there has been no ability to collate the data resulting from the clinical audit process. This has limited the utilization of clinical audits in the quality improvement process, dissemination of the information to improve quality of a broader perspective and development of standards to provide better benchmarking [11].

United States Perspective

The pathway to accreditation in the United States (US) has taken a different route as demonstrated in the comparative analysis outlined in Fig. 5.1. The accrediting bodies in the US are private nonprofit organizations independent of the societies,

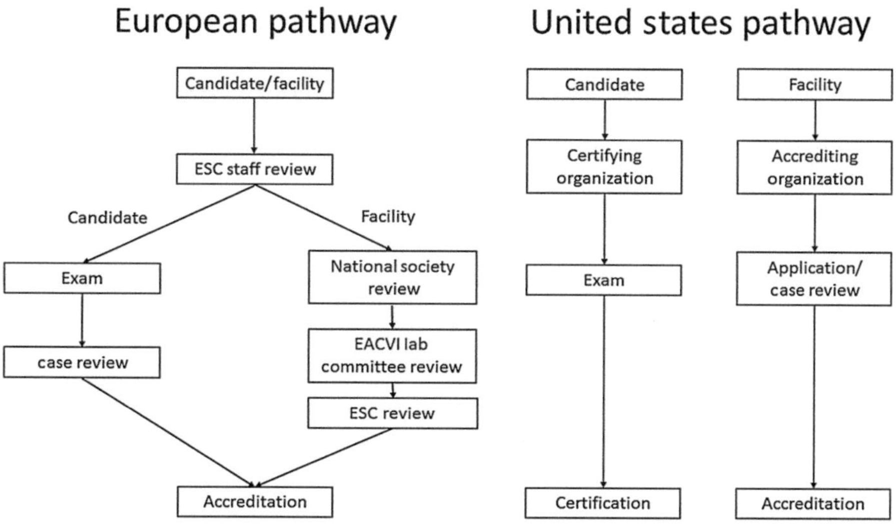

Fig. 5.1 Comparison of accreditation pathways in Europe and the United Sates

however, somewhat related to governmental authority. The Medicare Improvements for Patients and Providers Act (MIPPA) in 2008 required all advanced diagnostic imaging services to be accredited by a Centers for Medicare and Medicaid approved accrediting organization by 2012. This included nuclear medicine and positron emission tomography, computed tomographic and magnetic resonance imaging. Three organizations applied for and received certification from the federal government as being able to meet the comprehensive requirements set forth in the legislation. These included the American College of Radiology (ACR), Inter-societal Accreditation Commission (IAC) and The Joint Commission (TJC) for accreditation of hospitals. Each of these has taken a somewhat different approach to accreditation. Their approaches will be examined independently.

Accreditation with the American College of Radiology (ACR)

The ACR approach is primarily focused on image quality and the structure and process involved with obtaining images [11]. They began participation in the accreditation process in 1987 and are currently covering nine imaging modalities and radiation therapy. The standards utilized by the accreditation programs of the ACR are based upon literature and/or committees of experts within a certain modality. The focus of the ACR program has always been on providing education and guidance on meeting the standards.

The major areas of accreditation standards include personnel qualifications, equipment specifications and quality control and quality assurance procedures. Personnel have specific training and experience requirements with ongoing continuing education being an important aspect of ongoing training. Additionally, physicians are required to participate in a peer review program assessing accuracy and appropriateness. With regard to imaging, all equipment is assessed for its ability to perform up to standard and provide clinical images that are adequate for interpretation. Major areas of focus for adequate image quality include technique, artifacts, and appropriate demographic information. In addition to the clinical images, images of phantoms are required for each modality. Information is submitted electronically in the majority of cases and there is an on-site evaluation that can occur mid-cycle. This allows the assurance of compliance with the standards.

From an international perspective, the ACR has a presence either through partnering with other organizations or through a direct offer. The process is complicated by the degree and variability of governmental regulation. As a result, different standards may need to be applied to encompass the use of higher-end equipment, personnel requirements and to overcome cultural and language barriers. It has been observed that there is a lack of a tie of quality to study performance internationally with Canada and Australia the early exceptions to this pattern. This is most likely related to a difference in standards internationally. Such is not the case in the United States due to MIPPA resulting in a coalescence of standards.

The ACR accreditation programs have seen a decrease in new site applications recently while maintaining a similar number of reaccreditation applications. This may be due to increasing consolidation of the healthcare system in the United States. To further inform the ACR accreditation process regarding current practice and to drive standards that will continue to improve facility performance, the ACR is presently developing and growing registries in the imaging modalities. The data derived from these registries will be utilized to further refine standards leading to accreditation and thus complete the quality improvement cycle.

Accreditation with the Intersocietal Accreditation Commission (IAC)

The IAC began an accreditation program in the late 1980s as well. The initial effort was a multi-society approach to accreditation of noninvasive vascular facilities utilizing these societies as sponsors for the process. The first vascular facility was accredited in 1992 through this pathway. The IAC approached CMS at that time and were told that for accreditation to be part of federal regulation it would require an act of Congress. This was visionary on all parts given the implementation of MIPPA 16 years later. The IAC multi-societal approach was expanded to echocardiography in 1986 in partnership with the American Society of Echocardiography with the first facility accredited in 1997. Similarly with myocardial perfusion imaging and the American Society of Nuclear Cardiology partnership in 1997 with the first facility being accredited in 1998. The first program that was based on payment was with one of the major insurance companies in 1999 when they required accreditation for payments of magnetic resonance imaging studies. The IAC had a major reorganization in 2006 merging its multiple business lines into a single corporation with individual divisions addressing each imaging modality. At that time CT, and magnetic resonance imaging were added to the portfolio. This timeline of development is demonstrated in Fig. 5.2. IAC accreditation now includes dental, CT, carotid stenting and electrophysiology laboratories.

The IAC approach to accreditation has been similar with unique differences compared to the ACR approach [12]. Both organization's standards are based on implementation of societal guidelines with input from expert consensus panels as required. The societal approach is more of a focus for the IAC then for the ACR, the latter of which historically has been more consensus driven. With its reorganization in 2006, the IAC was able to provide a baseline single set of standards independent of modality that would apply to all facilities. These include areas with regard to infection control practices and policy and procedure regarding safety, training and general education. With these in place, specific standards for each modality are then developed. These standards address: personnel training including continuing education for both technologists and physicians; policy and procedures specific to the modality to ensure that the standards of current best practice are utilized throughout the performance of tests; review of clinical studies to ensure image quality and basic interpretive skills are present; and review of the reports to assess compliance with present standards regarding content and timeliness. The facility applies through an online process with an online review and feedback mechanism in place to provide the facility feedback regarding areas for improvement prior to accreditation. The IAC has a 3-year reaccreditation cycle with the ability to perform audits and/or on-site reviews between reaccreditation cycles.

The IAC has not pursued an international presence in facility accreditation unless the facility seeks this independently. Through use of its online application process, the IAC has a wealth of information regarding the facilities and the procedures and

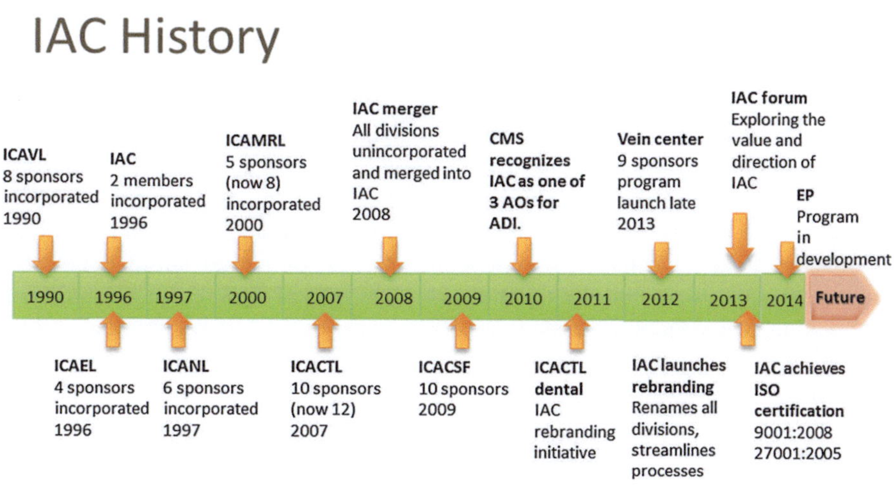

Fig. 5.2 The timeline for the development of the current IAC structure

processes of the facilities in acquiring images. This information has allowed the IAC to develop a separate research division and a funding mechanism for performance of studies utilizing the data to support and inform the accreditation process through research.

Over time the number of facilities seeking accreditation through the IAC pathway in all modalities has continued to grow. There was a significant impact of the implementation of MIPPA on the number of facilities seeking accreditation. This volume has remained fairly constant recently with relatively little change in the number of facilities seeking reaccreditation [13].

Accreditation with the Joint Commission (TJC)

The Joint Commission is a CMS certified accreditation organization for advanced diagnostic imaging. It has been certified for this activity since the program's inception in 2010. TJC has a long history of participating in accreditation of healthcare facilities beginning in 1975 with now greater than 2,000 facilities certified in a number of clinical settings. Accreditation in advanced diagnostic imaging is part of the long standing ambulatory care accreditation program. This program required the addition of only three elements of performance in order to meet the certification standards in 2010. The elements of performance become the evaluative criteria which are utilized by the on-site surveyors for every accreditation visit. There are numerous standards that remain under continuous evaluation and revision covering the spectrum of advanced diagnostic imaging. These include but are not limited to environment of care, emergency management, human resources, infection prevention and control, information management, leadership, medication management, provision of care, performance improvement, record of care, rights of the individual and required written documentation [14]. Through these standards they offer a comprehensive review of practices in the diagnostic imaging center. The most recent revisions to these standards were planned for implementation in a stepwise manner starting in 2014 with completion in 2015. This has since been delayed to a single implementation in 2015. The 2014 update focused on the environment of care with regard to magnetic resonance imaging and with ensuring image quality [15]. The full update includes the addition of 28 elements in response to TJC's belief that the quality bar had to be raised further when accrediting hospital and ambulatory imaging centers. This was independent of the advanced diagnostic imaging process, however, the additions were supported by a recent Government Accounting Office report assessing the effectiveness of the MIPPA program. All of the TJC accreditation requirements are carried out through an on-site surveyor, who may also be accompanied by an advanced diagnostic imaging specialist, usually an imaging technologist, providing expertise in the particular imaging modalities being surveyed. Following accreditation there is an ongoing focused standards assessment at 12 and 24 months with the submission of findings and corrective actions to ensure continued compliance with the standards throughout the 3-year accreditation [14].

Table 5.1 Characteristics of accreditation compared between European and United States based methodologies

Characteristic	European	United States
Mechanism of accreditation	Societal	Independent
Mandated for payment	No	Yes (CT, CMR, nuclear medicine, PET)
Modalities available		
Echocardiography	Yes	Yes – IAC
Nuclear medicine/PET	Yes	Yes – ACR, IAC, TJC
CMR	No	Yes – ACR, IAC, TJC
CT	No	Yes – ACR, IAC, TJC
Non-invasive vascular	No	Yes –IAC
Government regulation	Local and national regulations	Indirectly through MIPPA

PET positron emission tomography, *CMR* cardiac magnetic resonance, *CT* computed tomography, *IAC* Intersocietal Accreditation Commission, *ACR* American College of Radiology, *TJC* The Joint Commission, *MIPPA* Medicare Improvements for Patients and Providers Act

From an international perspective, The Joint Commission has an affiliated company performing accreditation in this setting. There is a division of this company focused on ambulatory care centers. There has been little if any interest in certification for advanced diagnostic imaging.

The TJC's approach to accreditation varies from the ACR and IAC approach in several important perspectives. TJC's approach is based completely on on-site review as a mechanism for assessing compliance with standards. A second important difference is that the site visit is focused on an organizational wide approach as opposed to one that is technology driven. As noted previously, the review process not only focuses on the imaging aspects but also includes an assessment of overall patient and staff safety, environment of care concerns and individual patient rights. This results in a profile of the usual participants being facilities with multiple modalities and or physical locations that are applying for accreditation. This approach has been a cornerstone of TJC methodology and is not expected to change.

The US accreditation process has developed into one that is more comprehensive based on pressures from the insurers and governmental regulations. Table 5.1 compiles the differences between the US and European accreditation programs that are in place currently. It remains unclear how this will evolve going forward.

Future Perspective

Moving forward, there has been a vision of the accreditation and reaccreditation process becoming more continuous and built into the daily operations of the facility. This would allow a continuous feedback with the accrediting organization and potentially serve as a source of data for other certification processes such as maintenance of certification and/or maintenance of licensure for individuals

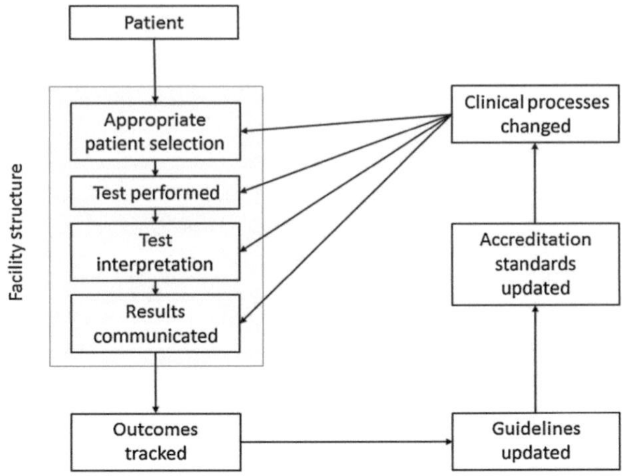

Fig. 5.3 The accreditation process improvement cycle

practicing in the facility [16]. Continued development of standards for facility accreditation will be based upon ongoing evolution of guidelines that will be better informed through research initiatives evaluating the impact of accreditation on patient care outcomes and through an improvement algorithm outlined in Fig. 5.3. Outcome-based research with regard to the performance of the current accreditation standards will be an essential part of the ongoing accreditation of all imaging modalities and facilities [17].

References

1. Joint Royal Colleges of Physicians Training Board. Specialty training curriculum for cardiology Aug 2010. [Internet]. 2010 [cited 2014 Jul 1]. Available from: http://www.jrcptb.org.uk/trainingandcert/ST3-SpR/Documents/2010(AUC)Cardiologycurriculum.pdf.
2. Shah BN, Lindsay AC, Nicol ED. What is the role of accreditation in the era of competency-based specialist training – a perspective from the United Kingdom. Int J Cardiol. 2012;160(2):79–81.
3. British Society of Cardiovascular Imaging. BSCI guidance for revalidation in cardiovascular CT, Version 1.0, Dec 2011. [Internet] 2011 [cited 2014 Jul 1]. Available from: www.bsci.org.uk/revalidation/category/6-bsci-documents?download=23:bscci-revalidation-document-revised-12-03-06
4. Nihoyannopoulos P, Fox K, Fraser A, Pinto F. EAE facility standards and accreditation. Eur J Echocardiogr. 2007;8(1):80–7.
5. Fox K, Popescu B, Janiszewski S, Nihoyannopoulos P, Fraser A, Pinto F. Report on the european association of echocardiography accreditations in echocardiography: december 2003 – september 2006. Eur J Echocardiogr. 2007;8(1):74–9.
6. Popescu B, Stefanidis A, Nihoyannopoulos P, Fox K, Ray S, Cardim N, Rigo F, Badano LP, Fraser AG, Pinto F, Zamorano JL, Habib G, Maurer G, Lancellotti P, Andrade MJ, Donal E, Edvardsen T, Varga A. Updated standards and processes for accreditation of echocardiographic facilities from the European Association of Cardiovascular Imaging. Eur Heart J Cardiovasc Imaging. 2014;15(7):717–27.
7. Plein S, Schulz-Menger J, Almeida A, Mahrholdt H, Rademakers F, Pennell D, Nagle E, Schwitter J, Lombardi M, Working Group on Cardiovascular Magnetic Resonance, European

Society of Cardiology. Training and accreditation in cardiovascular magnetic resonance in Europe: a position statement of the working group on cardiovascular magnetic resonance of the European Society of Cardiology. Eur Heart J. 2011;32(7):93–8.

8. Taylor J. ESC recommendations for individual certification and institutional cardiovascular magnetic resonance accreditation in Europe. Eur Heart J. 2010;31(21):2560–2.
9. Teunen D. The European Directive on health protection of individuals against the dangers of ionizing radiation in relation to medical exposure (97/43/EURATOM). J Radiol Prot. 1998;18(2):133–7.
10. European Commission. European Commission guidelines on clinical audit for medical radiological practices (diagnostic radiology, nuclear medicine and radiotherapy). Radiation Protection No 159. [Internet]. 2009 [cited 2014 Jul 14]. Available from: http://ec.europa.eu/energy/nuclear/radiation_protection/publications_en.htm.
11. Jarvinen H, Wilcox P. Clinical audit and practice accreditation. In: Lau L, Ng K, editors. Radiological safety and quality: paradigms in leadership and innovation. Netherlands: Springer; 2014.
12. Heller G, Katanick S, Sloper T, Garcia M. Accreditation for cardiovascular imaging: setting quality standards for patient care. JACC Cardiovasc Imaging. 2008;1(3):390–7.
13. Rose G, Weissman N. Demystifying imaging facility accreditation. JACC Cardiovasc Imaging. 2014;7(2):212–4.
14. 2014 Ambulatory care accreditation overview: a snapshot of the accreditation process. Oak Brook: Joint Commission Resources; 2014 [cited 2014 Jul 14]. Available from: http://www.jointcommission.org/assets/1/6/2014_AHC_Overview_Guide.pdf.
15. Joint Commission Resources. Revised timeline for implementation of The Joint Commission's new and revised diagnostic imaging standards. [Internet]. 2014 [cited 2014 Jul 14]. Available from: http://www.jointcommission.org/assets/1/18/S10.pdf.
16. Cohen M. Maintenance of certification and accreditation: a call for daily deeds rather than periodic paper pushing. J Nucl Cardiol. 2010;17(2):342–3.
17. Douglas P, Chen J, Gillam L, Hendel R, Hundley WG, Masoudi F, Patel M, Peterson E. Achieving quality in cardiovascular imaging II: proceedings from the second American College of Cardiology – Duke University Medical Center Think Tank on Quality in Cardiovascular Imaging. JACC Cardiovasc Imaging. 2009;2(2):231–40.

Part II
CT

Chapter 6
Clinical Applications of Cardiac CT

Amgad N. Makaryus and Seth Uretsky

Abstract Cardiac computed tomography (CCT) has become an important tool in the evaluation of structural heart disease, large vessel disease, and coronary atherosclerosis, covering a broad spectrum of cardiovascular disease. Recently, the clinical applications have increased dramatically as CCT technology has significantly improved. The improvement in technology and expanding clinical applications will be reviewed.

Keywords Cardiac computed tomography • Calcium scoring • Cardiac computed tomography angiography

Introduction

Cardiac computed tomography (CCT) has become a mainstream imaging tool for the assessment of coronary atherosclerosis and pathology resulting from pericardial, valvular and myocardial heart disease whether ischemic or non-ischemic. Spiral multi-detector CT scanning has increased spatial and contrast resolution, and results in a dramatic expansion of the use of CT for evaluation of patients with acquired and congenital heart disease. Further advances with dual-source scanning also improved on the temporal resolution capabilities of the current generation scanners. The

A.N. Makaryus, MD, FACC, FACP, FASE, FSCCT
Department of Cardiology, NuHealth, Nassau University Medical Center,
2201 Hempstead Turnpike, East Meadow, NY 11554, USA
e-mail: amakaryu@numc.edu

S. Uretsky, MD, FACC (✉)
Cardiovascular Fellowship Program, Atlantic Health System, Gagnon Cardiovascular Center,
100 Madison Avenue, Morristown, NJ 07960, USA
e-mail: seth.uretsky@atlantichealth.org

P.L. Tilkemeier et al. (eds.), *Quality Evaluation in Non-Invasive Cardiovascular Imaging*, DOI 10.1007/978-3-319-28011-0_6

adequate and appropriate use of CCT is central to its use in clinical practice and assures quality acquisition and reporting of results.

Technical developments in the field of computed tomography over the past 10 years have largely driven the expansion of the clinical applicability and utility of CCT for the evaluation of the cardiac patient. As the number of detectors has increased, the size of each detector has become smaller. Therefore, the length of the edge of a picture element resolved in a 256- or 320-detector scan is smaller than that obtained by a 16- or 64-detector scan, affording higher spatial resolution. Contrast resolution, the ability to differentiate between two shades of gray in adjacent picture elements, has also improved and is predicated upon reduced patient radiation exposure and the sensitivity of scanner detectors. Electrocardiographically (ECG) gated CT acquisition is routinely used to "freeze" cardiac motion and provide high temporal resolution images based on the improved speed of gantry rotation. These technological advancements have allowed for the expansion of the clinical applications derived from CCT into such areas as myocardial perfusion and coronary fractional flow assessment and have therefore improved the quality and utility of the images obtained [1–3].

Calcium Scoring

Coronary artery calcium (CAC) quantification is known to be a reliable and independent predictor of adverse cardiovascular events. Coronary calcification has been employed to help risk stratify patients, both symptomatic and asymptomatic, at risk for coronary artery disease (CAD) by using the score along with other stratification tools such as the Framingham risk score. The calcium score is also employed in guideline driven management of patients [4]. In subsets of patients with high calcium scores (particularly ≥400 Agatston units), the artifactual effects and scatter associated with radio-dense calcium deposits limit the specificity of cardiac CT angiography (CCTA) in delineating the extent of clinically significant CAD. Early studies comparing the diagnostic capabilities of CCTA with invasive coronary angiography often excluded patients with elevated baseline calcium scores as a result of the negative impact of high score on the scan accuracy or the inability to assess the presence or absence of stenosis with increased calcification [3, 5]. Similarly, studies which did include arterial segments with high levels of calcification, usually denoted a significant decline in the diagnostic accuracy of the CT scan [3]. With improving technologies, the limitations of calcium on the CCT images are improving and calcium scoring is used routinely in the assessment of CAD along with CCTA as a tool for risk assessment. CAC use in acute chest pain is not indicated. The clinical applications are addressed in greater detail in Chap. 7.

Cardiac Computed Tomography Angiography (CCTA)

Quality CCTA images are obtained when appropriate techniques, including hardware and software and trained individuals are employed. Images must be obtained as quickly as possible, using protocols that employ the use of contrast agent for visualization of the coronary tree. Patients must also be properly screened and prepared for the imaging procedure. Numerous studies have evaluated the utility of CCTA to define focal coronary stenoses and have shown reliability for ruling out disease in non-diseased patients. The sensitivity of CCTA is >90 % in most studies evaluating the diagnostic abilities of CCTA compared to the gold standard of invasive angiography, with a negative predictive value >95 % [1].

Cardiac Structural Assessment

Due to recent technological advancements, new CCT techniques are being employed for a more comprehensive appraisal of anatomic, structural, and functional aspects of heart disease. Structural analysis and quantification of gross cardiac anatomy is becoming an integral part of the assessment and treatment prior to structural heart therapies being employed for example in the percutaneous transcatheter replacement of stenosed aortic valves. CCT provides quantification of necessary measurements required for sizing as well as three-dimensional placement for delivery during these procedures. Additionally, hybrid software technologies that combine CCT images with other imaging techniques such as echocardiography and fluroroscopic images allow for ideal visualization and appropriate procedure execution [6]. Additional structural assessment applications include assessment of left atrial appendage and pulmonary vein anatomy prior to electrophysiology-based ablative procedures.

Myocardial Perfusion

CCT assessment of myocardial perfusion is performed based on the distribution of intravenously injected iodinated contrast material during its first pass through the myocardium denoting myocardial blood flow. Myocardial perfusion defects can be identified as areas of hypo-attenuation containing reduced amounts of contrast material. Attenuation followed over consecutive time points (initial first pass versus delayed or post-stress imaging) provides dynamic myocardial perfusion imaging. Furthermore, fractional flow reserve techniques employing CCTA are now also being evaluated for the indirect assessment of functional significance of stenosis within the coronary arteries [7]. While these techniques show promise, they are still undergoing development and refinement to allow for adequate mainstream clinical implementation. Furthermore, use of these techniques also needs refinement due to the drawbacks of increased radiation dose and multiple artifactual drawbacks that may limit the diagnostic accuracy of these methods and routine clinical use [8, 9].

References

1. Kohsaka S, Makaryus AN. Coronary angiography using noninvasive imaging techniques of cardiac ct and mri. Curr Cardiol Rev. 2008;4:323–30.
2. Makaryus AN, Henry S, Loewinger L, Makaryus JN, Boxt L. Multi-detector coronary ct imaging for the identification of coronary artery stenoses in a "real-world" population. Clin Med Insights Cardiol. 2014;8:13–22.
3. Makaryus JN, Makaryus AN. Coronary calcification: Achilles' heel in the assessment for coronary artery disease in patients with symptomatic angina? Int J Cardiovasc Imaging. 2009;25:855–7.
4. Watson K, Wilson PW, Eddleman KM, Jarrett NM, LaBresh K, Nevo L, Wnek J, Anderson JL, Halperin JL, Albert NM, Bozkurt B, Brindis RG, Curtis LH, DeMets D, Hochman JS, Kovacs RJ, Ohman EM, Pressler SJ, Sellke FW, Shen WK, Smith Jr SC, Tomaselli GF, American College of Cardiology/American Heart Association Task Force on Practice G. Acc/aha guideline on the treatment of blood cholesterol to reduce atherosclerotic cardiovascular risk in adults: a report of the American College of Cardiology/American Heart Association Task Force on Practice Guidelines. Circulation. 2014;129:S1–45.
5. Miller JM, Rochitte CE, Dewey M, Arbab-Zadeh A, Niinuma H, Gottlieb I, Paul N, Clouse ME, Shapiro EP, Hoe J, Lardo AC, Bush DE, de Roos A, Cox C, Brinker J, Lima JA. Diagnostic performance of coronary angiography by 64-row ct. N Engl J Med. 2008;359:2324–36.
6. Nasis A, Mottram PM, Cameron JD, Seneviratne SK. Current and evolving clinical applications of multidetector cardiac ct in assessment of structural heart disease. Radiology. 2013;267:11–25.
7. Min JK, Leipsic J, Pencina MJ, Berman DS, Koo BK, Mieghem C, Erglis A, Lin FY, Dunning AM, Apruzzese P, Budoff MJ, Cole JH, Jaffer FA, Leon MB, Malpeso J, Mancini GBJ, Park SJ, Schwartz RS, Shaw LJ, Mauri L. Diagnostic accuracy of fractional flow reserve from anatomic CT angiography. J Am Med Assoc. 2012;308(12):1237–45.
8. George RT, Arbab-Zadeh A, Miller JM, Vavere AL, Bengel FM, Lardo AC, Lima JA. Computed tomography myocardial perfusion imaging with 320-row detector computed tomography accurately detects myocardial ischemia in patients with obstructive coronary artery disease. Circ Cardiovasc Imaging. 2012;5:333–40.
9. George RT, Silva C, Cordeiro MA, DiPaula A, Thompson DR, McCarthy WF, Ichihara T, Lima JA, Lardo AC. Multidetector computed tomography myocardial perfusion imaging during adenosine stress. J Am Coll Cardiol. 2006;48:153–60.

Chapter 7
CT: Patient Selection

Steve W. Leung and Marcus Y. Chen

Abstract Proper patient selection is extremely important in all diagnostic testing. The potential benefit should outweigh the risk of the test. With cardiac CT, valuable information regarding coronary arteries and cardiac anatomy can be rapidly obtained in a non-invasive manner. Appropriate use criteria documents have been developed to help guide practitioners on whether a test is likely to be beneficial in making the correct diagnosis, providing prognostic information, or obtaining vital information prior to invasive procedures. Despite these potential benefits, there are risks related to cardiac CT including radiation and contrast agents, which should be minimized as much as possible. There are also patient factors that can influence the diagnostic quality of the cardiac CT exam, which can render the exam uninterpretable and not beneficial. Careful patient selection will help improve the benefit to risk ratio and maximize the usefulness of cardiac CT.

Keywords Cardiac CT • Radiation • Appropriate use • Coronary artery angiography

Patient Selection

Proper patient selection is extremely important in all diagnostic testing, whether it is a basic laboratory blood test or invasive diagnostic procedure. The potential benefit should outweigh the risk of the test. With cardiac CT, valuable information regarding coronary arteries and cardiac anatomy can be obtained rapidly in a non-invasive manner. However, there are factors that can influence the diagnostic quality of the cardiac CT exam, which can render the exam non-diagnostic and uninterpretable,

S.W. Leung, MD (✉)
Division of Cardiovascular Medicine, Departments of Medicine and Radiology, University of Kentucky, 900 S. Limestone St., CT Wethington Bldg, Rm 326, Lexington, KY 40536, USA
e-mail: steve.leung@uky.edu

M.Y. Chen, MD
Cardiovascular and Pulmonary Branch, National Heart, Lung, and Blood Institute, National Institutes of Health, 10 Center Drive, MSC 1061 Building 10, Room B1D416, Bethesda, MD 20892-1061, USA
e-mail: marcus.chen@nih.gov

P.L. Tilkemeier et al. (eds.), *Quality Evaluation in Non-Invasive Cardiovascular Imaging*, DOI 10.1007/978-3-319-28011-0_7

and thus provide no benefit to the patient. These factors can differ based on the indication for the tests.

In general, patients who have trouble staying motionless or holding their breath should not undergo a cardiac CT scan since motion artifacts cannot be corrected. Patients who are unable to raise their arms away from the thorax should avoid undergoing cardiac CT due to extra tissue and bone creating significant attenuation or artifacts rendering the images more difficult to interpret. For certain indications where ECG gating is necessary, patients who have electrical implants that can cause significant amount of electromagnetic interference, may not be able to undergo a gated cardiac CT. These interferences cause artifacts in the patient's electrocardiogram (ECG), which can cause the scanner to gate incorrectly and obtain non-diagnostic images. More importantly, however, is that the patient must have a slow and regular rhythm so as to gate the images. Therefore, frequent ectopy and rhythms such as atrial fibrillation are contraindications for the performance of CCTA.

Unfortunately, there are also potential risks related to this non-invasive procedure, which includes radiation exposure, infiltration of intravenous line causing compartment syndrome and exposure to contrast agents that can cause anaphylactic reactions or nephrotoxicity. Child-bearing age women should be evaluated for pregnancy to avoid radiation to the fetus. Although the uterus is not directly scanned, the scattered x-rays from the thorax can reach the fetus. Patients may also be exposed to medications that decrease their heart rate for the scan, which can cause heart block or bronchospasm, or nitroglycerin for vasodilation of the coronaries, which can cause severe hypotension. Though the potential risks are small, they are also avoidable risks. If the results of the test do not alter patient management or provide useful data for invasive procedure planning, the test should be avoided. In total, approximately one-third of patients being considered for CCTA should not undergo the procedure due to the risks noted above or the likelihood of an inadequate study.

Coronary Artery Calcium Scoring (CACS)

Coronary artery calcium scoring (CACS) is extremely helpful in the identification of coronary atherosclerosis. In addition to the detection of the presence of CAD, CACS is also a great prognostic indicator in determining a patient's risk for mortality and cardiovascular event [1–4]. Based on the Multi-Ethnic Study of Atherosclerosis (MESA) data, CACS can be used to assess the patient's relative calcium score compared to other patients matched for age, gender, and ethnicity. This data is applicable to patients who are between 45 and 84 years of age, and does not have diabetes mellitus (DM) or history of known CAD [5]. An online calculator can be used to calculate this percentile (http://www.mesa-nhlbi.org/Calcium/input.aspx) based on the patient's age, gender and ethnicity.

For CACS exams, patients should be asymptomatic and do not have known history of CAD, including previous coronary stenting or bypass operations. Without the use of contrast to perform coronary angiography, CACS cannot distinguish whether a patient has obstructive CAD or not, and thus would not be useful in symptomatic patients where obstructive CAD is being questioned. Patients who have no coronary calcium identified by CACS still have approximately 5 % likelihood of having obstructive CAD (non-calcified plaques) [6]. Patients with large amount of tissue in the chest area can cause significant amounts of image noise over the heart which are >130 Hounsfield units, and falsely be considered as coronary calcification. Patients with fast heart rates can cause significant coronary motion that would result in an inaccurate calcium score [7].

Coronary Computed Tomographic Angiography

Coronary computed tomographic angiography (CTA) has the highest specificity in the identification of obstructive CAD compared to other non-invasive diagnostic tests [8, 9]. Patients, who are at low to intermediate risk for CAD and experiencing symptoms that are suggestive of obstructive CAD, benefit the most from coronary CTA [10]. In patients who have high-risk features such as presenting with acute coronary syndrome (e.g. elevated cardiac enzymes or ST-elevation on electrocardiogram (ECG)) would benefit more from directly undergoing coronary angiography and potentially percutaneous intervention.

Since a large portion of coronary arteries are small structures ranging between 1 and 5 mm, to obtain optimal coronary CTA images for evaluation of CAD, patients must be able to follow commands, hold their breath and keep their body still. They should have slow heart rate, a regular rhythm, normal renal function, no history of reactions to iodinated contrast and reasonable body mass around the chest. Breathing and body movement can cause motion artifacts that are not correctable, and thus would result in uninterpretable images. Slow and regular heart rates are optimal for coronary CTA. Next generation scanners that can acquire images of the coronaries within a single heartbeat can potentially overcome the issue regarding irregular heart rhythm. Patients with faster heart rates can be slowed with oral and intravenous (IV) medications. In patients with renal insufficiency and history of anaphylactic reaction, since iodinated contrast is used to visualize coronary arteries, one must weigh the risk of the test vs the benefit, and make the appropriate preparations prior to the scan if the test is necessary.

Good IV access (able to sustain ≥5 mL/s contrast injection for the duration of the contrast injection) is necessary to the optimal opacification of the coronary arteries. These are generally 20 gauge or larger peripheral IV catheters placed in the antecubital area. Patients with poor IV access should not undergo coronary CTA as the image quality is likely to be non-diagnostic.

Although one can increase the radiation peak energy (kVp), number of photons (mAs), or use higher density iodinated-contrast agent to improve image quality in morbidly obese patients with body mass index (BMI) >40 kg/m^2, there is a limit to which the signal-to-noise and contrast-to-noise overwhelms the diagnostic quality of the image. In extreme cases, the patient would have received a significant amount of radiation and nephrotoxic contrast without the benefit of a diagnosis due to uninterpretable images. Other factors also include patients who are unable to raise their arms above their shoulders, which can cause significant x-ray attenuation throughout the chest from the humerus. Another potential problem includes patients with pacemaker or implantable cardioverter defibrillators, where streak artifacts from metallic leads can interfere with interpretation of the coronary arteries [11].

Cardiac Structures

Due to the high spatial resolution, cardiac CT is optimal in the assessment of cardiac structures that have minimal motion such as the left atrial appendage, pulmonary veins, coronary sinus, or vascular connections in complex congenital heart disease. Cardiac CT acquisitions are fast and can cover a larger area of the body compared to echocardiography, which is sometimes limited by echocardiographic windows. However, because of lower temporal resolution and radiation exposure, cardiac CT should only be used to assess valvular heart disease and ventricular function if echocardiography was suboptimal and patient cannot undergo cardiac MRI.

Similar to coronary artery evaluation, it would be optimal for the patient to be able to follow commands and hold their breath. If the exam is for the evaluation of small, mobile cardiac structures, slow heart rate, regular heart rhythm, good renal function and reasonable body habitus would also improve image quality. Good IV access is necessary for optimal contrast opacification of the cardiac structures of interest. In complex congenital heart disease, pre-procedure planning including the placement of peripheral IV catheter in the appropriate extremity is essential as vascular connections may not be typical and can interfere with optimal contrast opacification. Since most cardiac structures of interest are larger than coronary arteries, these restrictions are not as stringent to obtain diagnostic images.

Cardiac Perfusion

With the availability of faster scanners with lower radiation dose, stress cardiac perfusion has been evaluated to be feasible. Stress cardiac perfusion by CT has been demonstrated to correctly identify patients with obstructive CAD [12, 13]. Patients are generally first scanned at rest, which will include resting perfusion as well as anatomical data on the coronary arteries. Then, the patient will be started on a vasodilator such as adenosine infusion, which can increase the heart rate. A second contrast injection is given and stress perfusion scan performed.

In the CT perfusion trials, patients underwent adenosine stress, which required two IV access, one for the adenosine infusion and the other for contrast injection. Atrial fibrillation, body mass index >40 kg/m^2, high degree heart block and renal insufficiency were exclusion criteria in these studies. Currently, cardiac CT perfusion is not widely used and should be considered investigational.

Contraindications

In general, non-dialysis patients with renal dysfunction at risk of further renal damage from nephrotoxic contrast should consider avoiding coronary CTA or contrast-enhanced cardiac CT and undergo alternative method of testing, which may include invasive strategies such as cardiac catheterization, if indicated. Despite various techniques to reduce the risk of nephrotoxicity (e.g. low osmolality contrast and IV fluids), there is still a risk of worsening renal function [14–21].

Patients who do not have adequate IV access cannot undergo coronary CTA, since it requires high injection rates to achieve diagnostic opacification of coronary arteries.

Patients who have difficult to control heart rates (>80 bpm) despite beta blocker or calcium channel blocker administration should not undergo coronary CTA, as the rate of non-diagnostic study is high due to coronary motion artifacts and should be considered for alternative testing.

Patients with irregular heart rhythms should be evaluated and determine whether coronary CTA should be performed. In some facilities, where single heart beat scanning can be performed utilizing wide area detectors, slow irregular rhythm may not be a contraindication to the study. Otherwise, these patients should not have a coronary CTA as the result is likely to be a non-diagnostic study due to significant stitching (step) artifacts.

Patients who have significantly large body size or body mass index (BMI) should avoid coronary CTA due to the potentially high levels of noise in the image. These factors would have to be assessed on an individual patient basis since the distribution of weight, and actual body mass may play different roles towards image quality. For example, a patient with BMI >50 kg/m^2, 5-foot tall with most of the mass distributed in the abdomen and pelvis is likely to have less noise than one that is 6-foot tall with most of the mass distributed over the chest. Also, certain scanners can deliver higher dose of radiation or have iterative reconstruction capabilities, which may reduce noise and improve the diagnostic quality of the study. While using higher peak voltage (kVp), one must consider using higher iodine concentration contrast to improve contrast-to-noise within opacified coronaries as well, since higher kVp penetrate through lower contrast densities causing decreased contrast-to-noise ratio. Both of these factors increase overall radiation dose and contrast exposure to the patient, and higher likelihood of potential nephrotoxic effects.

Many of the contraindications related to coronary artery assessment may not apply to patients undergoing cardiac structural assessment. To be able to evaluate smaller structures such as the coronary arteries and potential obstructive disease require techniques that are less forgiving compared to assessment of larger structures (e.g. pulmonary veins). Patients with faster, irregular heart rhythms, higher BMIs can still have diagnostic imaging of the cardiac structures despite uninterpretable coronary arteries. However, to evaluate smaller/thinner structures such as valvular disease would still require regular heart rhythm and decreased heart rate.

Radiation Exposure

Although there are no prospective randomized controlled trials evaluating the effects of medical radiation on the risk of cancer, it is believed that there is a non-linear no threshold risk of cancer based on radiation exposure by atomic bomb survivors as published in the BEIR VII phase-2 report [22].

The optimal method of minimizing radiation exposure is to avoid performing unnecessary cardiac CT in patients that is unlikely to change management. However, when testing is necessary, ALARA (As Low As Reasonably Achievable) principle should be applied. There are methods of reducing radiation exposure without losing diagnostic quality of the images. The Society of Cardiovascular CT released a guideline in 2011 aimed at providing strategies, which can reduce radiation in cardiovascular CT without reducing quality [23].

It is common practice for CACS to be performed prior to coronary CTA; however, the benefit has not been demonstrated. The potential benefit of having CACS may include identification of heavy calcification that would preclude a diagnostic coronary CTA, and thus would avoid exposure of additional radiation and nephrotoxic contrast. By obtaining a CACS prior to coronary CTA, some may benefit from better localization of the coronary artery location, and thus can reduce the z-axis distance and radiation exposure or potential need for repeat scanning due to clipping of proximal coronaries. There is also potential benefit of determining whether the set tube current (mAs) is too much or too little for a given image quality, and optimize the protocol to obtain diagnostic coronary CTA images.

Patient preparation is key to minimizing radiation exposure. By obtaining good IV access, giving adequate breath holding instructions, informing the patient of the sensation after nitroglycerin administration and contrast injection, reducing heart rate with beta blockers or calcium channel blockers can help reduce the need for repeat scanning secondary to motion artifacts or inadequate opacification of coronary arteries (Fig. 7.1).

Specifics regarding reducing radiation dosimetry by adjusting acquisition and processing parameters will be addressed in detail in Chap. 9.

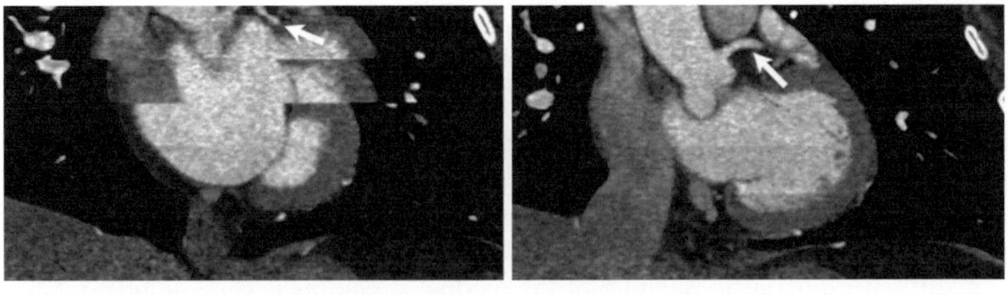

Fig. 7.1 Breathing artifacts. Both scans were performed at the same scout position. During the first scan (*left*), the patient did not start the breath hold until after the first beat acquisition resulting in significant step artifact. After better patient instruction, a repeat scan (*right*) was performed and the images were diagnostic. Note the position of the left main coronary artery (*arrows*), and the step artifacts from this prospectively gated scan

Appropriate Use Criteria

Appropriate use criteria (AUC) documents are based on available data and consensus amongst these experts to help guide practitioners on whether a test is likely to be beneficial in various clinical situations. In carefully selected populations, the results of the imaging tests can help practitioners regarding the next steps of patient management, which ultimately saves lives, reduce morbidity, improve quality of life and be cost effective.

AUC for CT were initially developed in 2007 and then revised in 2010 in order to help guide practitioners in the use of cardiac CT [24]. In addition, for patients with stable ischemic heart disease, a separate appropriate use criteria document was published in 2013 [10]. The appropriate use criteria are separated into three categories for each indication: appropriate, maybe appropriate or rarely appropriate. However, one needs to be mindful that even if a patient's indication for a particular test is considered appropriate, it does not mean that they should undergo testing. In contrast, a patient may benefit from a test for an indication that may be considered rarely appropriate (or inappropriate). These appropriate use criteria are general guidelines for practitioners and each patient should be assessed for appropriateness individually.

Coronary Artery Calcium Scoring (CACS)

CACS should only be performed on patients without symptoms clearly related to CAD, and may also be performed for risk stratification purposes. In patients who have low overall cardiovascular event risk, but have significant family history of early onset of CAD are also indicated to have CACS performed, if it changes management. In patients with intermediate cardiovascular risk and cannot determine whether statin therapy should be implemented, CACS can also help guide therapy. With the new Adult Treatment Panel IV cholesterol guidelines, patients without history of CAD and has DM <40 years of age or >75 years of age or LDL <70, or patients without history of CAD or DM with a <5 % 10-year atherosclerosis cardiovascular disease risk, age <40 years old, >75 years old and LDL <190, coronary calcium Agatston score of ≥300, or ≥75th percentile of matched age, gender and ethnicity may help patient and clinician decision making in whether to start statin therapy [25].

Coronary Computed Tomography Angiography

Evaluation of CAD in Asymptomatic Patient

Asymptomatic patients are rarely appropriate to undergo coronary CTA. Even if significant CAD is found, revascularization has not been shown to reduce the risk of myocardial infarction or death in patients who are not having active acute coronary syndrome [26]. The only benefit that revascularization or percutaneous coronary intervention has demonstrated in this population is reduction in symptoms, which would not be helpful for asymptomatic patients. Currently, there are no clinical trial evidence that treating asymptomatic patients with incidental stenosis can help reduce future cardiovascular events. Coronary CTA may be appropriate in asymptomatic heart transplant patients for evaluation of transplant vasculopathy [27]. Since transplanted hearts are not innervated in the recipient, patients may not have anginal equivalent symptoms. Although one should also be mindful that these patients generally have higher heart rates because they do not have baseline vagal tone suppression of the sinus node, and therefore heart rates can be difficult to control even with beta blockers to obtain a diagnostic scan.

Evaluation of CAD in Symptomatic Patient, Non-emergent Setting

Patients presenting in non-emergent situations with symptoms suggestive of CAD should be risk stratified based on their risk factors for having CAD. In patients with low to intermediate risk, coronary CTA is appropriate. In patients with intermediate risk, there remains a debate whether they should undergo physiologic stress testing or anatomic evaluation with coronary CTA. The results of the PROMISE trial demonstrate that CCTA is an effective alternative to stress imaging [28]. In patients with high risk for CAD, they should not undergo coronary CTA, and should be assessed with invasive coronary angiography.

Evaluation of CAD in Symptomatic Patient, Acute Setting

In the acute setting, coronary CTA has been demonstrated to be extremely useful in patients with low to intermediate risk for CAD [29–31]. Coronary CTA has a very high negative predictive value, and negative likelihood ratio. Patients with normal coronary CTA have a lower risk of cardiovascular events. Thus, patients with low to intermediate probability of having CAD are considered appropriate to undergo coronary CTA for further evaluation. Patients with high probability for CAD such as patients with elevated cardiac enzymes or ECG changes, will benefit from going directly to invasive coronary angiography, and avoid delays in diagnosis and potential treatment in addition to radiation and contrast from coronary CTA.

Evaluation of CAD in Patients with Prior Testing

In patients who have undergone stress testing for CAD (e.g. ECG, echocardiography, nuclear or cardiac MRI) which had equivocal results, further evaluation by coronary CTA is considered appropriate. In patients with moderate to severe ischemia findings should proceed with invasive coronary angiography rather than coronary CTA since the pre-test likelihood for CAD is not low. In patients with mild ischemic findings, they can consider coronary CTA for further evaluation, since it may represent a false positive result. In patients with continued symptoms despite normal ECG stress test (no imaging), they can be considered for coronary CTA for diagnosis of obstructive CAD.

Prior to coronary CTA, many institutions perform CACS. If the CACS demonstrate coronary calcification of >600–1000, it is reasonable to stop the test and recommend alternative method of diagnosis since the calcified plaque can cause blooming and beam hardening artifacts that obscure view of the coronary artery's true lumen. Patients with coronary calcium of <600 can proceed with coronary CTA portion of the test with minimal risk of non-diagnostic images due to dense calcification.

CAD with History of Coronary Stent Placement

Patients with a history of CAD and has had coronary stenting may still be considered appropriate to undergo coronary CTA if the stent is ≥3.0 mm in size. Due to the blooming artifact and beam hardening effects of the metallic struts, the lumen of smaller stent sizes are more difficult to assess. By utilizing a sharper/harder filter/kernel, these vessels can be assessed more accurately [32, 33].

CAD with History of Coronary Artery Bypass Grafting

In patients with a history of coronary artery bypass grafting and symptoms suggestive of obstructive disease, graft location and patency can be readily assessed with coronary CTA. These patients will need to have their heart scanned from a higher starting point to cover the origin of the internal mammary arteries, which is a common artery used in coronary artery bypass grafting. Also of note, this bypass graft can be performed via minimal invasive method and thus the patient may not have sternal wires.

One safety caveat to consider is that these scans cover from the clavicle down to the diaphragm. In patients who are pacemaker dependent, scanning over the pacemaker can cause electromagnetic interference that causes missensing of the pacemaker and inhibit pacing. Since coronary CTA are gated studies, there would be lack of gating during pacemaker inhibition, and the CT scanner will continue to scan at the same location while the patient remains pulseless.

Anomalous Coronary Artery

In patients with suspected anomalous coronaries, or identified anomalous coronary by cardiac catheterization, coronary CTA can identify the site of origin and course which can help guide downstream management such as surgical approach.

New Onset Heart Failure

Patients presented with new onset heart failure should undergo evaluation to determine whether ischemia from CAD is the cause of the cardiomyopathy. These patients generally present with systolic heart failure (decreased ejection fraction). Thus if they have a low to intermediate risk of CAD, coronary CTA is deemed appropriate. However, if they are at high risk for CAD, they should undergo cardiac catheterization for definitive diagnosis and potential therapy via stenting or bypass grafting. In patients who present with diastolic heart failure (preserved ejection fraction), it is uncertain whether coronary CTA can be beneficial as the likelihood of CAD causing diastolic heart failure is low.

Pre-operative Assessment

Pre-operative cardiac risk assessment is a complex topic. Patients can be risk stratified pre-operatively, but there are no clinical trial data that suggest these risks can be modified [34]. In patients undergoing non-coronary cardiac operation, they should undergo further testing for CAD if they are intermediate to high risk of having CAD. These patients can potentially undergo coronary artery bypass grafting during their non-coronary cardiac operation to avoid another sternotomy. It is appropriate to evaluate for CAD with coronary CTA in intermediate risk patients; however, for high-risk patients, the appropriateness remains uncertain as these patients may benefit from invasive coronary angiography as they are more likely to have CAD. In patients undergoing non-cardiac operations, the appropriateness of performing cardiac CTA in patients undergoing intermediate risk or vascular operations who are unable to perform four METS and has one or more clinical risk factors is considered uncertain.

Cardiac Structures

Pulmonary Venous Anatomy

Prior to atrial fibrillation ablation procedure, pulmonary venous anatomy should be evaluated. Pulmonary venous anatomy can vary between patients due to confluence of several pulmonary veins into a common vein prior to entering into the left atrium or accessory pulmonary vein [35]. The identification of pulmonary venous anatomy can help guide the electrophysiologist in determining areas that would require ablation, and potentially identify accessory pulmonary veins that are often missed [36].

Cardiac Venous Anatomy

The variability of cardiac venous anatomy makes it difficult for electrophysiologists to place the left ventricular lead in biventricular implantable cardioverter-defibrillator devices. The left ventricular lead is generally placed via the coronary sinus into a lateral cardiac vein. By performing a slightly delayed timing of coronary CTA relative to coronary artery assessment, the cardiac venous anatomy can be optimally visualized and provide a roadmap for the electrophysiologists.

Congenital Heart Disease

Congenital heart disease can be extremely complex to describe and image with CTA. It requires understanding of the surgical corrections, venous connections and IV placement, along with flow dynamics to be able to capture the complexity of congenital heart disease. Due to the risk of radiation exposure and nephrotoxic contrast, in patients who are unable to undergo cardiac MRI, cardiac CT would be an appropriate alternative.

Valvular Disease

Patients, who have valvular disease or prosthetic valves, which could not be adequately evaluated by echocardiography or cardiac MR, may be considered for cardiac CT for evaluation of valvular function to determine severity of stenosis or regurgitation, although this is far from the ideal modality. Since cardiac CT can only assess anatomical data, many of the parameters used to evaluate valvular function severity by echocardiography and cardiac MRI cannot be used (e.g. mean and peak gradients, regurgitant volume, regurgitant fraction). However, due to the high spatial resolution and 3D data set, anatomic planimetry can be performed to accurately assess the size of valvular stenosis or regurgitant orifice area.

With the increasing numbers of transcatheter aortic valve implantation procedures, the use of cardiac CT is essential in pre-procedure planning [37]. Cardiac CT can help in sizing the aortic annulus to determine the size of the valve necessary for the procedure, and reduce the incidence of post-implant peri-valvular leak and need for repeat dilation, which carries a fourfold increased risk of stroke [38]. Various complicating factors can be identified including annular calcification, coronary height, sinotubular junction size and calcification, potential transaortic and transapical access sites and route, approximate orientation of the valve deployment angle under fluoroscopy to reduce fluoroscopy time and contrast use in aortograms, and vascular access approach.

Pericardium

The assessment of the pericardium can be performed with cardiac CT. In patients with suspected constrictive pericarditis, a cardiac CT can identify areas of calcification of the pericardium and pericardial thickening.

Cardiac Mass

When there is suspected cardiac mass, cardiac CT is a useful tool to characterize the size, location and type of the mass when other imaging modalities are unable to evaluate it fully (e.g. echocardiogram or cardiac MRI). In certain instances, the combination of positron emission tomography/CT would be helpful to determine whether the mass is metabolically active.

Cardiac Function

Cardiac function, such as ventricular ejection fraction, can be evaluated by contrast-enhanced cardiac CT. Since CT scanners require at least 180° gantry rotation to have sufficient data to create an image, the temporal resolution depends heavily on gantry rotational speed. Most scanners have gantry rotational speed of at most 350 ms per rotation (i.e. temporal resolution is 175 ms). Even with dual source CT scanners where it only requires a quarter rotation, the temporal resolution remains at approximately 66–88 ms, which is more than two times slower compared to echocardiography and cardiac MRI.

To obtain cardiac function, a retrospective scan is required, which exposes the patient with significantly higher amount of radiation than a prospective scan. Due to the availability of other non-radiating methods and better temporal resolution, cardiac CT should be reserved for patients who do not have good echocardiographic windows or unable to undergo cardiac MRI. Since cardiac CT has high spatial resolution and is not limited by echocardiographic window, both ventricles can be easily imaged and seen. Thus contrast-enhanced cardiac CT can be used for evaluation of biventricular function. In patients with suspected arrhythmogenic right ventricular dysplasia (ARVD), cardiac CT is considered appropriate for evaluation of right ventricular morphology as well. Of note, the 2010 ARVD Task Force Criteria for the diagnosis of ARVD does not include the use of cardiac CT [39].

References

1. Blaha M, Budoff MJ, Shaw LJ, Khosa F, Rumberger JA, Berman D, et al. Absence of coronary artery calcification and all-cause mortality. JACC Cardiovasc Imaging. 2009;2(6):692–700.
2. Patel J, Blaha MJ, McEvoy JW, Qadir S, Tota-Maharaj R, Shaw LJ, et al. All-cause mortality in asymptomatic persons with extensive Agatston scores above 1000. J Cardiovasc Comput Tomogr. 2014;8(1):26–32.
3. Nasir K, Rubin J, Blaha MJ, Shaw LJ, Blankstein R, Rivera JJ, et al. Interplay of coronary artery calcification and traditional risk factors for the prediction of all-cause mortality in asymptomatic individuals. Circ Cardiovasc Imaging. 2012;5(4):467–73.
4. Greenland P, Alpert JS, Beller GA, Benjamin EJ, Budoff MJ, Fayad ZA, et al. 2010 ACCF/AHA guideline for assessment of cardiovascular risk in asymptomatic adults: a report of the American College of Cardiology Foundation/American Heart Association Task Force on Practice Guidelines. J Am Coll Cardiol. 2010;56(25):e50–103.

5. McClelland RL, Chung H, Detrano R, Post W, Kronmal RA. Distribution of coronary artery calcium by race, gender, and age: results from the Multi-Ethnic Study of Atherosclerosis (MESA). Circulation. 2006;113(1):30–7.
6. Kim YJ, Hur J, Lee HJ, Chang HJ, Nam JE, Hong YJ, et al. Meaning of zero coronary calcium score in symptomatic patients referred for coronary computed tomographic angiography. Eur Heart J Cardiovasc Imaging. 2012;13(9):776–85.
7. Brown SJ, Hayball MP, Coulden RA. Impact of motion artefact on the measurement of coronary calcium score. Br J Radiol. 2000;73(873):956–62.
8. Miller JM, Rochitte CE, Dewey M, Arbab-Zadeh A, Niinuma H, Gottlieb I, et al. Diagnostic performance of coronary angiography by 64-row CT. N Engl J Med. 2008;359(22): 2324–36.
9. Budoff MJ, Dowe D, Jollis JG, Gitter M, Sutherland J, Halamert E, et al. Diagnostic performance of 64-multidetector row coronary computed tomographic angiography for evaluation of coronary artery stenosis in individuals without known coronary artery disease: results from the prospective multicenter ACCURACY (Assessment by Coronary Computed Tomographic Angiography of Individuals Undergoing Invasive Coronary Angiography) trial. J Am Coll Cardiol. 2008;52(21):1724–32.
10. Wolk MJ, Bailey SR, Doherty JU, Douglas PS, Hendel RC, Kramer CM, et al. ACCF/AHA/ASE/ASNC/HFSA/HRS/SCAI/SCCT/SCMR/STS 2013 multimodality appropriate use criteria for the detection and risk assessment of stable ischemic heart disease: a report of the American College of Cardiology Foundation Appropriate Use Criteria Task Force, American Heart Association, American Society of Echocardiography, American Society of Nuclear Cardiology, Heart Failure Society of America, Heart Rhythm Society, Society for Cardiovascular Angiography and Interventions, Society of Cardiovascular Computed Tomography, Society for Cardiovascular Magnetic Resonance, and Society of Thoracic Surgeons. J Am Coll Cardiol. 2014;63(4):380–406.
11. Mak GS, Truong QA. Cardiac CT: imaging of and through cardiac devices. Curr Cardiovas Imaging Rep. 2012;5(5):328–36.
12. Rochitte CE, George RT, Chen MY, Arbab-Zadeh A, Dewey M, Miller JM, et al. Computed tomography angiography and perfusion to assess coronary artery stenosis causing perfusion defects by single photon emission computed tomography: the CORE320 study. Eur Heart J. 2014;35(17):1120–30.
13. George RT, Arbab-Zadeh A, Miller JM, Kitagawa K, Chang HJ, Bluemke DA, et al. Adenosine stress 64- and 256-row detector computed tomography angiography and perfusion imaging: a pilot study evaluating the transmural extent of perfusion abnormalities to predict atherosclerosis causing myocardial ischemia. Circ Cardiovasc Imaging. 2009;2(3):174–82.
14. Brar SS, Shen AY, Jorgensen MB, Kotlewski A, Aharonian VJ, Desai N, et al. Sodium bicarbonate vs sodium chloride for the prevention of contrast medium-induced nephropathy in patients undergoing coronary angiography: a randomized trial. JAMA. 2008;300(9):1038–46.
15. Briguori C, Airoldi F, D'Andrea D, Bonizzoni E, Morici N, Focaccio A, et al. Renal Insufficiency Following Contrast Media Administration Trial (REMEDIAL): a randomized comparison of 3 preventive strategies. Circulation. 2007;115(10):1211–7.
16. Merten GJ, Burgess WP, Gray LV, Holleman JH, Roush TS, Kowalchuk GJ, et al. Prevention of contrast-induced nephropathy with sodium bicarbonate: a randomized controlled trial. JAMA. 2004;291(19):2328–34.
17. Investigators ACT. Acetylcysteine for prevention of renal outcomes in patients undergoing coronary and peripheral vascular angiography: main results from the randomized Acetylcysteine for Contrast-induced nephropathy Trial (ACT). Circulation. 2011;124(11):1250–9.
18. Kay J, Chow WH, Chan TM, Lo SK, Kwok OH, Yip A, et al. Acetylcysteine for prevention of acute deterioration of renal function following elective coronary angiography and intervention: a randomized controlled trial. JAMA. 2003;289(5):553–8.
19. Marenzi G, Assanelli E, Marana I, Lauri G, Campodonico J, Grazi M, et al. N-acetylcysteine and contrast-induced nephropathy in primary angioplasty. N Engl J Med. 2006;354(26): 2773–82.

20. Han Y, Zhu G, Han L, Hou F, Huang W, Liu H, et al. Short-term rosuvastatin therapy for prevention of contrast-induced acute kidney injury in patients with diabetes and chronic kidney disease. J Am Coll Cardiol. 2014;63(1):62–70.
21. Leoncini M, Toso A, Maioli M, Tropeano F, Villani S, Bellandi F. Early high-dose rosuvastatin for contrast-induced nephropathy prevention in acute coronary syndrome: results from the PRATO-ACS Study (Protective Effect of Rosuvastatin and Antiplatelet Therapy On contrast-induced acute kidney injury and myocardial damage in patients with Acute Coronary Syndrome). J Am Coll Cardiol. 2014;63(1):71–9.
22. National Research Council (U.S.). Committee to assess health risks from exposure to low level of ionizing radiation. Health risks from exposure to low levels of ionizing radiation: BEIR VII phase 2. Washington, DC: National Academies Press; 2006. p. xvi. 406 p.
23. Halliburton SS, Abbara S, Chen MY, Gentry R, Mahesh M, Raff GL, et al. SCCT guidelines on radiation dose and dose-optimization strategies in cardiovascular CT. J Cardiovasc Comput Tomogr. 2011;5(4):198–224.
24. Taylor AJ, Cerqueira M, Hodgson JM, Mark D, Min J, O'Gara P, et al. ACCF/SCCT/ACR/AHA/ASE/ASNC/NASCI/SCAI/SCMR 2010 appropriate Use criteria for cardiac computed tomography. A report of the American College of Cardiology Foundation Appropriate Use Criteria Task Force, the Society of Cardiovascular Computed Tomography, the American College of Radiology, the American Heart Association, the American Society of Echocardiography, the American Society of Nuclear Cardiology, the North American Society for Cardiovascular Imaging, the Society for Cardiovascular Angiography and Interventions, and the Society for Cardiovascular Magnetic Resonance. J Cardiovasc Comput Tomogr. 2010;4(6):407.e1–33.
25. Stone NJ, Robinson JG, Lichtenstein AH, Bairey Merz CN, Blum CB, Eckel RH, et al. 2013 ACC/AHA guideline on the treatment of blood cholesterol to reduce atherosclerotic cardiovascular risk in adults: a report of the American College of Cardiology/American Heart Association Task Force on Practice Guidelines. Circulation. 2014;129(25 Suppl 2):S1–45.
26. Boden WE, O'Rourke RA, Teo KK, Hartigan PM, Maron DJ, Kostuk WJ, et al. Optimal medical therapy with or without PCI for stable coronary disease. N Engl J Med. 2007;356(15):1503–16.
27. Wever-Pinzon O, Romero J, Kelesidis I, Wever-Pinzon J, Manrique C, Budge D, et al. Coronary computed tomography angiography for the detection of cardiac allograft vasculopathy: a meta-analysis of prospective trials. J Am Coll Cardiol. 2014;63(19):1992–2004.
28. Douglas PS, Hoffmann U, Lee KL, Mark DB, Al-Khalidi HR, Anstrom K, et al. PROspective multicenter imaging study for evaluation of chest pain: rationale and design of the PROMISE trial. Am Heart J. 2014;167(6):796–803.e1.
29. Goldstein JA, Chinnaiyan KM, Abidov A, Achenbach S, Berman DS, Hayes SW, et al. The CT-STAT (Coronary Computed Tomographic Angiography for Systematic Triage of Acute Chest Pain Patients to Treatment) trial. J Am Coll Cardiol. 2011;58(14):1414–22.
30. Goldstein JA, Gallagher MJ, O'Neill WW, Ross MA, O'Neil BJ, Raff GL. A randomized controlled trial of multi-slice coronary computed tomography for evaluation of acute chest pain. J Am Coll Cardiol. 2007;49(8):863–71.
31. Litt HI, Gatsonis C, Snyder B, Singh H, Miller CD, Entrikin DW, et al. CT angiography for safe discharge of patients with possible acute coronary syndromes. N Engl J Med. 2012;366(15):1393–403.
32. Seifarth H, Raupach R, Schaller S, Fallenberg EM, Flohr T, Heindel W, et al. Assessment of coronary artery stents using 16-slice MDCT angiography: evaluation of a dedicated reconstruction kernel and a noise reduction filter. Eur Radiol. 2005;15(4):721–6.
33. Ehara M, Kawai M, Surmely JF, Matsubara T, Terashima M, Tsuchikane E, et al. Diagnostic accuracy of coronary in-stent restenosis using 64-slice computed tomography: comparison with invasive coronary angiography. J Am Coll Cardiol. 2007;49(9):951–9.
34. McFalls EO, Ward HB, Moritz TE, Goldman S, Krupski WC, Littooy F, et al. Coronary-artery revascularization before elective major vascular surgery. N Engl J Med. 2004;351(27):2795–804.

35. Kato R, Lickfett L, Meininger G, Dickfeld T, Wu R, Juang G, et al. Pulmonary vein anatomy in patients undergoing catheter ablation of atrial fibrillation: lessons learned by use of magnetic resonance imaging. Circulation. 2003;107(15):2004–10.
36. Jongbloed MR, Bax JJ, Lamb HJ, Dirksen MS, Zeppenfeld K, van der Wall EE, et al. Multislice computed tomography versus intracardiac echocardiography to evaluate the pulmonary veins before radiofrequency catheter ablation of atrial fibrillation: a head-to-head comparison. J Am Coll Cardiol. 2005;45(3):343–50.
37. Achenbach S, Delgado V, Hausleiter J, Schoenhagen P, Min JK, Leipsic JA. SCCT expert consensus document on computed tomography imaging before transcatheter aortic valve implantation (TAVI)/transcatheter aortic valve replacement (TAVR). J Cardiovasc Comput Tomogr. 2012;6(6):366–80.
38. Jilaihawi H, Kashif M, Fontana G, Furugen A, Shiota T, Friede G, et al. Cross-sectional computed tomographic assessment improves accuracy of aortic annular sizing for transcatheter aortic valve replacement and reduces the incidence of paravalvular aortic regurgitation. J Am Coll Cardiol. 2012;59(14):1275–86.
39. Marcus FI, McKenna WJ, Sherrill D, Basso C, Bauce B, Bluemke DA, et al. Diagnosis of arrhythmogenic right ventricular cardiomyopathy/dysplasia: proposed modification of the task force criteria. Circulation. 2010;121(13):1533–41.

Chapter 8
Computed Tomography: Quality Control

James A. Case

Abstract Cardiovascular CT has the potential to deliver very high resolution images of the coronary artery system with minimal radiation dosage and study time. To achieve diagnostic quality images, CT acquisitions must be acquired using appropriate protocols, an appropriate scanner instrumentation and data processed correctly. Technologists should be aware of the trade-offs in acquisition parameters and understand optimal processing techniques. Physicians should also be able to recognize high quality cardiac CT studies and identify image artifacts as well as acquisition/processing errors when present.

Keywords Cardiac CT • Quality control • Data processing • CT radiation • Artifact recognition

History of CT

In 1973, the invention of x-ray computed tomography was announced which revolutionized medical imaging by allowing high resolution, high contrast, non-invasive volumetric images of internal anatomy [1, 2]. The combination of CT and contrast enhanced angiography open the door to volumetric imaging of the cardiovascular system. Despite this theoretical possibility, several practical considerations remained. First, the vessels to be imaged are small (<3 mm), second, many of the lesions of the coronaries have comparable density to soft tissue (fat = –40 Hounsfield Units (HU), blood and muscle = 10 HU, and fibrous tissue = 70 HU). By far, the greatest challenge is the fact the heart is constantly in motion.

In a typical cardiac cycle of 60 beats/min, the blood vessels will move 20 mm giving them an average speed of 20 mm/s. In 1983, Imatron released the first commercial electron beam based computed tomography system (EBCT). Unlike traditional CT scanners, the Imatron system used a small linear accelerator to create

J.A. Case, PhD
Technical Director, Technical Director, Cardiovascular Imaging Technologies, Kansas City, MO, USA
e-mail: jcase@cvit.com

P.L. Tilkemeier et al. (eds.), *Quality Evaluation in Non-Invasive Cardiovascular Imaging*, DOI 10.1007/978-3-319-28011-0_8

a beam of electrons that could be steered around the patient. These electrons were swept across a system of targets to create an arc of x-rays necessary to produce tomographic images. Because this system did not require any moving parts, it could achieve extremely fast temporal resolution (~50 ms), capable of imaging the entire cardiac cycle at very high precision [3–5].

Despite the success in temporal resolution, the Imatron scanner could never achieve the spatial and contrast resolution necessary for CT angiography. Beginning in 1998, scanners enabled a true 'freezing' of a slice of the heart within a single heart beat. This scanner was quickly validated for coronary calcium screening and also opened up the door to contrast enhanced vascular studies [6–10].

Today, state of the art cardiovascular CT, typically performed on a >64 slice system with very high rotation speed (>240/min) allows these systems to freeze the heart in the cardiac cycle.

The X-Ray Tube

At the heart of the multi-slice CT scanner is the X-ray tube. The x-ray tube consists of two ends of an electric potential: the cathode and the anode (see Fig. 8.1). When the cathode is heated and high enough voltage is applied to the anode radiation is created that we commonly refer to as x-ray.

The parameters that describe the performance of the X-ray tube are:

- kVp = kilovolt potential. This represents the accelerating electric potential across the cathode and anode. The higher the voltage, the higher energy photons that can be produced.
- mAs = milliamp seconds. This is a measure of the total electron flux across the potential. This number will directly relate to the signal to noise ratio in the final transmission image.

Photons produced from an x-ray tube will produce a continuous distribution of photon energy distributed from 0 keV to the energy of the incedent electrons (kVp) (See Fig. 8.2).

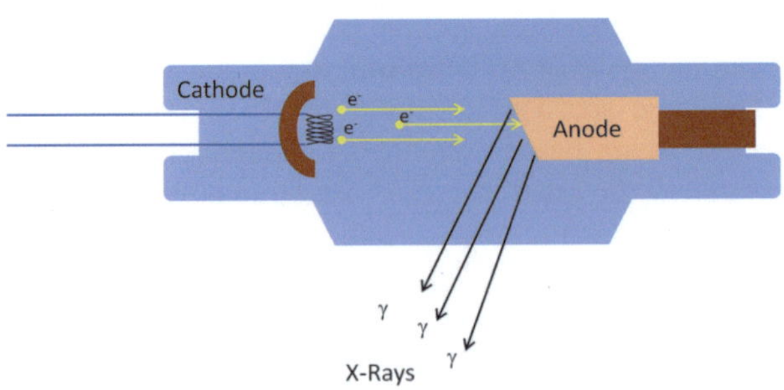

Fig. 8.1 The X-ray tube consists of a negatively charged cathode and a positively charged anode. Electrons are accelerated across a potential (V) where they then collide with the anode (typical tungsten). As they decelerate in the material, bremsstrahlung x-rays are emitted

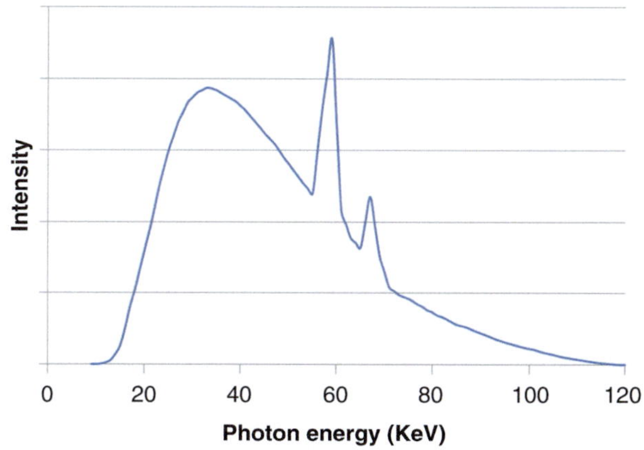

Fig. 8.2 Above is a typical spectrum from a 120 kVp x-ray tube using a tungsten target. Bremsstrahlung x-rays are emitted in a continuum from the incident electron energy downward. Characteristic x-rays can also be seen in the spectrum

Multi-slice CT

The image quality in X-Ray computed tomography is driven primarily by two characteristics: resolution and contrast. High resolution is critical to detect the size and shape of coronary lesions and to assess coronary anatomy. To achieve this high resolution, scanners must be capable of high temporal and spatial resolution to "freeze" the moving heart in time and space.

Image contrast is essential for tissue differentiation. This is directly related to the number of photons used and thus the radiation dosage. It is also influenced by the energy of the x-ray tube (kVp), the choice of the field of view of the scanner, image reconstruction technique and the spatial resolution itself. Optimizing image contrast for each patient and protocol is essential for minimizing patient radiation dosage. For example, lower kVp can result in higher contrast images at lower radiation dosage. However, in large patients, the lower kVp can also result in unacceptably noise images in large patients. Similarly, mAs requirements are typically higher for coronary CTA studies when compared with coronary calcium studies. The impact on patient dosage is summarized in Table 8.1.

Isotropy in coronary CT imaging is important because of the often torturous route the coronaries make as they traverse the epicardium. In order to assess the presence of coronary plaques, resolution and angulation variations can change the appearance of the lesion significantly (see Fig. 8.3). Comparisons of sensitivity and specificity in a coronary CTA multi-center trial demonstrated unacceptably high numbers of segments of the vessels that could not be evaluated [11–13] when using 16 slice scanners. However, when 64 slice systems are used, the number of segments that cannot be evaluated is significantly reduced [14]. These differences are well appreciated and national accreditation guidelines have adopted 16 slices as the minimum standard for coronary calcium screening and 64 slices as the minimum

Table 8.1 Varying acquisition parameters can impact the image quality and radiation dosage delivered to the patient

Parameter	Effect on dosage
mAs	Linear increase
length of scan	Linear increase
pitch	Linear decrease
kVp	Increase

Reducing dosage can often times be achieved without sacrificing overall image quality

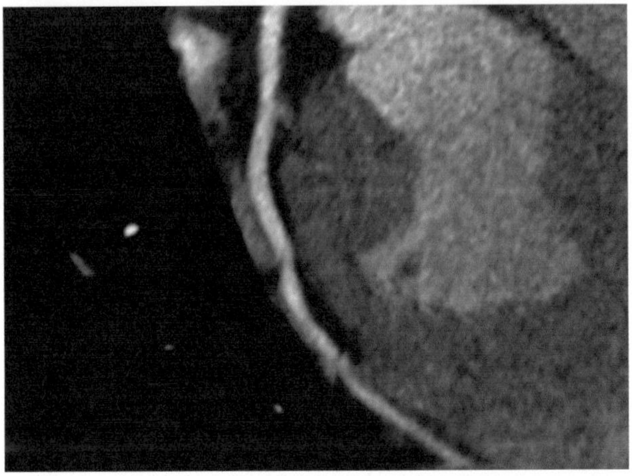

Fig. 8.3 Cardiac motion artifacts can appear as coronary lesions where the beginning and end of volumes to not completely align. This effect is made worse the fewer slices available in the scanner

standard for coronary CTA [15]. In a small recent study (36 patients) with 256 slice systems using very low dosage (0.29 mSv) and iterative reconstruction demonstrated very high sensitivity (100 %) and specificity (85 %) when compared with interventional angiography [16].

Patient Centered Imaging

Medical imaging must balance the need for protocol standardization and patient specific adaptations to improve individual image quality, while at the same time reduce patient radiation dosage and improve patient comfort. In practicing patient centered imaging, it is essential that choices do not undermine the diagnostic power of the test or introduce the chance of a technical error in favor of, for example radiation exposure Several techniques can be provide a high quality, reproducible test, that is also optimized to the clinical question and the patient [17].

Most CT systems have the capability to acquire data in a step and shoot, sequential fashion (prospective ECG triggering) or in a spiral rotational mode. The prospective ECG triggering acquisition mode (sometime referred in cardiac applications as "sequential acquisition") acquires the CT data by acquiring a complete tomographic volume before moving to the next volume. In cardiac applications this has several advantages for cardiac CT. First, the scanner is only acquiring during the diastolic phase, thereby minimizing dosage [18–21]. A second advantage to sequential imaging is the CT arc is the same at each step. This may result in improvements in diagnostic accuracy and image quality [22–24]. Prospective ECG triggering disadvantages are more serious on lower slice systems, such that the breath holds can be prohibitively long, and image quality can suffer when multiple CT rotations must be combined to cover the entire cardiac volume. Evidence suggests that for most cardiac applications (with the exception of calcium scoring), prospective triggering should only be used with 64 slice or higher CT systems [25–28].

A second approach to cardiac CT imaging is to allow the system to continuously acquire in spiral mode, acquiring data only during the diastolic phase of the cardiac cycle (retrospective ECG gating). In this mode, the CT scanner continuously spins around the patient while the table feeds the patient through the scanner. This has the advantage of providing an efficient, volumetric scan of the patient. The drawback of this approach is unnecessary radiation dosage during times where the scanner is not acquiring data: overlapping slices, outside of the diastolic ECG window.

Several approaches have been proposed to reduce the radiation dosage from spiral applications. The most effective dose reduction technique is to vary the X-Ray tube current during the acquisition. This technique varies the dosage during the ECG phase to reduce the tube current during systolic phases and then increase the tube current during the diastolic phase. More modern implementations use z axis modulation as well; lowering tube current as the scanner passes over the lung regions and then increasing it over the abdomen regions (Automatic Exposure Control, AEC). This can result in additional reductions in radiation exposure of up to 14–38 % [29, 30]. Additional radiation reduction can also be achieved by limiting the field of view of the acquisition to the target organ, using appropriate slice thicknesses and minimizing slice overlap [24].

Advances in reconstruction techniques have also resulted in reductions in the dosage needed to achieve certain image quality. These reconstruction techniques have existed since the early days of computed tomography [31]. Reduction of the reconstruction times was not achieved until ordered subsets techniques could be applied to computed tomography [32]. Other techniques have also been investigated for improving signal to noise, contrast and resolution [33].

Reconstruction and Filtering

The reconstruction of CT data is typically accomplished using a filtered back projection (FBP) reconstruction algorithm. This algorithm is based on the Radon transform, which assumes that counts received at the detector are equal to the sum of all of the counts along the line of the detector.

The quantity that is displayed in CT imaging is the Hounsfield Unit (HU). This unit is based on a semi empirical linear scale where water attenuation is defined as 0 and air attenuation is defined as −1000. All other materials are determined by mapping their measured attenuation coefficient onto this scale (see Table 8.2 for representative HU for various materials). The useful attenuation range for CT data is different depending on the organ being imaged. For example, lung fields are typically imaged with a width of 1000 HU centered on −700 HU. For coronary CTA, typical parameters center on 200 HU with a width of 600 (see Fig. 8.4).

Imaging Protocols

The CT procedures that can be performed today play an important role in the diagnosis of disease, risk management, evaluation of cardiac symptoms and in the post-evaluation of interventional procedures.

Table 8.2 Representative HU units for common tissue types

Tissue type	Hounsfield units
Air	−1000
Lung	−500
Fat	−100 to −50
Water	0
Blood	30–45
Muscle	10–40
Bone	700–3000

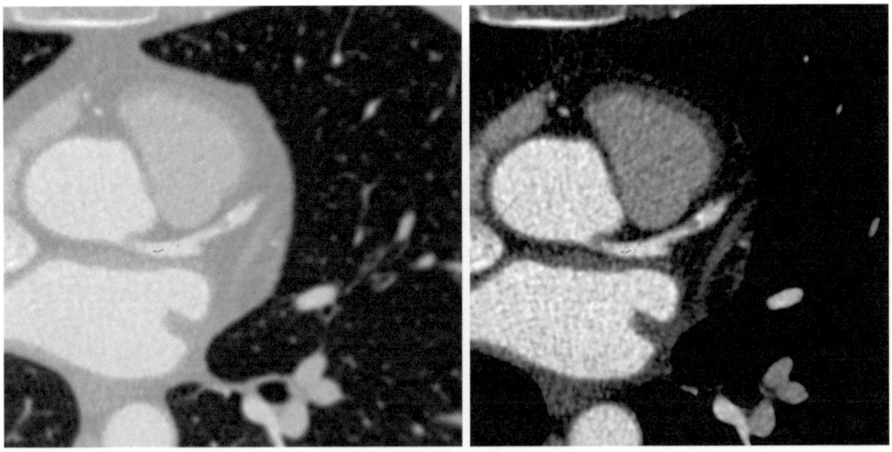

Fig. 8.4 Correct contrast windowing is essential for performing an accurate assessment. The above image on the left uses a lung windowing (−700 HU center, 1000 HU width), and the – image uses chest angiography window (200 HU center, 600 HU width)

CA Scoring

Coronary calcium screening is a non-contrast enhanced CT imaging procedure used to detect the presence of significant calcium deposits in the coronary arteries and thoracic vasculature associated with atherosclerosis (Fig. 8.5).

Quantitative assessment of coronary plaque was first proposed by Agatston [5] in 1990. This risk model relied on the measurement of the degree of calcification (described as a weighting factor) and its volume determined from a thresholding procedure applied to the CT images.

Coronary CTA Acquisition Setup

Coronary CTA is a rapid and efficient tool for imaging the coronary arteries. Current guidelines for performing coronary CTA are flexible, owing to the rapidly changing hardware and software environment. Despite this, minimum standards have been established. The Intersocietal Commission on Accreditation of Computed Tomography Laboratories (ICACTL) has taken the position that the data is not supportive of accreditation for CT machines with less than 64 slices and slower than 500 ms rotation speed [34].

As with any angiographic study, proper patient preparation and exclusions due to contraindications is crucial. Kidney tolerance of the contrast and location and abundance of metallic objects in the thorax, are all important considerations. Iodine allergy, though common, may not represent an absolute contraindication. It is commonly accepted that patients with high heart rates should have their heart rate reduced to less than 60 bpm using beta blockers [35, 36]. Use of nitrates can also improve vascular size, improving image quality.

ECG gating is essential in all coronary CTA studies to freeze the coronaries in time. This is accomplished at the time of least cardiac motion: typically diastole. The best diastolic phase can often be found at 75 % of the RR interval, however, this is not an absolute rule for all patients. Several authors recommend examining 65 %, 75 % and 85 % of the RR interval to be reconstructed and presented to the interpreting physician and the "best diastolic phase" be selected from those three. Another confounding problem with the selection of the best diastolic phase is that it may not be the same for all three vessels [37] (see Fig. 8.6).

Routinely, technologists provide the interpreting physician with at least three reconstructions and the interpreter chooses the best phase for each vessel. These reconstructions should create a volume transaxial stack of CTA data with isotropic resolution in all three directions, cubic voxel size with less than 1 mm on each side, and adequate noise filtering. The physician should inspect all three reconstructions and select the best reconstruction for each vessel.

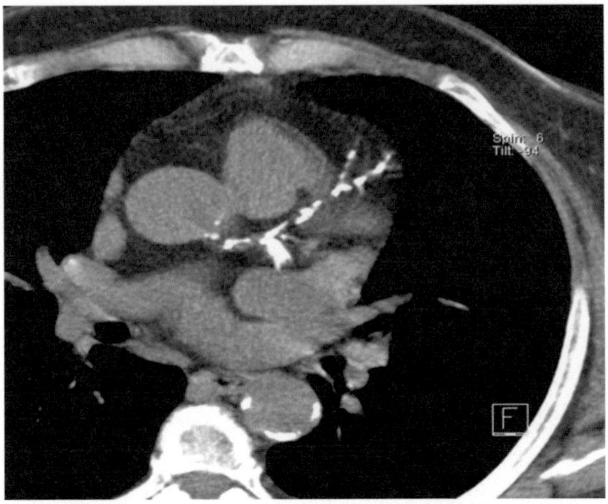

Fig. 8.5 Coronary calcium can easily be recognized in low dosage CT studies. These studies do not require contrast or high mAs to quantitate coronary calcium burden

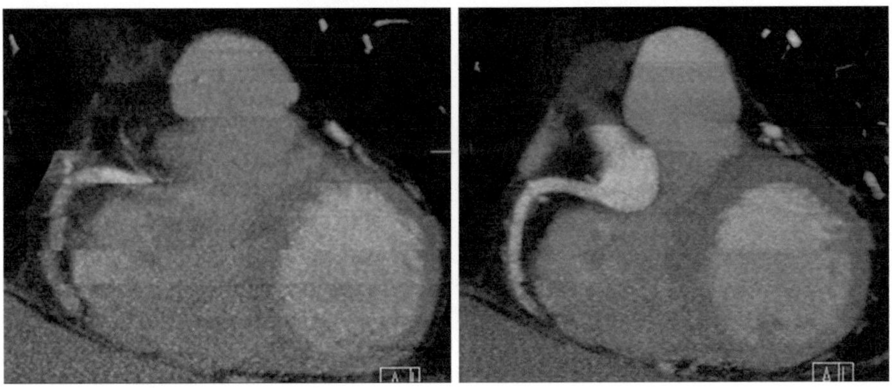

Fig. 8.6 Multi-slice spiral imaging can be rendered un-interpretable in the presence of patient motion (*left*). Technologist must carefully inspect images for patient motion and reprocess using the optimal RR window or reimage when necessary (*right*)

Artifacts

The quality of patient studies is dependent on many factors beyond the performance of the imaging system. Breathing, heart rate, beam hardening, metal artifacts all can play a role in determining the quality of the final CT image. Breathing artifacts in cardiac CT can occur in coronary CTA studies that exceed a comfortable breath hold of a patient (typically 10 s). When this occurs, there can be a repeating effect in the data in which the same tissue may be seen twice in a single slice. This can easily be detected in a coronal view of the patient as a discontinuity in the surface of the mediastinum (Fig. 8.7).

Beam hardening artifacts occur when the lower energy photons of the x-ray beam are disproportionately removed and can be worse with metal or calcium. The resulting beam has higher average energy, giving it better penetrating power than the

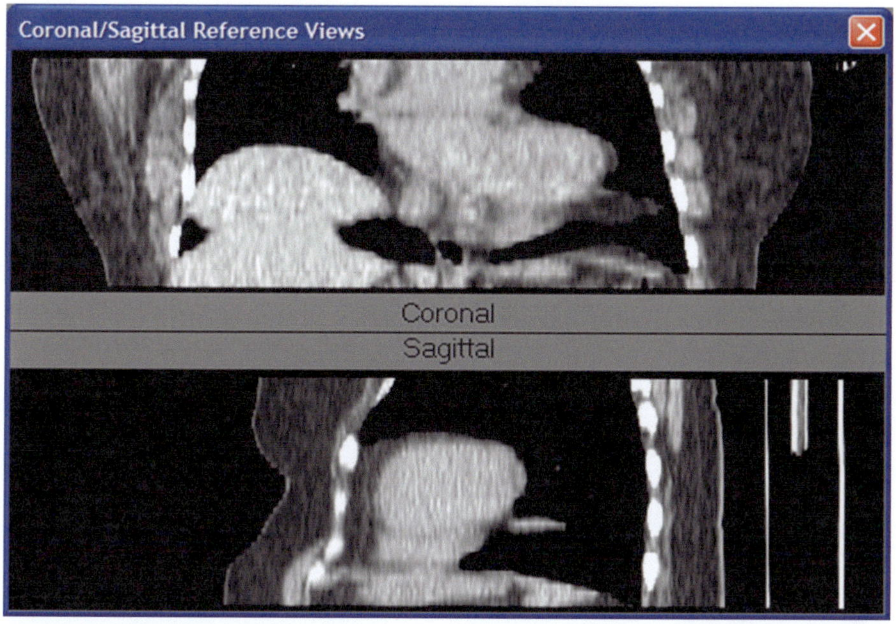

Fig. 8.7 Breathing artifacts are caused when the patient cannot hold their breath throughout the entire scan. This results in a "double counting" of slices. In extreme causes, organs can be duplicated vertically in a scan. This problem is made worse for scanners with fewer slices

original beam. The result is lower attenuation values (or HU) and dark streaks through the image originating from or near these dense structures. In chest CT studies, this is often caused by the sternum, large coronary calcifications or breast shields (see Fig. 8.8). Though not as common as in peripheral studies of the hips or head, beam hardening can limit the quantitative accuracy of studies. Beam hardening can be detected by changing the imaging display window to amplify image contrast in the transaxial views. Beam hardening effects can be reduced by using a higher kVp tube voltage and starting with a harder beam. An extreme example of beam hardening can occur with metal artifacts such as with pacemakers, implanted defibrillators and surgical clips. In this case, all photons are removed from the beam leaving no detected counts at the detector. This has the effect of introducing singularities into the reconstruction which cause bright streaking appearances in the images.

Display Formats

The most common display is the transaxial image display. This projection display format will be used in all interpretation schemes because it has the least amount of geometric and projection distortions. If lesions cannot be confirmed on the transaxial slices, they are unlikely to be real. Reconstruction of the transmission data is typically performed by a vendor specific algorithm that models system 3D geometry, scatter correction, beam hardening, etc.

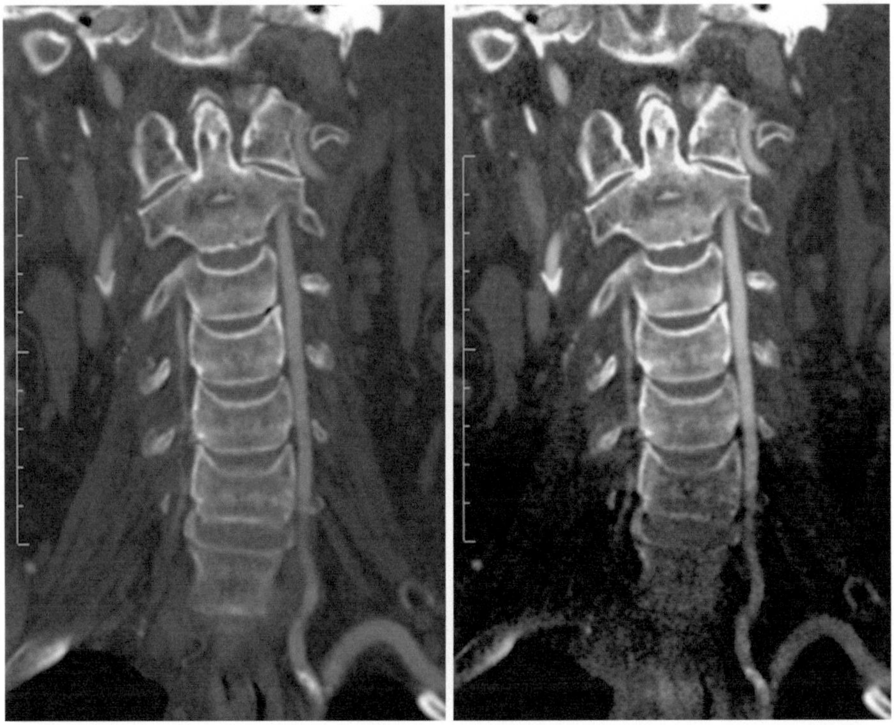

Fig. 8.8 Beam hardening occurs when low energy x-rays are preferentially removed from the beam by metals or calcium. As the beam is hardened, it can penetrate the tissue more easily giving the appearance of less attenuation. At high tube voltages (140 kVP, *left*) this problem is less than at low tube voltages (80 kVP, *right*)

For calcium screening procedures, the scoring is performed on the image transaxial data. In these types of studies, it may not be necessary to use isotropic voxel dimensions (3 mm slice thickness) with 0.75 mm in plane resolution is very common in coronary Ca screening procedures. For high resolution, 3D studies, such as coronary CTA, isotropic spatial resolution is crucial and slice thickness must match the in-plane pixel sizes.

The maximum intensity projection, or MIP, is another common display format. This technique creates a planar two dimensional image from a finite slab of slices. To create the projection, the user will define a slab thickness and the CT workstation will then determine a MIP from that slab by taking the maximum intensity value along a line of sight towards the user (see Fig. 8.9). This has the effect of greatly improving the signal to noise ration while preserving the image contrast and boundary resolution (which would normally be sacrificed in a conventional blurring technique). A disadvantage of the MIP is that it can obscure real lesions depending on the viewing angle. If there is an area of high contrast between a soft lesion and the user, the MIP will take the values of the contrast, and the lesion will be lost.

Another important tool is the curved multi-planar reformat (curved MPR). In this view, the vessel will be projected onto a set of views that will create a virtual "stack"

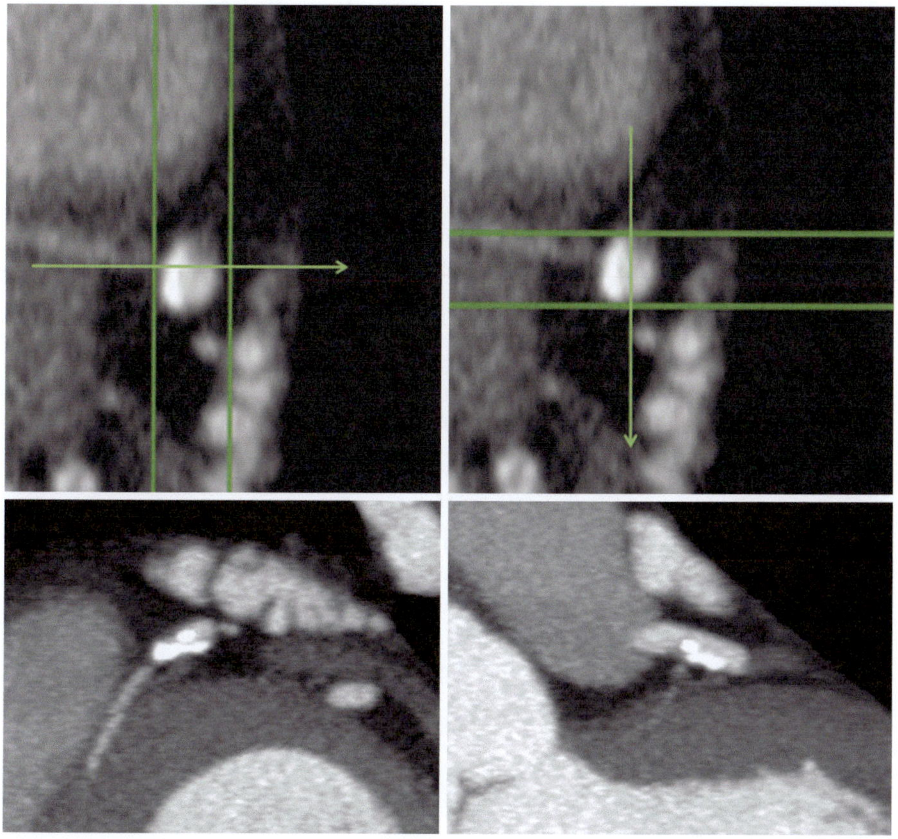

Fig. 8.9 Maximum intensity projection (MIP) images are created by taking the maximum count along a line of site within a finite slab of tissue. Though high resolution, high contrast images are obtain, care must be taken to insure the three dimensional nature of smaller lesion is not lost. On the left, a partially calcified plaque in a coronary artery can look completed occluded in one MIP projection (*left*), and only partially occlude in an orthogonal projection (*right*)

of cross sections of the vessel. First, a centerline is defined through the vessel (Fig. 8.10). Then, by defining a set of orthogonal planes to the centerline, a stack of cross sections are created. In these views, lesion size and composition can be assessed quantitatively. However, the problem with the curved MPR is that the resampling can mask artifacts and create spatial distortions that resemble soft plaques.

Conclusion

Coronary computed tomography represents one of the most powerful additions to the tools that are available to the practicing cardiologist for accurate, non-invasive diagnosis of CAD, peripheral artery disease and patient management. Advancements in the field also open up the possibility of using this technique for the assessment of plaque vulnerability and composition.

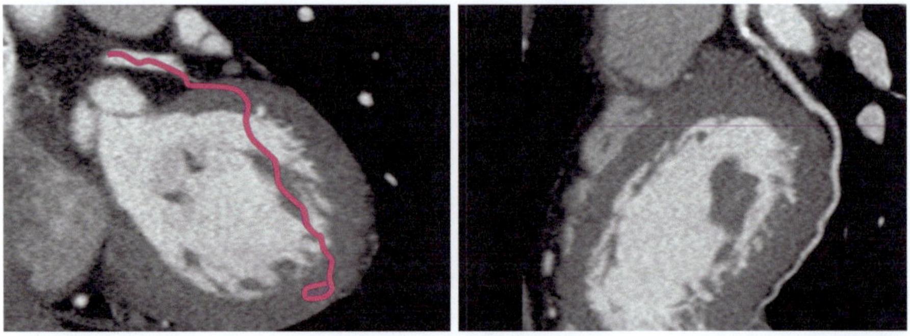

Fig. 8.10 The curved multi-planar reformat (MPR) image allows the clinician to appreciate the entire length of a vessel by taking the twists and turns out and reprojecting the vessel as if it were straight, though this is a convenient view to assess the entire vessel in a single view geometric distortions can exaggerate some feature and mask others. Careful review of transaxial views should also be performed to confirm any finding on the MPR images

Considerable work remains to allow for this modality to achieve it potential, including accurate outcomes data to better define appropriate indications for this technique, reduced radiation exposure to take advantage of its capability of imaging patients earlier in the evolution of their atherosclerosis and patient management models that demonstrate to practitioners and payers the value of this modality.

References

1. Cormack AM. Reconstruction of densities from their projections, with applications in radiological physics. Phys Med Biol. 1973;18(2):195–207.
2. Hounsfield GN. Computerized transverse axial scanning (tomography)—part 1 description of the system. Br J Radiol. 1973;46:1016–22.
3. Wang S, Detrano RC, Tang W, Doherty TM, Puentes G, Wong N, Brundage BH. Detection of coronary calcification with electron beam computed tomography: evaluation of inter-examination reproducibility and comparison of three image acquisition protocols. Am Heart J. 1996;132:550–8.
4. Mahaisavariya P, Detrano RC, Kang X, Garner D, Vo A, Georgiou D, Molloi S, Brundage BH. Quantitation of in vitro coronary artery calcium using ultrafast computed tomography. Cathet Cardiovasc Diagn. 1994;32:387–93.
5. Agatston AS, Janowitz WR, Hildner FJ, Zusmer N, Viamonte M, Detrano RC. Quantification of coronary artery calcium using ultrafast computed tomography. J Am Coll Cardiol. 1990;15:827–32.
6. McCollough C, Zink F. Performance evaluation of a multi-slice CT system. Med Phys. 1999;26:2223–30.
7. Nieman K, Oudkerk M, Rensing BJ, et al. Coronary angiography with multi-slice computed tomography. Lancet. 2001;357(9256):599–603.
8. Hoffmann U, Moselewski F, Cury RC, et al. Predictive value of 16- slice multidetector spiral computed tomography to detect significant obstructive coronary artery disease in patients at high risk for coronary artery disease: patient-versus segment-based analysis. Circulation. 2004;110(17):2638–43.

9. Raff GL, Gallagher MJ, O'Neill WW, et al. Diagnostic accuracy of noninvasive coronary angiography using 64-slice spiral computed tomography. J Am Coll Cardiol. 2005;46(3):552–7.
10. Budoff MJ, Dowe D, Jollis JG, et al. Diagnostic performance of 64- multidetector row coronary computed tomographic angiography for evaluation of coronary artery stenosis in individuals without known coronary artery disease: results from the prospective multicenter ACCURACY (Assessment by Coronary Computed Tomographic Angiography of Individuals Undergoing Invasive Coronary Angiography) trial. J Am Coll Cardiol. 2008;52:1724–32.
11. John M. Boone, Anthony Seibert: an accurate method for computer-generating tungsten anode X-ray spectra from 30 to 140 kV. Med Phys. 1997;24(11):1661–70.
12. Sun Z, Jiang W. Diagnostic value of multislice computed tomography angiography in coronary artery disease: a metaanalysis. Eur J Radiol. 2006;60(2):279–86.
13. Achenbach S, Ropers D, Pohle FK, et al. Detection of coronary artery stenoses using multi-detector CT with 16 × 0.75 collimation and 375 ms rotation. Eur Heart J. 2005;26(19):1978–86.
14. Sun Z, Lin C, Davidson R, et al. Diagnostic value of 64-slice CT angiography in coronary artery disease: a systematic review. Eur J Radiol. 2008;67(1):78–84.
15. Abdulla J, Abildstrom SZ, Gotzsche O, et al. 64-multislice detector computed tomography coronary angiography as potential alternative to conventional coronary angiography: a systematic review and meta-analysis. Eur Heart J. 2007;28(24):3042–50.
16. Stehli J M.D., Fuchs TA M.D., Bull S M.D., Clerc OF M.D., Possner M M.D., Buechel RR M.D., Gaemperli O M.D., Kaufmann PA M.D. Accuracy of coronary CT angiography using a submillisievert fraction of radiation exposure comparison with invasive coronary angiography. J Am Coll Cardiol. 2014;64(8):772–80.
17. Russell MT, Fink JR, Rebeles F, Kanal K, Ramos M, Anzai Y. Balancing radiation dose and image quality: clinical applications of neck volume CT. AJNR Am J Neuroradiol. 2008;29:727–31.
18. Husmann L, Valenta I, Gaemperli O, et al. Feasibility of low-dose coronary CT angiography: first experience with prospective ECG-gating. Eur Heart J. 2008;29:191–7.
19. Herzog BA, Wyss CA, Husmann L, et al. First head-to-head comparison of effective radiation dose from low-dose 64-slice CT with prospective ECG-triggering versus invasive coronary angiography. Heart. 2009;95:1656–61.
20. Schoenhagen P. Back to the future: coronary CT angiography using prospective ECG triggering. Eur Heart J. 2008;29:153–4.
21. Hong YJ, Kim SJ, Lee SM, et al. Low-dose coronary computed tomography angiography using prospective ECG-triggering compared to invasive coronary angiography. Int J Cardiovasc Imaging. 2011;27:425–31.
22. Shuman WP, Branch KR, May JM, et al. Prospective versus retrospective ECG gating for 64-detector CT of the coronary arteries: comparison of image quality and patient radiation dose. Radiology. 2008;248:431–7.
23. Pontone G, Andreini D, Bartorelli AL, et al. Diagnostic accuracy of coronary computed tomography angiography: a comparison between prospective and retrospective electrocardiogram triggering. J Am Coll Cardiol. 2009;54:346–55.
24. DeFrance T, Dubois E, Gebow D, et al. Helical prospective ECG-gating in cardiac computed tomography: radiation dose and image quality. Int J Cardiovasc Imaging. 2010;26:99–107.
25. Hlaihel C, Boussel L, Cochet H, et al. Dose and image quality comparison between prospectively gated axial and retrospectively gated helical coronary CT angiography. Br J Radiol. 2011;84:51–7.
26. Feng Q, Yin Y, Hua X, et al. Prospective ECG triggering versus low-dose retrospective ECG-gated 128-channel CT coronary angiography: comparison of image quality and radiation dose. Clin Radiol. 2010;65:809–14.
27. Duarte R, Fernandez G, Castellon D, et al. Prospective coronary CT angiography 128-MDCT versus retrospective 64-MDCT: improved image quality and reduced radiation dose. Heart Lung Circ. 2011;20:119–25.

28. Qin J, Liu LY, Meng XC, et al. Prospective versus retrospective ECG gating for 320-detector CT of the coronary arteries: comparison of image quality and patient radiation dose. Clin Imaging. 2011;35:193–7.
29. Mulkens TH, Bellinck P, Baeyaert M, et al. Use of an automatic exposure control mechanism for dose optimization in multi-detector row CT examinations: clinical evaluation. Radiology. 2005;237:213–23.
30. Kalra MK, Rizzo S, Maher MM, et al. Chest CT performed with z-axis modulation: scanning protocol and radiation dose. Radiology. 2005;237:303–8.
31. Gordon R, Bender R, Herman GT. Algebraic reconstruction techniques (ART) for three-dimensional electron microscopy and x-ray photography. J Theor Biol. 1970;29:471–82.
32. Manglos SH, Gagne GM, Krol A, Thomas FD, Narayanaswamy R. Transmission maximum-likelihood reconstruction with ordered subsets for cone beam CT. Phys Med Biol. 1995;40:1225–41.
33. Beister M, Kolditz D, Kalender WA. Iterative reconstruction methods in x-ray CT. Phys Med. 2012;29(2):94–108.
34. The IAC Standards and Guidelines for CT Accreditation. 2014. Intersocietal Accreditation Commission. http://www.intersocietal.org/ct/standards/IACCTStandards2014.pdf.
35. Shim SS, Kim Y, Lim SM. Improvement of image quality with beta-blocker premedication on ECG-gated 16-MDCT coronary angiography. AJR Am J Roentgenol. 2005;184:649–54.
36. Shapiro M, Pena A, Nichols JH, Worrell S, Bamberg F, Dannemann N, et al. Efficacy of pre-scan b-blockade and impact of heart rate on image quality in patients undergoing coronary multidetector computed tomography angiography. Eur J Radiol. 2008;66:37–4.
37. Leschka S, Husmann L, Desbiolles LM, Gaemperli O, Schepis T, Koepfli P, Boehm T, Marincek B, Kaufmann PA, Alkadhi H. Optimal image reconstruction intervals for non-invasive coronary angiography with 64-slice CT. Eur Radiol. 2006;16(9):1964–72.

Chapter 9
Reporting and Accreditation of Cardiac CT

Amgad N. Makaryus and Seth Uretsky

Abstract Reporting of cardiac CT scans is a process involving the appropriate indications, patient characteristics, description of protocols, recognition of artifacts and concise communication regarding findings at the conclusion of the test. The necessary elements for successful reporting will be reviewed. The utilization of standards with regard to these reports will be emphasized. Available resources to improve successful reporting are noted. Just as as appropriate test selection and patient preparation are important aspects of a quality laboratory, the report is the final element of this process.

Accreditation of laboratories performing cardiac CT scans is an important marker of quality. As with all modalities, qualified personnel, adherence to protocols and accurate reporting are all important aspects of accreditation by any of the qualified organizations.

Keywords Laboratory accreditation • Cardiac computed tomography • Structured reporting • Key reporting elements • Agatston score

CT Reporting: Background

The information submitted to the referring health care person can be the most important part of the process. Failure to convey results in a timely, concise and accurate means can substantially reduce the value of the testing procedure even if the images and protocols are superb. While there have been significant changes in the scope and utilization of CCT, essential components for the adequate use of CT report results remain. Additionally, there continues to be wide expansion of clinical

---

A.N. Makaryus, MD, FACC, FACP, FASE, FSCCT
Department of Cardiology, NuHealth, Nassau University Medical Center,
2201 Hempstead Turnpike, East Meadow, NY 11554, USA
e-mail: amakaryu@numc.edu

S. Uretsky, MD, FACC (✉)
Cardiovascular Fellowship Program, Atlantic Health System, Gagnon Cardiovascular Center,
100 Madison Avenue, Morristown, NJ 07960, USA
e-mail: seth.uretsky@atlantichealth.org

P.L. Tilkemeier et al. (eds.), *Quality Evaluation in Non-Invasive Cardiovascular Imaging*, DOI 10.1007/978-3-319-28011-0_9

applications of CCT as well as the development of new techniques. Recommendations for CCT reporting were developed as an educational tool for practitioners to continue to improve the care for patients and to follow systematic standards of practice for CCT based on the best available data and expert consensus [1].

The CCT report (Fig. 9.1) should give the complete interpretation of the CCT and include all of the required key elements based on recommended image post-

Hospital Cardiovascular Imaging Laboratory
Amgad N. Makaryus MD, FACC, FASE, FSCCT, Director of Cardiovascular Imaging

CARDIOVASCULAR COMPUTED TOMOGRAPHY REPORT

Patient Name:	JOHN SMITH	Patient Age:	52 years	Study date:	5/17/2015
Patient ID #:	123456	Height:	68.0 in	Gender:	M
		Weight:	192.0 lb	Blood Press:	130/80 mmHg
		BSA:	2.01 m^2	Pt. Location:	1161A

Referring Physician: DOE, JANE **Technician:** AB

Interpreting Physician(s): Amgad Makaryus MD, Cardiologist/John Doe MD, Radiologist

Indication(s): Chest pain -786.50

History: 59 year old man with a history hypertension and chest pain on exertion with prior equivocal nuclear stress test performed three weeks ago.

Procedures (CPT Codes) performed: CT Coronary Angiography (CCTA 75574). Informed consent was obtained from the patient and there were no complications during the procedure. ECG prospectively-gated 320-detector CT pre- and post-contrast images (Omnipaque 350: 80 cc) of the heart were obtained. The patient was pretreated with 50 mg of PO metoprolol one half hour before exam and 0.4 mg of sublingual nitroglycerin just prior to the contrast portion of the exam; heart rate at time of the examination was 62 beats/min and regular. Axial two dimensional and three-dimensional images were reconstructed using an analysis workstation.

Estimated effective radiation dose from this study: 150 mGy·cm (~2.1 mSv)

Study Quality: Image quality for this study is adequate.

FINDINGS:

Non-Cardiac:

The visualized lung fields are clear. There is no significant mediastinal adenopathy. The visualized osseous structures are grossly unremarkable. No thoracic aortic dissection is noted in the visualized thoracic aorta. No pulmonary embolus is noted within the visualized central pulmonary arteries. Visualized portions of the upper abdominal structures demonstrate no abnormality.

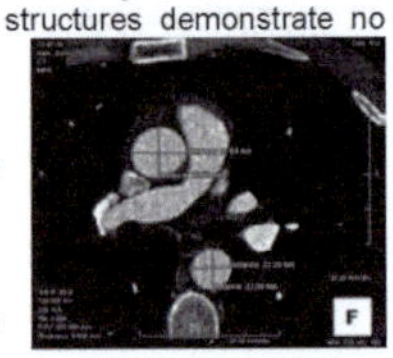

Cardiac:

Normal chamber sizes. Normal pericardium without pericardial effusion. SVC/IVC normal. Main PA and proximal branches free of filling defect. Ascending aorta size= 3.2 cm x 2.9 cm.

Coronary:

Coronary Calcium Score = 0 Agatston Units (0 percentile) for subjects of the same age, gender, and race/ethnicity who are free of clinical cardiovascular disease and treated diabetes.

The left main coronary artery is patent. The anterior descending artery demonstrates no focal luminal narrowing. A ramus branch is patent. Two diagonal branches are patent. The circumflex artery is widely patent. An obtuse marginal branch is patent. The right coronary artery, a dominant vessel, demonstrates no focal luminal narrowing. The PDA and posterolateral branch are patent.

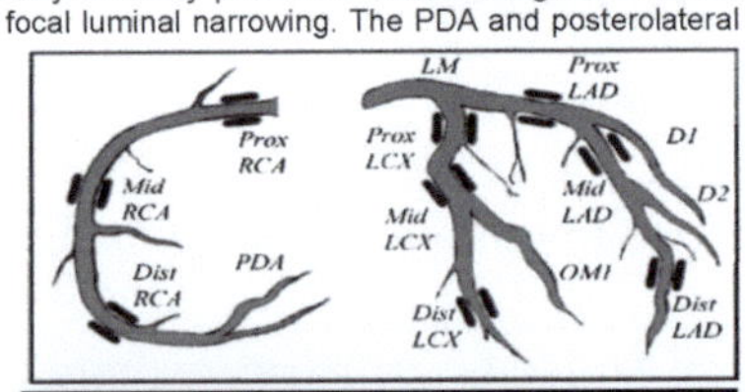

CT Coronary Angiography shows:

Artery	Stenosis/Location/Dominance	Calcium Score
LM	Widely Patent	0
LAD	Widely Patent	0
LCX	Widely Patent	0
RCA	Dominant; Widely Patent	0

IMPRESSIONS AND CONCLUSION:

1. Normal coronary arteries without coronary atherosclerosis.
2. Risk factor modification and CAD primary prevention recommended.

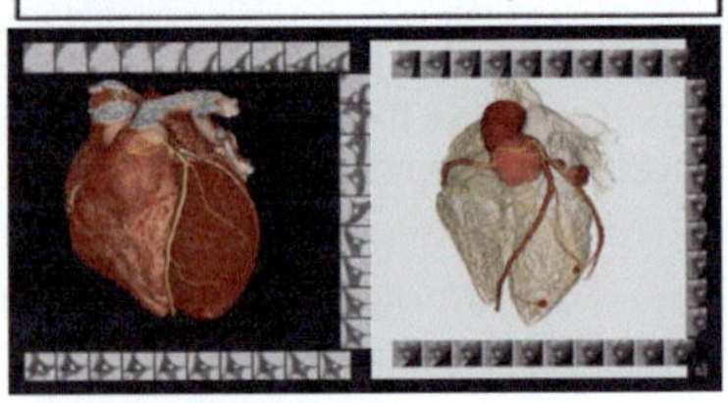

Amgad Makaryus MD, Attending Cardiologist
John Doe MD, Attending Radiologist
Dictated on: 5/17/2015 at 10:21:32 AM
Electronically signed on: 5/17/2015 at 10:21:32 AM

Final

Fig. 9.1 Example of a CCT report

processing formats. The recommended formats include axial image review, multi-planar reformation image review, maximum intensity projection image review, curved multi-planar reformation image review and possibly volume-rendered reconstructions for certain circumstances. Interpretation should be made on three-dimensional cardiac-specific interpretation software equipped to display the recommended image reconstruction formats; however, customization of image reconstructions for the particular case being examined may be necessary on a per-case basis. Artifacts in the dataset must be identified so as not to confuse the interpretation. Non-contrast sequences in the study should be reviewed before the contrast portion(s). The coronary tree should be examined systematically using standard coronary tree labeling and nomenclature. Lesions should be assessed for extent of stenosis, quality, location, and morphology of the plaque. And finally, extra-coronary cardiac and thoracic anatomy should be examined within the cardiac field of view. Further quantification and assessment of cardiac anatomy is also performed as indicated by the study indication [1].

CT Reporting: Key Elements

The CCT report should be a comprehensive report including analysis of all the views and components of the acquired study including the non-contrast as well as contrast portions of the study. A report starts with clinical data about the patient being studied such as symptoms, risk factors, relevant diagnostic test results, and the indication or reason for the CCT. The standard demographics including procedure date, patient name, date of birth, sex, and referring clinician is also required. It is also recommended to include the patient's height, weight, and body mass index. The next essential portion of the report relays the procedure and equipment data including a description of the test type (e.g., coronary CT angiography, calcium scoring, ventricular function, etc.) and scanner type with respect to the number of detectors (and number of x-ray sources if applicable). The SCCT also recommends noting the amount of radiation exposure (dose-length product; DLP). Medications employed such as beta-blockers, nitroglycerin, as well as type and volume of contrast used should also be reported. Heart rate, heart rhythm other than sinus rhythm, and arrhythmia, if present should be documented [1].

The next portion of the exam relates the findings of the scan. The body of the report starts with an assessment of the technical quality of the scan and the possible presence and type of artifact and effect on the interpretation. An Agatston score for the total study (sum of four vessels) with the score percentile based on age and sex nomogram (representative cohort for population being evaluated) is provided. Optionally, an Agatston score for each vessel may also be provided. Coronary anatomy including coronary dominance, anomalies (origins and course), dilation/aneurysms, benign anatomical variants, and myocardial bridging is noted. If present, stenosis location and severity (obstructive/non-obstructive) is required to be documented along with stenosis plaque type (calcified, predominantly calcified, non-calcified, and predominantly non-calcified). Additionally, stenosis extent with respect to length, ostial, or branch involvement, positive remodeling, and tortuosity should be documented. It is important to note that the term "normal" in reference to the coronary arteries should be used only when there is no evidence of any coronary artery disease with a normal lumen and no plaque whether calcified or non-calcified. Any segment containing non-obstructive atherosclerotic plaque should not be labelled as normal. Non-coronary vessel abnormalities of the aorta, vena cavae, pulmonary arteries, and pulmonary veins, if present, should also be noted in the report [1].

Further cardiovascular findings including presence of calcium in the aortic wall, aortic valve, mitral annulus/valve, pericardium, chambers and abnormalities of wall thicknesses, and myocardium are noted. Left ventricular ejection fraction and volumes may also be reported if functional data is obtained. Prosthetic valves and other devices such as pacemakers/defibrillators should be documented. The body of the report should also document the non-cardiac structures (lungs, mediastinum, esophagus, bony structures, chest wall and any visualized abdominal structures) [1].

The report should end with an "Impressions and Conclusion" section including statements where the coronary findings are interpreted and possibly correlated with the clinical background and prior studies if available. Any significant abnormal non-cardiac findings should also be summarized. Further clinical recommendations may optionally be provided and representative images of identified pathology/findings may also be provided [1]. The common reasons for incomplete reports includes: No Date of Signature, no signature, indication(s) missing, missed findings (after IAC review), reports not standardized (individual laboratory including use of SCCT terminology) and timeliness of report completion.

Date of report finalization with an electronic or physical signature should be included in the report. All potentially life-threatening findings are reported to the referring physician on the same date of the study and a record of a verbal communication with respect to these findings may be included in the report. Generally, reports of emergency studies should be issued within 24 h, and elective studies should generally be reported with 24–48 h of the exam [1, 2].

CT Reporting: Summary

The report is a key element of the quality of a CCT laboratory. It is vital to provide an accurate, concise report with detail on the patient undergoing the test, indications, test performed and any problems encounter. The body of the report should include all abnormal findings, including non-cardiac and cardiac with enough detail to provide the referring healthcare provider with enough information to render a clinical decision, and in a timely fashion. The conclusion should be concise and state whether normal or abnormal. Provision of a high quality report is a marker of an excellent laboratory.

Laboratory Accreditation

The Medicare Improvements for Patients and Providers Act of 2008 (MIPPA) required all non-hospital CT facilities to become accredited by January 1, 2012 as a condition of reimbursement by CMS. Thus, currently, all out-patient facilities that perform CCT must be accredited by one of three organizations approved by CMS: Intersocietal Accreditation Commission (IAC), American College of Radiology (ACR) or The Joint Commission (TJC) [3]. The IAC-CT accreditation process is generally favored by cardiology groups as the IAC also accredits other cardiovascular procedures such as echocardiography, nuclear cardiology, vascular medicine and MR. The application processes are similar, thus providing efficiency for the applying institution. Of the three accreditation bodies (IAC, ACR, JACHO), the IAC-CT division is the only one requiring evaluation of reports. Failure to provide reports with the recommended fields is the second most common cause of "delay" for accreditation. The key elements for IAC-CT accreditation are listed in Table 9.1. The ACR or TJC pathway may be preferable to many performing cardiac CT in a hospital based laboratory as it may be beneficial to apply as part of a larger facility based application. Each accrediting organization's requirements should be evaluated by a laboratory applying for accreditation to find the one best suited to their needs. An excellent overview of

Table 9.1 Key elements required for IAC-CT report

1	Date of the examination
2	Clinical indications leading to the performance of the examination
3	Patient date of birth or age
4	Patient ID or name;
5	Name of the examination;
6	Protocol used in the examination
7	Quality of the study performed
8	Details of drug and/or medication administration (include the name, dose administered and route)
9	Administration of contrast, if used (include the name, type, and amount of IV contrast administered)
10	An overview of the results of the examination including pertinent findings
	Comment: This must include localization and quantification of abnormal findings (where appropriate)
11	A summary of the test findings; reports must be typewritten
12	Physician signature line (the printed name of the interpreting physician)
13	Manual and/or electronic interpreting physician signature
14	Date of interpreting physician signature and/or verification
15	Referring physician name
16	Name and address of institution performing the test

Source: Intersocietal Accreditation Commission (IAC) CT Standards and Guidelines, updated 08/2012

the history of the accreditation process and the differences between the accrediting organizations philosophies and methodologies can be found in Chaps. 5 and 24 of this book.

Although these accreditation standards can be helpful in establishing a high quality cardiac CT program, practice guidelines published through the imaging societies offer current "best practices" for protocols and procedures [4–6]. In managing a cardiac CT program, both resources should be closely and regularly reviewed to insure current best practices are used.

Training Requirements

The performance of cardiovascular CT requires considerable training. Technologists must be certified by a national society, usually the American Registry of Radiologic Technologists (ARRT) and often must be licensed in the state they are practicing in. In addition to the primary registration as a radiological technologist, a post primary specialization in computed tomography is often required.

The primary pathway requirement for the ARRT at the time of this publication is an associate's degree or higher in an acceptable program and a formal education program in radiography [7]. In addition, candidates for certification must complete a specific number of procedures to meet the competency requirements [8]. Post certification in computed tomography requires the candidate demonstrate additional competency in computed tomography [9]. Although there is no requirement for specific cardiovascular training, however, technologists should obtain specific training in CT tomography with and without contrast, ECG gating, and processing of cardiac and cardiovascular studies [10]. After registration, maintaining the registration requires a minimum of 24 h per biennium of acceptable continuing education [9]. Technologists should review educational programs to insure the applicability of the program to meeting this requirement.

Physician training is also rigorous with defined training criteria for fellows in training by the American College of Cardiology Foundation. There is a certification examination available through the Certification Board of Cardiovascular Computed Tomography. The certification is time limited and there are clinical requirements for ongoing certification. Details regarding the certification process can be located on their website at http://www.cccvi.org/cbcct.

References

1. Leipsic J, Abbara S, Achenbach S, Cury R, Earls JP, Mancini GJ, Nieman K, Pontone G, Raff GL. Scct guidelines for the interpretation and reporting of coronary ct angiography: a report of the society of cardiovascular computed tomography guidelines committee. J Cardiovasc Comput Tomogr. 2014;8:342–58.

2. Abbara S, Arbab-Zadeh A, Callister TQ, Desai MY, Mamuya W, Thomson L, Weigold WG. Scct guidelines for performance of coronary computed tomographic angiography: a report of the society of cardiovascular computed tomography guidelines committee. J Cardiovasc Comput Tomogr. 2009;3:190–204.
3. Payment Policies, Intersocietal Accreditation Commission, http://intersocietal.org/iac/reimbursement/policies/IACCT_PaymentPolicies.pdf.
4. ACR–NASCI–SPR practice parameter for the performance and interpretation of cardiac Computed Tomography (CT), Resolution 39. 2014. http://www.acr.org/~/media/ACR/Documents/PGTS/guidelines/CT_Cardiac.pdf.
5. Abbara S, Arbab-Zadeh A, Callister TQ, Milind Y, Desai MY, Mamuya W, Thomson L, Weigold G. SCCT guidelines for performance of coronary computed tomographic angiography: a report of the Society of Cardiovascular Computed Tomography Guidelines Committee. J Cardiovasc Comput Tomogr. 2009;3:190–204.
6. Radiation protection in newer medical imaging techniques: cardiac CT, 2008, IAEA, Dafety Report Series No. 60.
7. Primary certification: didactic and clinical competency requirements, American Registry of Radiologic Technologists. 2012. https://www.arrt.org/pdfs/Disciplines/Competency-Requirements/RAD-Competency-Requirements.pdf.
8. Structured education and clinical experience requirements, American Registry of Radiologic Technologists. 2011. https://www.arrt.org/pdfs/Disciplines/Clinical-Experience/CT-Clinical-Experience.pdf.
9. ARRT continuing education requirements. 2014. https://www.arrt.org/pdfs/Governing-Documents/Continuing-Education-Requirements.pdf.
10. Pelberg R, Budoff M, Goraya T, Keevil J, Lesser J, Litwin S, Newton C, Ridner M, Rumberger J, Teague S, Winkler M. Training, competency, and certification in cardiac CT: a summary statement from the Society of Cardiovascular Computed Tomography. J Cardiovasc Comput Tomogr. 2011;5:279–85.

Part III
MRI

Chapter 10
MRI: Clinical Applications

Ibrahim M. Saeed and Ryan Longmore

Abstract Cardiac magnetic resonance imaging is a technique that can assist in a broad array of clinical applications. These include functional assessments that allow both ventricular as well as valvular function to be addressed, as well as characterization of metabolic function and perfusion. Structural assessment can be used to identify cardiomyopathies, congenital abnormalities, myocarditis, pericardial disease, cardiac masses or anomalous coronary vasculature. Assessment of myocardial viability following a myocardial infarction is also a particular strength of cardiac magnetic resonance imaging. Finally, the field of stress cardiac magnetic resonance imaging will be discussed including the multimodality appropriate use criteria and their application to MRI.

Keywords Cardiac magnetic resonance imaging • Functional imaging • Structural imaging • Perfusion imaging • Appropriate use criteria

Prologue: Common and Not-So Common Uses of Cardiovascular Magnetic Resonance (CMR)

Even with the first cardiac studies using magnetic resonance, it became clear that CMR provides both high quality images and outstanding endocardial definition. This was initially in the setting of advanced congenital heart disease, particularly after complex surgical corrections, that it found its role. Evaluating anatomy, surgical baffles and shunts, and quantifying their flows was routine.

Figure 10.1 reflects the subtleties of CMR. A three-chambered view of the heart suggests significant mitral regurgitation. The thinning of the basal inferolat-

I.M. Saeed, MD, FACC, FAAP (✉)
Saint Luke's Mid America Heart Institute Cardiovascular Consultants, University of Missouri, Kansas City, MO, USA
e-mail: isaeed@saint-lukes.org; imsaeed@gmail.com

R. Longmore, DO
Department of Cardiology, Saint Luke's Hospital, Kansas City, MO, USA
e-mail: ryan.longmore@gmail.com

P.L. Tilkemeier et al. (eds.), *Quality Evaluation in Non-Invasive Cardiovascular Imaging*, DOI 10.1007/978-3-319-28011-0_10

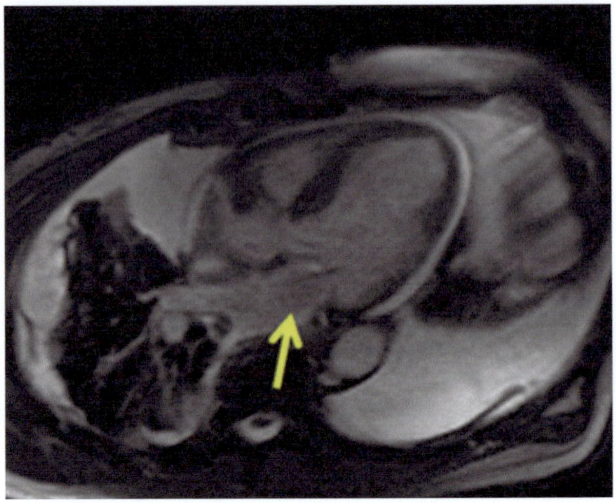

Fig. 10.1 Three chamber view of mitral regurgitation (*arrow*). Noted in this view are bilateral pleural effusions, small circumferential pericardial effusion. The basal-to-mid inferolateral wall is thin. Taken together, this gentleman with dyspnea is in heart failure, and the mitral regurgitation appears to be ischemic in etiology

eral wall suggests that the etiology is from an infarcted myocardium and that this valve disease is ischemic in etiology. The pleural and pericardial effusions show that this patient is in heart failure. This one snapshot provides a clue as to how CMR can provide hemodynamic data, the metabolic data of infarction, and the overall anatomy as would be seen in a chest CT. This is one of many sequences, and although this is a still frame, a movie of serial images also provides additional functional data.

It was the power of tissue characterization that highlighted the potential role of Cardiac MRI. In a landmark paper in 1999, Kim [1] and his colleagues highlighted the ability of retained gadolinium to enhance and delineate scar tissue in the myocardium. The following year, the same group revealed its utility in identifying viable tissue and predicting its chances for recovering myocardial contractility after revascularization [2]. Patterns of late gadolinium enhancement were then used to identify other causes of heart failure, particularly the non-ischemic cardiomyopathies (especially those that have an arrhythmic potential), intra-cardiac masses, and pericardial diseases. Valve disease continues to be studied. And although imaging coronary arteries (both atherosclerotic and anomalous) can be challenging, stress perfusion cardiac MRI allows the potential for both stress testing in the magnet while concomitantly imaging for viable tissue. Much of this is with the use of gadolinium, which, as of this writing, is still not approved by the United States Food and Drug Administration (FDA) for the use of cardiac imaging. However, in April 2005, the FDA approved MR imaging studies immediately after implantation of drug eluting stents, which is now reflected in their respective package instructions.

The excitement associated with CMR must be tempered with some realities. There is an increased cost for each facility as they use any MRI for any indication. It is not as portable as echocardiography, and there are precautions, contraindications, and safety concerns [3]. It is not as efficient as a CT scan and has slower through-put.

The prognostic data is not as well established as it has been in other modalities, particularly in the realm of nuclear stress testing. On the other hand, once a patient can get in the scanner, exquisite anatomical, hemodynamic and physiologic data can be obtained that is unparalleled without the concerns of poor acoustical windows seen in echocardiography, lack of photon penetration that can be a concern in CT, and the ionizing radiation concerns that CT and nuclear cardiology inherently have. Regardless, in the near future, each individual patient, clinician, and group practice will likely have to coordinate to determine which modality provides the most information that efficiently answers the clinical question.

With so many possible uses of cardiovascular MRI, and so many other competing technologies, in 2006, multiple imaging societies and stakeholders created appropriateness criteria [4]. The purpose of these next sections is to review these criteria and how it may apply to the use of cardiovascular MRI in your laboratory, as well as up and coming, intriguing uses. Formal protocols are described in Chap. 12.

Function

LV function is assessed by identifying end-systole and end-diastole in a slice of myocardium. By measuring slices of ventricles throughout to get an area, and then stacking those slices, one obtains a stroke volume and an ejection fraction. Limits include artifacts and arrhythmias. The following are appropriate uses of cardiovascular MRI, based on published 2006 appropriate use criteria, for the assessment of ventricular and valvular function.

1. **Evaluation of LV function following myocardial infarction OR in heart failure patients in the setting of technically limited images from an echocardiogram**, is considered appropriate. However, without a prior echocardiogram, it is considered Uncertain
2. **Quantification of LV function, particularly those in whom discordant information that is clinically significant from prior tests**. This data may help in determining left ventricular ejection fraction and the appropriateness of an implantable cardioverter defibrillator (ICD). Some centers have used the presence of scar location for electro-anatomical planning of ablation procedures, particularly if there is a concern for subsequent ventricular tachy-arrhythmias [5]. In our center, it is not uncommon to have a 3 month follow up evaluation of severe LV dysfunction with a CMR to evaluate EF and scar burden, or identify alternative etiologies in the setting of non-ischemic cardiomyopathies, particularly when standard heart failure therapies have been unsuccessful.
3. **Evaluation and characterization of native and prosthetic cardiac valves – including planimetry of stenotic disease and quantification of regurgitant disease, especially in patients with technically limited images from transthoracic or transesophageal echocardiography**. Echocardiography is, in general,

the standard tool for both initial and repeated assessment of valvular heart disease, specifically stenosis or regurgitation. Velocity, or the distance precessing protons travel over time, can be measured in the magnet, and as a result, so can flow. Stenosis is determined by assessing peak velocity across the valve and correlating either that to a peak gradient (modified Bernoulli equation of ~$4v^2$) or by planimetry (which is usually done with transesophageal echocardiography). The mean gradient is then quantified from the Doppler envelope. It is not unusual for a patient to go on to have a left and/or right heart cardiac catheterization to measure the gradients particularly if there are concerns regarding the veracity of the data in echocardiography.

In CMR, peak velocities are easy to obtain without any concerns for acoustic windows, but take time. Reasonable comparisons with echocardiography have been published that are based on small studies using either peak velocities on transthoracic echocardiography or planimetry on transesophageal echocardiography [6].

The amount of valvular regurgitation in echocardiography is assessed by either quantitation of regurgitant volume or regurgitant fraction, and on details of the proximal jet. Although this can be done in CMR, focus is now more on volumetrics.

For the aortic valve, both forward flow and reverse flow can be measured and therefore calculated. Although this has been validated in small studies [6], a recent study with clinical outcomes was also published with respect to aortic regurgitation [7]. This technique can also be used for the pulmonic valve, in combination with functional information about the right ventricle, and is often used for planning surgical timing in the setting of congenital heart disease (see 4. below).

For the mitral valve, there are several ways to quantify regurgitation. These include techniques such as measuring difference in volume that enters the ventricle from the mitral valve (diastolic inflow), and then exits the aortic valve (forward flow); or alternatively, using the difference between the left ventricular stroke volume from the aortic forward flow [8]. Some newer post-processing software allows direct measurement of regurgitation. It should be mentioned that currently, valve disease assessment may be quite involved from a scanner time and post-processing standpoint.

4. **Assessment of complex congenital heart disease, including anomalies of coronary circulation, great vessels, and cardiac chambers and valves**. These may include LV/RV mass and volumes, MR angiography, quantification of valvular disease, and contrast enhancement. These are often the longest exams. Younger children may require sedation and/or general anesthesia.

The greatest interest often lies in the function of the right ventricle. Furthermore, recent guidelines suggest that in the setting of Tetralogy of Fallot, this modality is “ideally suited for longitudinal follow-up”, is used “selectively during the first decade of life”, and assumes “a routine role in older patients.” This comprehensive examination also includes assessment of pulmonary regurgitation, branch PAs, etc. [9, 10].

Structural

Again, the power of MR is its capacity for tissue characterization. In that regard, identifying viable tissue, inflammatory tissue, characterizing masses, etc., is not as well performed by other modalities.

1. **Evaluation of specific cardiomyopathies (infiltrative [amyloid, sarcoid], HCM, or due to cardiotoxic therapies), which often include delayed enhancement**. The World Health Organization has created a classification of the non-ischemic cardiomyopathies [11]. The evaluation of these other potential etiologies of a cardiomyopathy has tremendous potential for specific therapy for an underlying disease process rather than the standard heart failure medications [12]. There are several of these potential cardiomyopathies, but some of the more common are listed here.

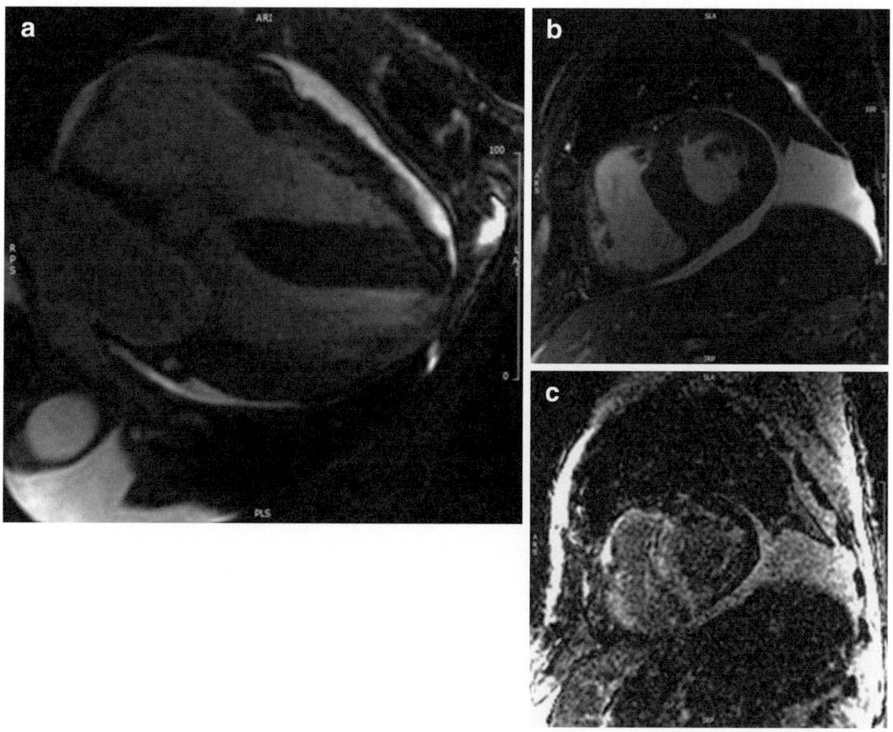

Fig. 10.2 (**a**) Steady state free precession (SSFP) image: biventricular hypertrophy, biatrial enlargement, and small circumferential pericardial effusion can be seen in the setting of cardiac amyloidosis. (**b**, **c**) MRI performed after patient's fat pad biopsy was negative for amyloid process. Top image (SSFP) is a short axis view of (**a**). Same position short axis late gadolinium enhancement. Diffuse subendocardial LGE involving the left ventricle in a non-coronary pattern, both left and right sides of the interventricular septum, and the right ventricle as well. This is a common pattern seen in cardiac amyloidosis

Cardiac amyloidosis is a condition where there is an abnormal amount of amyloid protein deposited in the ventricles. It can be associated with multiple myeloma. The classic echocardiographic description reveals biventricular hypertrophy and bi-atrial enlargement, and predominantly causes restrictive cardiomyopathy. Tissue characterization by late gadolinium enhancement cardiac MRI has implications for prognosis and therapy (see Fig. 10.2) [13, 14].

Sarcoidosis is a common process that involves non-caseating granulomas, predominantly in the lungs, but can affect any organ system. Although pulmonary sarcoidosis is the most common manifestation, it is unclear how common this is a cardiac manifestation based on either clinical (5 %) or post-mortem studies (20–30 %) [15, 16]. There is an increased potential for both assessing arrhythmias, or in changing immunosuppressive therapies, possibly defibrillator implantation or transplantation if arrhythmias cannot be suppressed (Fig. 10.3). As a result, Cardiac MRI is part of both the updated Japanese Ministry of Health and Welfare Guidelines [17] and the Heart Rhythm Society guidelines [18].

Hypertrophic cardiomyopathy (HCM) can be a challenging diagnosis, and has tremendous implications for sudden death. CMR can confirm the diagnosis if not well seen on echocardiography. The classic risk factors for sudden death in the setting of HCM are (1) prior cardiac arrest; (2) family history of sudden cardiac

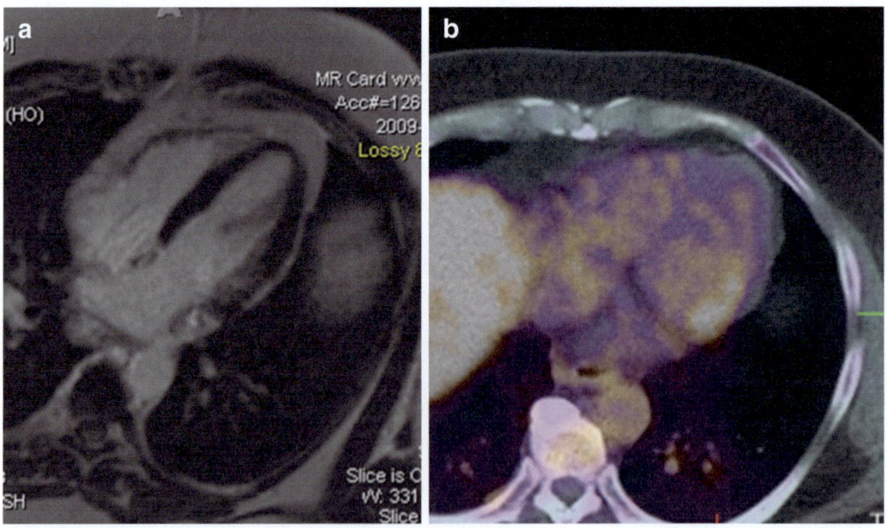

Fig. 10.3 (**a, b**) Patient presented with ventricular tachycardia storm. Late gadolinium enhancement in a focal area of the inferolateral wall, sub-epicardially, in the mid-ventricle, was felt to be in a non-coronary distribution. A special protocol with fluorodeoxyglucose using positron emission tomography shows avid uptake in the same distribution. Taken together, this is likely not infarction but expansion of the extracellular volume from inflammation. The patient received a diagnosis of cardiac sarcoid

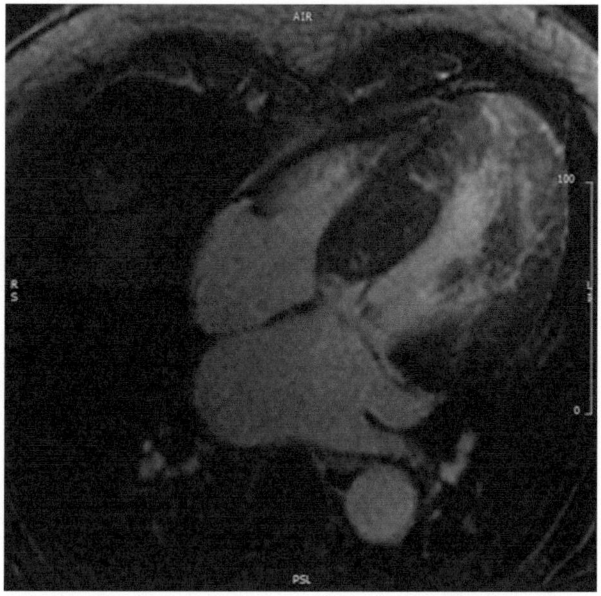

Fig. 10.4 Echocardiography revealed marked left ventricular hypertrophy in the absence of hypertension. This pattern is also diffuse and Anderson-Fabry was suggested, a glycogen storage disorder. This was confirmed on endomyocardial biopsy

death; (3) left ventricular wall >30 mm; (4) non-sustained ventricular tachycardia; (5) abnormal BP response to exercise; and (6) syncope. Cardiac MRI does not have the acoustic limitations of echocardiography and can assess the thickness of the ventricle. It can also quantify the amount of left ventricular outflow tract obstruction (similar to the way one can assess aortic stenosis) and differentiate it from mitral regurgitation. It can identify infiltrative etiologies of hypertrophy (Fig. 10.4). Furthermore, late gadolinium enhancement has been associated with non-sustained VT retrospectively, but it is still not clear if this is a separate prognostic marker over and above the standard risk factors [19, 20]. Some have advocated its use as an arbiter in the setting of unclear risk factors [21]. Alternatively, some feel that this is a marker instead for increased heart failure (either by admissions, New York Heart Association functional class, or heart-failure related death) [22].

Iron overload syndromes is another potential tool that does not necessitate the use of contrast. Whether in the setting of anemias (most commonly thalassemia major) or hemochromatosis, there are variations in iron deposition most common in the liver and heart. Iron can be quantified with excellent accuracy, can potentially forego the need for biopsy, and is useful in the setting of monitoring treatment with chelation (Fig. 10.5) [23].

2. **Evaluation for arrhythmogenic right ventricular cardiomyopathy (ARVC), or in patients presenting with syncope or ventricular arrhythmias**. ARVC is a condition that often involves fibrofatty replacement of at least the right ventricle. Since the power of MR is tissue characterization, the natural assumption is that MRI is uniquely capable of determining this diagnosis. However, recent consensus statements [24] suggest that the RV is thin-walled and likely does not

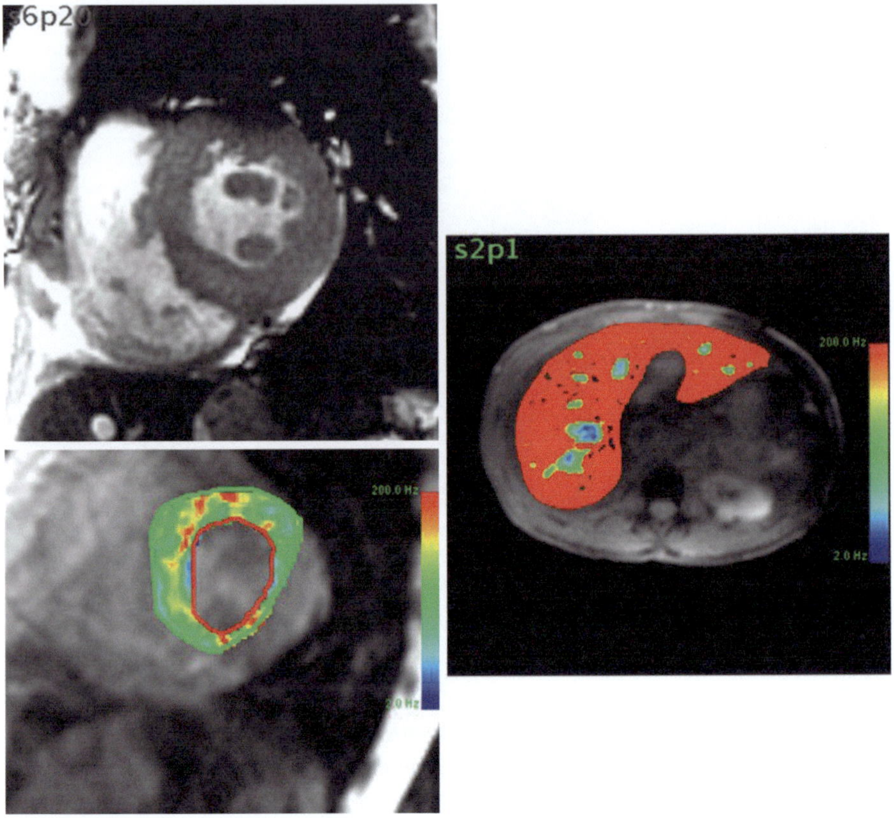

Fig. 10.5 *Upper left* corner. Normally the liver has an appearance similar to the myocardium on standard myocardial imaging with balanced steady state free precession (bSSFP). However, in this situation, it appears darker. Quantification performed with mapping suggests minimal iron deposition in the myocardium (*lower left* corner), and mild-to-moderate deposition in the liver (*below*)

have the spatial resolution to identify these findings. The criteria are now more dependent on RV volumetrics and wall motion. This, too, is problematic, as it raised specificity but potentially at the cost of reducing sensitivity, especially when reviewed retrospectively in patients with known disease [25]. Furthermore, the RV volumes suggested are very close to published normal values [26].

It is not uncommon for a referral for ventricular arrhythmias to be referred for MRI. It is strongly suggested that if a patient presents to your CMR with an indication of "R/O ARVC", that contrast be given. Although not necessary for the MR criteria for ARVC, there are other conditions that can present with VT in the setting of inflammatory etiologies such as sarcoidosis or myocarditis [12].

3. **Evaluation of myocarditis or myocardial infarction with normal coronary arteries, particularly those with cardiac enzymes without obstructive atherosclerosis on angiography**. There are usually three considerations in the

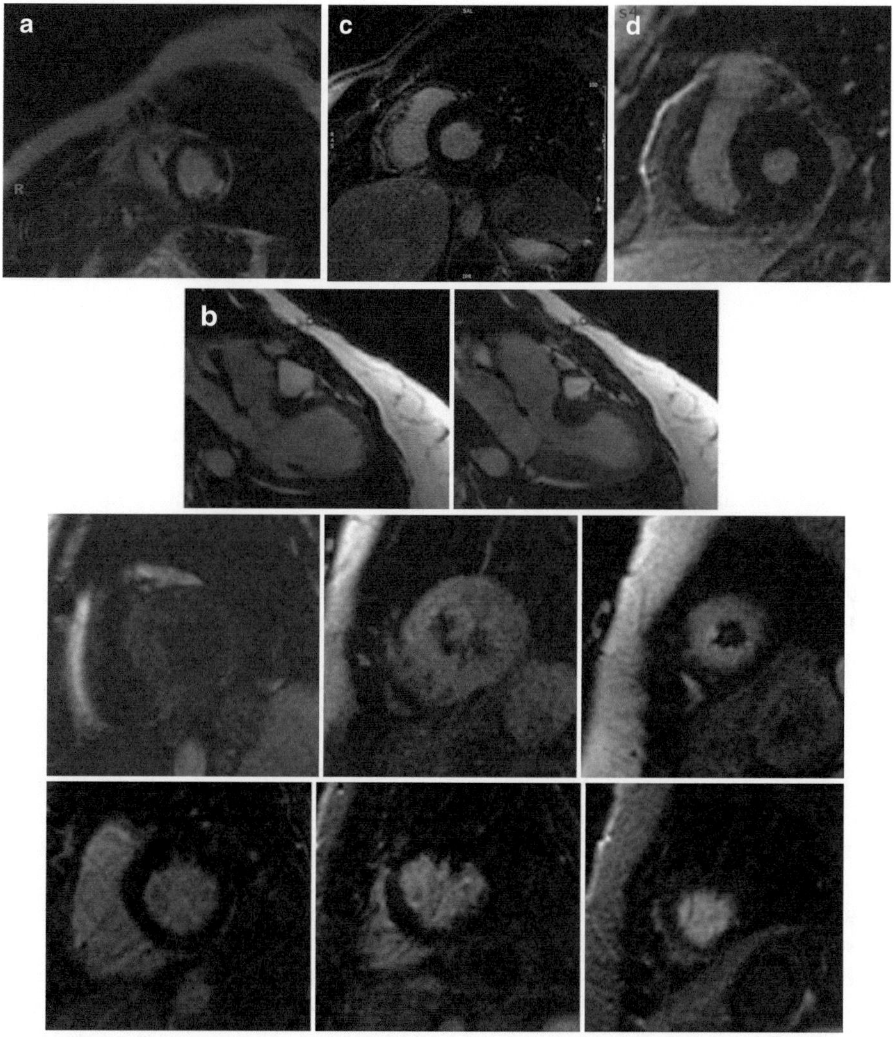

Fig. 10.6 (**a**) Patient presented with acute chest pain while smoking, but no other risk factors, resolved quickly with one nitroglycerin. Elevated troponins consistent with nSTeMI. Invasive coronary angiography with out any atherosclerotic disease. Cardiac MRI with contrast revealed a focal area of transmural late gadolinium enhancement in the basal-to-mid inferolateral wall consistent with myocardial infarction. Patient likely had vasospasm while smoking, which resolved with nitroglycerin. (**b**) *Top row* with diastole and systole showing typical apical akinesis seen in Tako Tsubo (stress cardiomyopathy). *Middle row* (basal, mid, and apical) with edema-based imaging showing progressive edema towards the apex. *Bottom row* (basal, mid, and apical) without late gadolinium enhancement showing that no clinically significant myocardial infarction is noted. (**c**) Twenty-eight year old man without coronary artery disease risk factors presents with chest pain, nonspecific EKG changes, and elevated troponins. Cardiac MRI shows sub-epicardial presence of late gadolinium enhancement consistent with a diagnosis of myocarditis. (**d**) Marked late gadolinium enhancement and thickening is noted of the pericardium

differential of elevated enzymes with normal coronary angiography. These include a myocardial infarction (with spontaneous clot lysis or vasospasm), myocarditis, or pericarditis (Fig. 10.6a). Each of these pathologies suggests different treatment paradigms. If there is late gadolinium enhancement in a coronary distribution, than this was likely a myocardial infarction (from vasospasm, spontaneous clot lysis, or perhaps labeled as Tako tsubo (stress catecholamine) cardiomyopathy, etc.) then aggressive coronary artery disease risk factor modification is recommended (Fig. 10.6a, b). If this is myocarditis, then further testing to assess arrhythmic potential or aggressive heart failure therapy (beta-blockade, afterload reduction) is suggested (Fig. 10.6c). If this is pericarditis, it may be clinically prudent to confirm the diagnosis prior to starting the potentially long cycle of non-steroidal anti-inflammatory agents, colchicine, and/or steroids (Fig. 10.6d).

4. **Evaluation of cardiac mass (suspected tumor or thrombus), which may often use perfusion and enhancement**. Different pulse sequences and algorithms are suggested to try to identify masses if they contain fat (as in a lipoma), water (as in a cyst), vascular like a tumor, limited gadolinium uptake as in a thrombus, etc. Again the power of MRI is tissue characterization, which can give strong clues, but not confirm the histopathological characteristics [27, 28].
5. **Evaluation of pericardial conditions**. Pericardial masses are similar to cardiac masses as above with a different differential. Determining fluid, prominent pericardial fat, cysts, or tumors can easily be performed with basic sequences.

   Constrictive pericarditis can often manifest as heart failure and is a challenging diagnosis that often involves multi-modality imaging. Interventricular interdependence is a finding seen with constrictive pericarditis, and is the finding that echocardiography or simultaneous left- and right-heart cardiac catheterization attempts to elucidate. This can also be seen with real-time imaging with CMR. In addition, exciting pilot data suggests late gadolinium enhancement (LGE) is a good marker for the potential for resolution with medications without the use of surgical stripping (Fig. 10.6d) [29].
6. **Evaluation for aortic dissection**. This is particularly helpful in identifying the etiology of chest pain in the ED. It has good accuracy [30–32], and can compete with CT for speed of diagnosis [33, 34]. Although gadolinium is not needed, it is typically used. This has the added benefit of not using CT contrast in a patient that may go on to have iodinated contrast for other procedures such as coronary angiography.
7. **Evaluation of pulmonary veins prior to radiofrequency ablation for atrial fibrillation**.

   The left atrial and pulmonary venous anatomy, including dimensions of veins for mapping purposes can be performed analogous to CT [35]. Another up and coming potential utility of CMR in the guidance of atrial fibrillation ablation is enhanced visualization of the left atrium with respect to scar and injury particularly in the setting of ablation therapies. It is well known that the development of atrial fibrosis leads to the development of atrial fibrillation [36]. Additionally, it has been shown that atrial fibrosis leads to an increased atrial fibrillation burden in these patients [37]. The high temporal and spatial resolution of CMR, as well as its ability to allow characterization of tissue composition, has made it a desirable potential modality for the imaging of these fibrotic changes in the left atrium. Most recently, the degree of pre-procedural atrial fibrosis estimated by delayed enhancement MRI was independently associated with likelihood of recurrent arrhythmia in patients undergoing ablation for atrial fibrillation [38, 39]. This could prove to be invaluable to electrophysiology specialists as they attempt to select patients for ablation that will have the lowest rates of atrial fibrillation recurrence after ablation.

CMR could also prove to be helpful post-procedurally as has been found to be effective in the visualization of radiofrequency-induced scar in the left atrial wall after AF ablation [40]. Success rates of AF ablation vary significantly, with recurrence rates ranging from 25 to 60 % after initial ablation [41]. This lack of consistency has been attributed in part to difficulty in assessing the extent and durability of left atrial wall injury induced by ablation. CMR has been used to identify gaps or recovered sites within ablation lesions that can be targeted during repeat procedures, suggesting a potential that this information could be used by electrophysiologists to avoid additional procedures by quickly and accurately closing all lesion sets during the repeat ablation [42].

8. **Symptomatic patients for the assessment of suspected coronary anomalies**. There are several techniques to evaluate this, but these are technically complicated, require time, and are often done at academic centers. Although not as rapid as CT angiography, it has the benefit of using non-ionizing radiation, an issue of particular importance to the pediatric and young adult population [43].

Viability

Viability imaging has been the main work horse for CMR imaging over the last decade and a half. Several concerns occur in the setting of a myocardial infarction. The left ventricular ejection fraction is typically assessed with echocardiography, which is also commonly used to assess for related mechanical complications. However, it is not unusual to have a question of whether or not percutaneous coronary intervention (PCI) was successful, in particular if TIMI Grade 3 flow is not established. Finally, in the setting of multivessel disease and significant left ventricular dysfunction, deciding the course of either aortocoronary bypass graft surgery vs PCI is also important, bringing into question the role of viability. More and more, CMR and its use of LGE are felt to be the gold standard for assessing viability.

1. **To determine viability prior to revascularization, especially as it may establish the likelihood of recovery of function with revascularization (PCI or CABG) or medical therapy** or when viability assessment by SPECT or dobutamine echo has provided "equivocal or indeterminate" results, continues to be an appropriate indication. In a sub-study of the recent Surgical Treatment for Heart

Disease Trial (STICH), a cohort of patients with CAD and LV dysfunction who were enrolled in a randomized trial of medical therapy with or without aorto-coronary bypass graft surgery, using either SPECT, dobutamine echocardiography, or both to assess myocardial viability, viable myocardium was associated with a greater likelihood of survival in patients with CAD and LV dysfunction, but felt to not be significant after adjustment for other baseline variables such as age, gender, race, prior MI, CAD risk factors, prior revascularization, etc. [44]. However, there has been controversy with these results in particular because this was a sub-study, and not the primary objective in the original study design and implementation. Furthermore, FDG PET and CMR that have improved spatial resolution over other standard modalities were not used [45]. Some have advocated the use of low-dose dobutamine (similar to echocardiographic techniques) to improve identification of viable tissue in addition to LGE to enhance the decision-making process that would suggest the likelihood of recovery [46].

2. **To determine the location and extent of myocardial necrosis including "no reflow" regions, particularly post-acute myocardial infarction**. It is estimated that "no-reflow" is present in as much as 40 % of primary PCI without complete myocardial reperfusion despite re-opening the infarct related artery. This carries tremendous weight in terms of prognosis [47]. However, appropriateness to detect post PCI myocardial necrosis remains uncertain.
3. **T1 mapping**. T1 mapping of myocardial fibrosis is another promising application of CMR that is presently under development. Myocardial fibrosis has been identified in conditions such as hypertensive heart disease, hypertrophic cardiomyopathy and idiopathic dilated cardiomyopathy [48]. This remodeling of the extracellular matrix (ECM) has been associated with impaired relaxation, development of arrhythmia, and decreased contractile reserve [49, 50]. Identifying diffuse myocardial fibrosis early in a patient's course is important for diagnosis and therapy, but other imaging modalities have been found to be inadequate as an alternative to endomyocardial biopsy. T1 mapping is a novel technique that has the potential to become a reliable modality for the quantitation of diffuse myocardial fibrosis. This approach would have a wide variety of clinical applications encompassing a wide variety of cardiac disease states.

For example, aldosterone excess in type II diabetes has been found to be associated with ECM expansion [51]. It is possible that identifying these patients early and treating them aggressively could slow progression of this fibrosis. It may also help to identify patients with extensive fibrotic changes for whom medical therapy may have less effect [48]. T1 mapping may eventually be used in the surveillance of patients with adult congenital heart disease as a relationship has been demonstrated between increased ECM and worsening volumetric parameters in these patients [52]. In patients with Takotsubo cardiomyopathy or other non-infarction related processes resulting in myocardial edema, T1 mapping has been shown to have the potential of quantifying both the extent and severity of these myocardial diseases [53]. Additionally, this same research team demonstrated that in patients with myocardial infarction, increased T1 values at the time of infarction correlated with decreased functional recovery at 6 months [54]. Finally, T1 mapping may have utility in determining timing of interventions in valvular disorders such as aortic stenosis as the degree of myocardial fibrosis pre-op has been shown to have a profound impact on long-term prognosis after aortic valve replacement [55].

The hope is to be able to have tissue characterization with respect to fibrosis that allows quantification without necessitating the use of contrast. With these and other potential applications, myocardial T1 mapping is likely to gain increasing clinical use in the future. Limits are vendor variations, but there is a working group amongst the relevant cardiac MRI societies that are actively working on resolving this. However, for now, it is not mentioned in the appropriateness guidelines.

Stress Perfusion

Vasodilator perfusion CMR uses predominantly adenosine, regadenoson, and on occasion dipyridamole. Although there are a few academic centers that perform stress perfusion CMR with exercise, guidelines in the management of stable ischemic heart disease, both in the US and in Europe, focus primarily on vasodilator stress perfusion CMR [56, 57]. Dobutamine Stress Functional CMR is similar to echocardiography in that wall motion abnormalities are ascertained at higher doses. Hypokinesis/akinesis of a wall segment is felt to be the result of ischemia. However, stress perfusion CMR with adenosine has been shown in multiple trials to have excellent sensitivity and specificity with receiver operator curves that are similar to SPECT and Stress Echocardiography [58, 59]. The largest of these trials was the CE-MARC trial that screened 4065 patients, of which 752 were randomly assigned to CMR vs SPECT to assess ischemia [60]. Although criticisms of the trial include the type of SPECT used, the sensitivity to assess ischemia was 86.5 %, and a negative predictive value of 90.5 %, each with a p value that was <0.0001.

With this basis in mind, the guidelines are listed below, and are similar for vasodilator SPECT.

1. **It is APPROPRIATE to evaluate the symptomatic patient with**:
   (a) Chest Pain and suspected CAD
      (i) Intermediate pre-test probability
      (ii) ECG uninterpretable OR unable to exercise.
   (b) Symptomatic with coronary angiography (CT or cath) suggesting stenosis of unclear severity.
2. **It is INAPPROPRIATE to use this to detect CAD in the following SYMPTOMATIC patients**:
   (a) Low-pretest probability of CAD, ECG interpretable AND able to exercise
   (b) Intermediate pre-test probability of CAD, ECG interpretable and able to exercise

(c) Intermediate pre-test probability of CAD, ECG un-interpretable OR able to exercise
(d) High pre-test probability of CAD
(e) Acute Chest Pain with high pre-test probability of CAD, ECG – ST-segment elevation and/or positive cardiac enzymes
(f) It is advisable that these patients should likely proceed to cardiac catheterization without the use of non-invasive testing.

3. **It is INAPPROPRIATE to use this for Risk assessment**

   (a) With Prior Test Results

      (i) Normal prior stress test (exercise, nuclear, echo, MRI)
      (ii) High CHD Framingham risk
      (iii) Within 1 year of prior stress test

   (b) Preoperative Evaluation for low-risk Non-Cardiac Surgery with intermediate peri-operative risk predictors
   (c) Detection of CAD Post-revascularization (PCI or CAG) in the valuation of Chest Pain Syndrome with the use of MR coronary angiography.

      (i) Evaluating bypass grafts
      (ii) History of percutaneous revascularization with stents
      (iii) An attempt was made to evaluate the coronaries in CE-MARC, and native CAD was seen only 55 % [60]. Furthermore, surgical clips and stents often have significant artifact surrounding them, precluding assessment of lumen severity.

4. **The role of stress perfusion CMR is UNCERTAIN in the following indications**:

   (a) Chest pain syndrome, and the detection of CAD in SYMPTOMATIC patients with:

      (i) Intermediate pre-test probability of CAD; and ECG interpretable AND able exercise
      (ii) Or high pre-test probability of CAD

   (b) Acute chest pain, and the detection of CAD in SYMPTOMATIC patients with

      (i) Intermediate pre-test probability of CAD; and no ECG changes; and serial cardiac enzymes are negative

   (c) Risk Assessment if prior stress test was equivocal (exercise, stress SPECT, or stress echocardiography), and intermediate CHD Framingham risk
   (d) Risk Assessment for Preoperative Evaluation for Non-Cardiac Intermediate or High-Risk Surgery with intermediate perioperative risk predictors
   (e) Asymptomatic or Stable Symptoms in the setting of stable ischemic heart disease have a Class IIa indication of stress testing, with either Nuclear MPI,

echocardiography, or CMR, with either exercise or pharmacological stress, which is felt to be useful for follow-up assessment at 2-year or longer intervals in patients with the above and prior evidence of silent ischemia or who are at high risk for a recurrent cardiac event and are

(i) Unable to exercise to an adequate workload
(ii) Have an uninterpretable ECG, or
(iii) Have a history of incomplete coronary revascularization [57].

Summary

In summary, CMR has tremendous potential to improve sub-endocardial definition of ventricles, valves, and vessels; to identify hemodynamic, physiologic, and metabolic data; and has support for its use through established guidelines. It has growing utility for morphology and function, ventricular and valvular, and has the potential role of identifying resting, ischemic, infarcted, and viability data in one 45 min session. In the next chapter, patient selection will be discussed.

References

1. Kim RJ, Fieno DS, Parrish TB, Harris K, Chen EL, Simonetti O, et al. Relationship of MRI delayed contrast enhancement to irreversible injury, infarct age, and contractile function. Circulation. 1999;100(19):1992–2002.
2. Kim RJ, Wu E, Rafael A, Chen EL, Parker MA, Simonetti O, et al. The use of contrast-enhanced magnetic resonance imaging to identify reversible myocardial dysfunction. N Engl J Med. 2000;343(20):1445–53.
3. International A. Standard practice for marking medical devices and other items for safety in the magnetic resonance environment. West Conshohocken: ASTM International2013. Report No.: ASTM F2503-13 Contract No.: ASTM F2503-13.
4. Beller GA. A proposal for an advanced cardiovascular imaging training track. J Am Coll Cardiol. 2006;48(7):1299–303.
5. Gupta S, Desjardins B, Baman T, Ilg K, Good E, Crawford T, et al. Delayed-enhanced MR scar imaging and intraprocedural registration into an electroanatomical mapping system in post-infarction patients. JACC Cardiovasc Imaging. 2012;5(2):207–10.
6. Cawley PJ, Maki JH, Otto CM. Cardiovascular magnetic resonance imaging for valvular heart disease: technique and validation. Circulation. 2009;119(3):468–78.
7. Myerson SG, d'Arcy J, Mohiaddin R, Greenwood JP, Karamitsos TD, Francis JM, et al. Aortic regurgitation quantification using cardiovascular magnetic resonance: association with clinical outcome. Circulation. 2012;126(12):1452–60.
8. Uretsky S, Gillam L, Lang R, Chaudhry FA, Argulian E, Supariwala A, et al. Discordance between echocardiography and MRI in the assessment of mitral regurgitation severity: a prospective multicenter trial. J Am Coll Cardiol. 2015;65(11):1078–88.
9. Valente AM, Cook S, Festa P, Ko HH, Krishnamurthy R, Taylor AM, et al. Multimodality imaging guidelines for patients with repaired tetralogy of fallot: a report from the AmericanSsociety of Echocardiography: developed in collaboration with the Society for

Cardiovascular Magnetic Resonance and the Society for Pediatric Radiology. J Am Soc Echocardiogr. 2014;27(2):111–41.
10. Geva T. Repaired tetralogy of Fallot: the roles of cardiovascular magnetic resonance in evaluating pathophysiology and for pulmonary valve replacement decision support. J Cardiovasc Magn Reson. 2011;13:9.
11. Richardson P, McKenna W, Bristow M, Maisch B, Mautner B, O'Connell J, et al. Report of the 1995 World Health Organization/International Society and Federation of Cardiology Task Force on the Definition and Classification of cardiomyopathies. Circulation. 1996;93(5):841–2.
12. O'Hanlon R, Prasad SK, Pennell DJ. Evaluation of nonischemic cardiomyopathies using cardiovascular magnetic resonance. J Nucl Cardiol. 2008;15(3):400–16.
13. Syed IS, Glockner JF, Feng D, Araoz PA, Martinez MW, Edwards WD, et al. Role of cardiac magnetic resonance imaging in the detection of cardiac amyloidosis. JACC Cardiovasc Imaging. 2010;3(2):155–64.
14. Austin BA, Tang WH, Rodriguez ER, Tan C, Flamm SD, Taylor DO, et al. Delayed hyper-enhancement magnetic resonance imaging provides incremental diagnostic and prognostic utility in suspected cardiac amyloidosis. JACC Cardiovasc Imaging. 2009;2(12):1369–77.
15. Silverman KJ, Hutchins GM, Bulkley BH. Cardiac sarcoid: a clinicopathologic study of 84 unselected patients with systemic sarcoidosis. Circulation. 1978;58(6):1204–11.
16. Iwai K, Tachibana T, Hosoda Y, Matsui Y. Sarcoidosis autopsies in Japan. Frequency and trend in the last 28 years. Sarcoidosis. 1988;5(1):60–5.
17. Sarcoidosis and granulomatous disorders [database on the Internet]. Japanese Ministry of Health & Welfare. [cited 2015]. Available from: http://www.mhlw.go.jp/english/.
18. Birnie DH, Sauer WH, Bogun F, Cooper JM, Culver DA, Duvernoy CS, et al. HRS expert consensus statement on the diagnosis and management of arrhythmias associated with cardiac sarcoidosis. Heart Rhythm. 2014;11(7):1305–23.
19. Moon JC, McKenna WJ, McCrohon JA, Elliott PM, Smith GC, Pennell DJ. Toward clinical risk assessment in hypertrophic cardiomyopathy with gadolinium cardiovascular magnetic resonance. J Am Coll Cardiol. 2003;41(9):1561–7.
20. Adabag AS, Maron BJ, Appelbaum E, Harrigan CJ, Buros JL, Gibson CM, et al. Occurrence and frequency of arrhythmias in hypertrophic cardiomyopathy in relation to delayed enhancement on cardiovascular magnetic resonance. J Am Coll Cardiol. 2008;51(14):1369–74.
21. Maron MS. Contrast-enhanced CMR, in HCM: what lies behind the bright light of LGE and why it now matters. JACC Cardiovasc Imaging. 2013;6(5):597–9.
22. O'Hanlon R, Grasso A, Roughton M, Moon JC, Clark S, Wage R, et al. Prognostic significance of myocardial fibrosis in hypertrophic cardiomyopathy. J Am Coll Cardiol. 2010;56(11):867–74.
23. Pennell DJ, Porter JB, Piga A, Lai YR, El-Beshlawy A, Elalfy M, et al. Sustained improvements in myocardial T2* over 2 years in severely iron-overloaded patients with beta thalassemia major treated with deferasirox or deferoxamine. Am J Hematol. 2015;90(2):91–6.
24. Bamberg F, Marcus R, Sommer W, Schwarz F, Nikolaou K, Becker CR, et al. Diagnostic image quality of a comprehensive high-pitch dual-spiral cardiothoracic CT protocol in patients with undifferentiated acute chest pain. Eur J Radiol. 2012;81(12):3697–702.
25. Vermes E, Strohm O, Otmani A, Childs H, Duff H, Friedrich MG. Impact of the revision of arrhythmogenic right ventricular cardiomyopathy/dysplasia task force criteria on its prevalence by CMR criteria. JACC Cardiovasc Imaging. 2011;4(3):282–7.
26. Hudsmith LE, Petersen SE, Francis JM, Robson MD, Neubauer S. Normal human left and right ventricular and left atrial dimensions using steady state free precession magnetic resonance imaging. J Cardiovasc Magn Reson. 2005;7(5):775–82.
27. O'Donnell DH, Abbara S, Chaithiraphan V, Yared K, Killeen RP, Cury RC, et al. Cardiac tumors: optimal cardiac MR sequences and spectrum of imaging appearances. AJR Am J Roentgenol. 2009;193(2):377–87.

28. Motwani M, Fairbairn TA, Larghat A, Mather AN, Biglands JD, Radjenovic A, et al. Systolic versus diastolic acquisition in myocardial perfusion MR imaging. Radiology. 2012;262(3):816–23.
29. Feng D, Glockner J, Kim K, Martinez M, Syed IS, Araoz P, et al. Cardiac magnetic resonance imaging pericardial late gadolinium enhancement and elevated inflammatory markers can predict the reversibility of constrictive pericarditis after antiinflammatory medical therapy: a pilot study. Circulation. 2011;124(17):1830–7.
30. Nienaber CA, von Kodolitsch Y, Nicolas V, Siglow V, Piepho A, Brockhoff C, et al. The diagnosis of thoracic aortic dissection by noninvasive imaging procedures. N Engl J Med. 1993;328(1):1–9.
31. Sommer T, Fehske W, Holzknecht N, Smekal AV, Keller E, Lutterbey G, et al. Aortic dissection: a comparative study of diagnosis with spiral CT, multiplanar transesophageal echocardiography, and MR imaging. Radiology. 1996;199(2):347–52.
32. Di Cesare E, Giordano AV, Cerone G, De Remigis F, Deusanio G, Masciocchi C. Comparative evaluation of TEE, conventional MRI and contrast-enhanced 3D breath-hold MRA in the post-operative follow-up of dissecting aneurysms. Int J Card Imaging. 2000;16(3):135–47.
33. Pereles FS, McCarthy RM, Baskaran V, Carr JC, Kapoor V, Krupinski EA, et al. Thoracic aortic dissection and aneurysm: evaluation with nonenhanced true FISP MR angiography in less than 4 minutes. Radiology. 2002;223(1):270–4.
34. Pennell DJ, Sechtem UP, Higgins CB, Manning WJ, Pohost GM, Rademakers FE, et al. Clinical indications for cardiovascular magnetic resonance (CMR): Consensus Panel report. Eur Heart J. 2004;25(21):1940–65.
35. Tops LF, Schalij MJ, Bax JJ. Imaging and atrial fibrillation: the role of multimodality imaging in patient evaluation and management of atrial fibrillation. Eur Heart J. 2010;31(5):542–51.
36. Allessie MA. Atrial electrophysiologic remodeling: another vicious circle? J Cardiovasc Electrophysiol. 1998;9(12):1378–93.
37. Everett TH, Olgin JE. Atrial fibrosis and the mechanisms of atrial fibrillation. Heart Rhythm. 2007;4(3 Suppl):S24–7.
38. Oakes RS, Badger TJ, Kholmovski EG, Akoum N, Burgon NS, Fish EN, et al. Detection and quantification of left atrial structural remodeling with delayed-enhancement magnetic resonance imaging in patients with atrial fibrillation. Circulation. 2009;119(13):1758–67.
39. Marrouche NF, Wilber D, Hindricks G, Jais P, Akoum N, Marchlinski F, et al. Association of atrial tissue fibrosis identified by delayed enhancement MRI and atrial fibrillation catheter ablation: the DECAAF study. JAMA. 2014;311(5):498–506.
40. McGann CJ, Kholmovski EG, Oakes RS, Blauer JJ, Daccarett M, Segerson N, et al. New magnetic resonance imaging-based method for defining the extent of left atrial wall injury after the ablation of atrial fibrillation. J Am Coll Cardiol. 2008;52(15):1263–71.
41. McGann C, Kholmovski E, Blauer J, Vijayakumar S, Haslam T, Cates J, et al. Dark regions of no-reflow on late gadolinium enhancement magnetic resonance imaging result in scar formation after atrial fibrillation ablation. J Am Coll Cardiol. 2011;58(2):177–85.
42. Badger TJ, Daccarett M, Akoum NW, Adjei-Poku YA, Burgon NS, Haslam TS, et al. Evaluation of left atrial lesions after initial and repeat atrial fibrillation ablation: lessons learned from delayed-enhancement MRI in repeat ablation procedures. Circ Arrhythm Electrophysiol. 2010;3(3):249–59.
43. Bluemke DA, Achenbach S, Budoff M, Gerber TC, Gersh B, Hillis LD, et al. Noninvasive coronary artery imaging: magnetic resonance angiography and multidetector computed tomography angiography: a scientific statement from the american heart association committee on cardiovascular imaging and intervention of the council on cardiovascular radiology and intervention, and the councils on clinical cardiology and cardiovascular disease in the young. Circulation. 2008;118(5):586–606.
44. Bonow RO, Maurer G, Lee KL, Holly TA, Binkley PF, Desvigne-Nickens P, et al. Myocardial viability and survival in ischemic left ventricular dysfunction. N Engl J Med. 2011;364(17):1617–25.

45. Jha S, Flamm SD, Kwon DH. Revascularization in heart failure in the post-STICH era. Curr Heart Fail Rep. 2013;10(4):365–72.
46. Scott AE, Semple SI, Redpath TW, Hillis GS. Low-dose dobutamine adds incremental value to late gadolinium enhancement cardiac magnetic resonance in the prediction of adverse remodelling following acute myocardial infarction. Eur Heart J Cardiovasc Imaging. 2013;14(9):906–13.
47. Galasso G, Schiekofer S, D'Anna C, Gioia GD, Piccolo R, Niglio T, et al. No-reflow phenomenon: pathophysiology, diagnosis, prevention, and treatment. A review of the current literature and future perspectives. Angiology. 2014;65(3):180–9.
48. Jellis CL, Kwon DH. Myocardial T1 mapping: modalities and clinical applications. Cardiovasc Diagn Ther. 2014;4(2):126–37.
49. Sugihara N, Genda A, Shimizu M, Suematsu T, Kita Y, Minamoto M, et al. Diastolic dysfunction and its relation to myocardial fibrosis in essential hypertension. J Cardiol. 1988;18(2):353–61.
50. McLenachan JM, Dargie HJ. Ventricular arrhythmias in hypertensive left ventricular hypertrophy. Relationship to coronary artery disease, left ventricular dysfunction, and myocardial fibrosis. Am J Hypertens. 1990;3(10):735–40.
51. Rao AD, Shah RV, Garg R, Abbasi SA, Neilan TG, Perlstein TS, et al. Aldosterone and myocardial extracellular matrix expansion in type 2 diabetes mellitus. Am J Cardiol. 2013;112(1):73–8.
52. Broberg CS, Chugh SS, Conklin C, Sahn DJ, Jerosch-Herold M. Quantification of diffuse myocardial fibrosis and its association with myocardial dysfunction in congenital heart disease. Circ Cardiovasc Imaging. 2010;3(6):727–34.
53. Ferreira VM, Piechnik SK, Dall'Armellina E, Karamitsos TD, Francis JM, Choudhury RP, et al. Non-contrast T1-mapping detects acute myocardial edema with high diagnostic accuracy: a comparison to T2-weighted cardiovascular magnetic resonance. J Cardiovasc Magn Reson. 2012;14:42.
54. Dall'Armellina E, Piechnik SK, Ferreira VM, Si QL, Robson MD, Francis JM, et al. Cardiovascular magnetic resonance by non contrast T1-mapping allows assessment of severity of injury in acute myocardial infarction. J Cardiovasc Magn Reson. 2012;14:15.
55. Weidemann F, Herrmann S, Stork S, Niemann M, Frantz S, Lange V, et al. Impact of myocardial fibrosis in patients with symptomatic severe aortic stenosis. Circulation. 2009;120(7):577–84.
56. Fox K, Garcia MA, Ardissino D, Buszman P, Camici PG, Crea F, et al. Guidelines on the management of stable angina pectoris: executive summary: the Task Force on the Management of Stable Angina Pectoris of the European Society of Cardiology. Eur Heart J. 2006;27(11):1341–81.
57. Fihn SD, Gardin JM, Abrams J, Berra K, Blankenship JC, Dallas AP, et al. 2012 ACCF/AHA/ACP/AATS/PCNA/SCAI/STS Guideline for the diagnosis and management of patients with stable ischemic heart disease: a report of the American College of Cardiology Foundation/American Heart Association Task Force on Practice Guidelines, and the American College of Physicians, American Association for Thoracic Surgery, Preventive Cardiovascular Nurses Association, Society for Cardiovascular Angiography and Interventions, and Society of Thoracic Surgeons. J Am Coll Cardiol. 2012;60(24):e44–164.
58. Cury RC, Cattani CA, Gabure LA, Racy DJ, de Gois JM, Siebert U, et al. Diagnostic performance of stress perfusion and delayed-enhancement MR imaging in patients with coronary artery disease. Radiology. 2006;240(1):39–45.
59. Klem I, Heitner JF, Shah DJ, Sketch Jr MH, Behar V, Weinsaft J, et al. Improved detection of coronary artery disease by stress perfusion cardiovascular magnetic resonance with the use of delayed enhancement infarction imaging. J Am Coll Cardiol. 2006;47(8):1630–8.
60. Greenwood JP, Maredia N, Younger JF, Brown JM, Nixon J, Everett CC, et al. Cardiovascular magnetic resonance and single-photon emission computed tomography for diagnosis of coronary heart disease (CE-MARC): a prospective trial. Lancet. 2012;379(9814):453–60.

Chapter 11
MRI Patient Selection

Ibrahim M. Saeed and Ryan Longmore

Abstract The appropriate selection of patients for magnetic resonance imaging is key to success of the test. There are numerous indications for testing, the most important concept being realization of the diagnostic capabilities of magnetic resonance to answer specific clinical questions. It is important to ensure that case selection is consistent with appropriate use criteria and the contraindications for the test which will be outlined in this chapter. Additionally appropriate patient preparation is necessary to ensure success. This includes addressing things such as claustrophobia, arrhythmias and inability to hold ones breath for the required amount of time. As gadolinium may be required, it is important to understand the potential side effects and reactions to this which will be discussed. Other important patient conditions such as implanted metallic devices will be discussed. Appropriate preparation for pharmacologically induced stress will also be reviewed.

Keywords Appropriate use criteria • Contraindications • Patient preparation • MRI contrast • Pharmacologic stress agents

Patient Selection and Preparation

Patient Selection

As discussed in the previous chapter, there are many appropriate indications for the use of cardiac MRI (CMR). The potential underutilization of CMR mandates continuous education of cardiologists and radiologists, cardiothoracic surgeons, and partner specialties including General Medicine and Pediatrics, Family Practitioners,

I.M. Saeed, MD, FACC, FAAP (✉)
Saint Luke's Mid America Heart Institute Cardiovascular Consultants, University of Missouri, Kansas City, MO, USA
e-mail: isaeed@saint-lukes.org; imsaeed@gmail.com

R. Longmore, DO
Department of Cardiology, Saint Luke's Hospital, Kansas City, MO, USA
e-mail: ryan.longmore@gmail.com

P.L. Tilkemeier et al. (eds.), *Quality Evaluation in Non-Invasive Cardiovascular Imaging*, DOI 10.1007/978-3-319-28011-0_11

and sub-specialties. These are some examples of potential educational opportunities to identify those patients that may benefit:

1. A mass in the left atrium is seen by a cardiologist. It is not uncommon for a TEE to be recommended as a result. Yet only the stalk may be visualized, and occasionally power Doppler may be used to assess vascularity.
2. A cardiac surgeon is debating whether the mitral regurgitation is moderate or severe.
3. An internist has received discordant data from a SPECT and an echocardiogram with respect to the left ventricular systolic function and ejection fraction.
4. A family practitioner notices a description of left ventricular hypertrophy on an echocardiogram, yet there is no evidence of hypertension, raising the suspicion for an infiltrative cardiomyopathy.
5. A pulmonologist is considering an echocardiogram to rule out cardiac sarcoidosis in one his patients with pulmonary sarcoidosis.
6. An oncologist is considering serial echocardiograms requiring echo-contrast to identify changes in left ventricular function before the next round of chemotherapy.
7. A rheumatologist orders an echocardiogram looking for serositis, myo- or pericarditis in one of her lupus patients.

Furthermore, there are other considerations. There is no ionizing radiation such as with nuclear cardiology or CT, and therefore ideal for younger patients who may be more susceptible to such exposures. It is a longer exam than the latter studies, so patient comfort needs to be assessed. Often there are arrhythmias. These are discussed under the relative and absolute contraindications.

Patient Preparation

This occurs either in clinic or prior to scheduling the relative and absolute contraindications as described below. We also prepare them for the time involved and whether or not the study will require an IV. Depending on the study, viability may take as little as 20 min, or a complex congenital can take 90 min. Specific areas of concern and relative and absolute contraindications will be addressed in the following subsections.

Appropriate Use Criteria

These are highlighted in the prior chapter (Chap. 10). A consensus statement has also been published [1].

Contraindications: Relative and Absolute

Consensus statements regarding MRI safety are found at the American College of Radiology website [2] as well as MRSafety.com. The following is not meant to be an all-inclusive statement, but are highlights.

Claustrophia

The potential for the patient to develop claustrophobia is assessed prior to scheduling the test to allow for appropriate preparation for the study. Patients with a history of claustrophobia have a relative contraindication for CMR, but this may be managed with light sedation, so as to permit cooperation with breath-holds and minimize abrupt motion that may occur in a somnolent patients. Outpatients who receive sedation should bring someone who can help drive them home. Rarely intubation is necessary, although this is more common for pediatric exams.

Arrhythmias

Establishing proper ECG gating prior to examination cannot be over-emphasized. It is invaluable. The classic "movie" pictures with bright appearing blood, (e.g., steady-state free-precession sequences), often requires averaging multiple cardiac segments. Lack of adequate gating can bring poor resolution, limiting ability to assess ejection fraction, late gadolinium enhancement, valve assessment, or some of the inversion recovery sequences, much like it does in CT, nuclear cardiology, and echocardiography. While there are "arrhythmia rejection" options on many scanners, these are often problematic and may not function well in the setting of a large burden of PVCs. One option is to do free breathing studies, but this can deteriorate temporal and spatial resolution.

Inability to Breath-Hold

Although there are free-breathing sequences, they are limited in spatial and temporal resolution. As many factors that can improve breath hold are recommended. For example, a patient with heart failure and bilateral pleural effusions should be diuresed and offered supplemental oxygen.

Gadolinium Considerations

Renal Failure and Nephrogenic Systemic Fibrosis

Gadolinium based contrast agents (GBCA) are different from the standard CT contrast agents. In the setting of poor renal clearance, gadolinium can be retained in tissues causing a local reaction. Nephrogenic systemic fibrosis (NSF, also known as nephrogenic fibrosing dermopathy) is a syndrome manifested by fibrosis of the skin, joints, and eyes that resembles scleromyxedema. There is no known cure. That being said, there are a total of 380 cases in the International Center for Nephrogenic Systemic Fibrosis Registry as of the date of this writing [3].

It has been shown that a small subset of patients with significant renal disease may be at risk of developing NSF after the administration of GBCA [4]. It is estimated that patients with ESRD (Chronic Kidney Disease (CKD stage V, estimated GRF <15 ml/min/1.73 m^2) or severe CKD (Stage IV, eGFR 15–29 ml/min/1.73 m^2) have between a 1 and 7 % chance of developing NSF after exposure to GBCA; however, most patients who developed NSF had ESRD and were on dialysis at the time of exposure [2]. Between 12 and 20 % of confirmed cases of NSF have occurred in patients with acute kidney injury; however, this is frequently superimposed on chronic kidney disease [2].

NSF is believed to occur most often when patients receive high doses of GBCA or multiple doses over months to years [5]. It is important to note that many GBCAs have not been strongly associated with the development of NSF. The American College of Radiology (ACR) has recently published an updated manual on the use of contrast media [6]. Regarding use of GBCAs they have provided a table listing these agents, with Group I agents conferring the greatest risk of development of NSF (see Table 11.1). The ACR recommends avoiding use of GBCAs in patients with ESRD on chronic dialysis, and if pursued, Group I agents would be contraindicated. There is limited data for group III agents, although, to date, few, if any, unconfounded cases of NSF.

Table 11.1 Classification of gadolinium-based contrast agents

Group I: Agents associated with the greatest number of NSF cases:
Gadodiamide (Omniscan ® – GE Healthcare)
Gadopentetate dimeglumine (Magnevist® – Bayer HealthCare Pharmaceuticals)
Gadoversetamide (OptiMARK® – Covidien)
Group II: Agents associated with few, if any, unconfounded cases of NSF:
Gadobenate dimeglumine (MultiHance® – Bracco Diagnostics)
Gadoteridol (ProHance® – Bracco Diagnostics)
Gadoteric acid (Dotarem® – Guerbet [as of this writing not FDA-approved for use in the U.S.]
Gadobutrol (GadavistR – Bayer HealthCare Pharmaceuticals)
Group III: Agents that have only recently appeared on the market:
Gadofosveset (Ablavar® – Lantheus Medical Imaging)
Gadoxetic acid (Eovist® – Bayer HealthCare Pharmaceuticals)

Allergic Reactions

NSF could be considered a delayed reaction. True, immediate, allergic reactions are extremely rare [7]. It is incumbent that all MR technologists are knowledgeable about the assessment of management of hypersensitivity reactions as pertains to gadolinium, and that they are aware of the crash cart and resuscitative medications. In addition, although a physician need not be present for a non-contrast MRI, it is mandated that a physician be on site (personally and immediately available) during administration of GBCA [2]. While there is a role for pre-medication in patients with a prior allergic reaction to GBCA using histamine blockers and steroids, it should be noted no clinical studies have unequivocally demonstrated prevention of contrast reactions using short-term IV corticosteroids.

Is Contrast Needed?

GBCA agents are not typically needed for general cardiovascular imaging that looks at morphology and function. Figures 10.1 and 11.1 are examples of non-contrast images. GBCA are often used to enhance tissue characterization and/or enhance efficiency and visualization with respect to vascular imaging. Examples are in Fig. 11.2. Figure 11.2 (top) is an example of a study for viability after an acute myocardial infarction who was re-vascularized within 3 h of onset of symptoms.

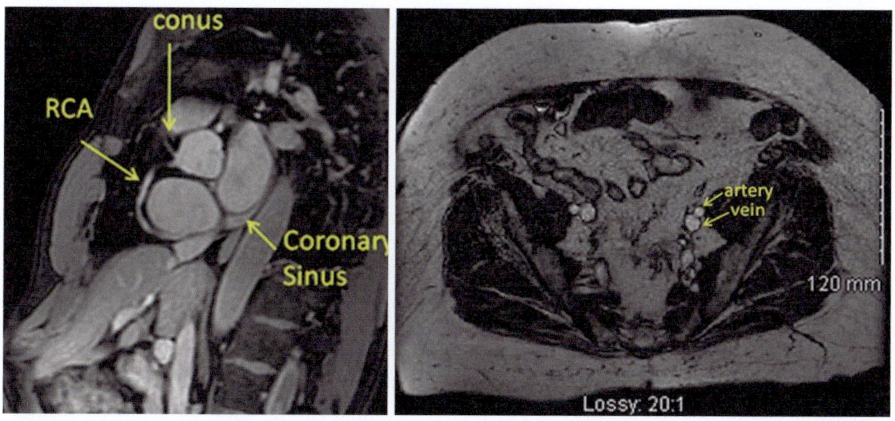

Fig. 11.1 (*Left*) Oblique stack in the short axis view to evaluate for any potential coronary anomalies. It took several minutes to acquire while this patient is free-breathing young patient. No contrast was necessary to visualized cardiac chambers, venous structures (the coronary sinus), Right coronary artery (RCA) with its conus branch. Not labeled but visible are the aorta and inferior vena cava. (*Right*) Iliac vessels for a patient being considered for transaortic valve replacement. Stack acquired without breath-hold as the diaphragm rarely interferes with image acquisition below the kidney. This was one slice of many that took about 15 s. Knowledge of arterial and venous anatomy is necessary to not confuse the two without the use of contrast; alternatively, contrast may be used to take advantage of the arterial or venous phase

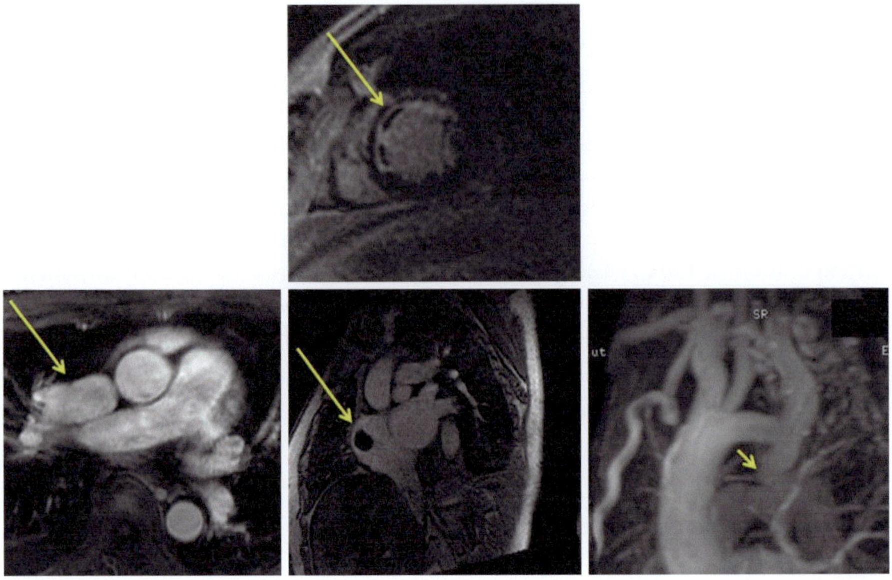

Fig. 11.2 (*Top*) Is an example of a study for viability after an acute myocardial infarction who was revascularizaed within 3 h of onset of symptoms. Although there is infarct, a dark area suggests areas of "no-reflow" likely representing microvascular obstruction. (*Bottom left*) Is an example where contrast was used for a faster assessment of the vasculature and a volume-set that is easier to manipulate on a workstation. In this case, there is an anomalous pulmonary vein coming into the SVC. (*Bottom center*) Is a case of a mass. Although GBCA is not needed to determine fat vs water (which is based off of T1 vs T2 characteristics), but it does help with identifying tumor vs thrombus. This "myxoma" was felt to be thrombus on MR because of the lack of contrast uptake suggesting no vascularity, and was confirmed on pathology. Finally (*bottom right*) is a 3-D view of the vasculature in a patient with aortic coarctation that can assist the surgeon prior to surgical repair

Although there is infarct, a dark area suggests areas of "no-reflow" likely representing microvascular obstruction. Figure 11.2 (bottom left) is an example where contrast was used for a faster assessment of the vasculature and a volume-set that is easier to manipulate on a workstation. In this case, there is an anomalous pulmonary vein coming into the SVC. Figure 11.2 (bottom center) is a case of a mass. Although GBCA is not needed to determine fat vs. water (which is based off of T1 vs. T2 characteristics), but it does help with identifying tumor vs. thrombus. This "myxoma" was felt to be thrombus on MR because of the lack of contrast uptake suggesting no vascularity, and was confirmed on pathology. Finally Fig. 11.2 (bottom right) is a nice 3-D view of the vasculature in a patient with aortic coarctation that can assist the surgeon prior to surgical repair.

In summary, discussions between the ordering and interpreting physician, MR technologist, and a patient are important if there are any concerns about the use of GBCA.

Metallic Implants

A screening form is available at MRIsafety.com [8], Metallic objects that were initially contraindicated are now felt to be reasonably safe; furthermore, newer implants are being designed that are less ferromagnetic. Common terms include MR safe, MR conditional, and MR unsafe as defined in Table 11.2.

It is not uncommon that after coronary stenting, a cardiac MRI may be indicated. Multiple papers have suggested that these devices are either MR safe or MR conditional [8–10]. Nevertheless although sternal wires and prosthetic valves are generally safe, there are still exceptions that are detailed on screening forms. These may include asking about brain clips for aneurysms, or a history of welding (metallic shrapnel in the eye remains an absolute contraindication.)

Pacemakers (PMS) and/or Implantable Cardioverter Defibrillators (ICDS)

In general, these MR exams are discouraged. There is potential for device or lead movement, asynchronous pacing, programming changes including activation of tachyarrhythmia therapies and/or inhibition of pacing output, inducing currents in the leads or causing stimulation, arrhythmia, death, and/or permanent dysfunction of the device and/or battery depletions necessitating a generator change. Nevertheless, increasing data suggests that it may still be safe if there is an appropriate indication in the setting of an institution with expertise in MR imaging and electrophysiology [2, 9].

In general, MR examination of non–pacemaker-dependent patients is discouraged and should only be considered in cases in which there is a strong clinical indication and in which the benefits clearly outweigh the risks. MR examination of pacemaker-dependent patients should not be performed unless there are highly compelling circumstances and when the benefits clearly outweigh the risks. There are MR conditional pacemakers that involve the presence of a device representative to change the mode. Similarly, MR examination of patients with ICDs should not be performed

Table 11.2 MR safety definitions [9]

MR safe	An item that poses no known hazards in any MR environment in that they are nonconducting, nonmetallic, and/or nonmagnetic items
MR conditional	An item that has been demonstrated to pose no known hazards in a specified MR imaging environment with specified conditions of use, such as static magnetic field strength, spatial magnetic gradient, radiofrequency fields and related systemic absorption rates, etc.
MR unsafe	An item that is known to pose hazards in all MR environments

unless there are highly compelling circumstances and when the benefits clearly outweigh the risks. As of the date of this writing, there are no "MR conditional" ICDs.

If scanning is performed, it should be done at experienced centers with MR imaging and electrophysiology expertise. Prior to this, a written informed consent reviewing the risks (which includes but is not limited to those listed above), benefits, and alternatives is important. In addition, a physician or physician designee with ACLS and pacemaker/ICD expertise should decide whether reprogramming the pacemaker/ICD before the MR examination is necessary and should be in attendance for the entire study. A person with expertise in MR physics and safety should be involved with the scan to optimally plan the scan to minimize risk, and consideration should be given to using scanning sequences that minimize study risk. These involve pre-scanning steps (interrogating the device to assess pre-test functions, and setting to asynchronous mode for those who are pacemaker dependent, disabling therapies planned by an ICD including therapy tachycardia/bradycardia modes);continuous monitoring of the heart rhythm and vital signs during the MRI, having available equipment for a sentinel event. After the MR examination, devices should be re-interrogated and reprogrammed to original settings by those with MR and electrophysiological expertise. Furthermore, a follow-up device-related clinic visit may also be necessary.

Preparation for Stress Testing

Stress testing for CMR is exclusively pharmacologic [11]. Dobutamine ± atropine, which increase myocardial oxygen demand (MVO_2); or adenosine vs. regadenoson, which are vasodilators, are the predominant agents. Patient preparation involves informed consent for the stress test.

Fasting is not mandatory but recommended because of the common adverse effect of nausea and vomiting, made more difficult by the supine nature of the exam in the relatively restrictive area of the MR chamber.

Dobutamine

Contraindications to dobutamine include severe systemic hypertension (blood pressure ≥220/120 mmHg) unstable angina pectoris, severe aortic valve stenosis, complex cardiac arrhythmias (including uncontrolled atrial fibrillation), hypertrophic cardiomyopathy, active inflammation (e.g., myocarditis, endocarditis, or pericarditis), or decompensated heart failure. Contraindications to atropine include narrow-angle glaucoma, myasthenia gravis, obstructive uropathy or gastrointestinal disorders. Finally avoidance of ß-blockers from 12 to 24 h in advance is recommended.

At high doses, chest pain and palpitations are common. Rare but severe complications include myocardial infarctions, as well as tachy-arrhythmias such as ventricular fibrillation or sustained ventricular tachycardia.

Vasodilator Stress

The vasodilators have similar contraindications as when they are used in standard stress testing, including second or third degree atrioventricular blocks or significant sinus node dysfunction, sinus bradycardia (heart rate <40 bpm), hypotension (systolic blood pressure <90 mmHg), active bronchoconstriction or bronchospastic disease that requires the regular use of inhalers, or known hypersensitivity to these agents. Patients are counseled 12- to -24 h in advance that food, beverages, or medications that contains caffeine, or the use of theophylline or dipyridamole, are not recommended. The same is also true of nicotine products.

With the use of adenosine, two intravenous lines (IVs) are required, preferentially antecubital. As adenosine is being infused, first pass perfusion with gadolinium is assessed and needs to be given in the second IV. Typically, this arm is used for blood pressure assessment as the adenosine infusion cannot be interrupted during the stress portion of the study. Only one IV is required for dipyridamole or regadenoson.

Common symptoms associated with dipyridamole, adenosine and regadenoson are flushing, chest pain, palpitations and breathlessness. More adverse and potentially serious complications include bronchospasm or transient heart block, hypotension, or sinus tachycardia.

Summary

Much more goes into preparing and selecting the patient adequate for MR examination than many other imaging techniques. Coordinated efforts between physicians, schedulers, and technologists are critical to maximize safety, comfort, through-put, and diagnostic capacity.

References

1. Hendel RC, Patel MR, Kramer CM, Poon M, Carr JC, Gerstad NA, et al. ACCF/ACR/SCCT/SCMR/ASNC/NASCI/SCAI/SIR 2006 appropriateness criteria for cardiac computed tomography and cardiac magnetic resonance imaging: a report of the American College of Cardiology Foundation Quality Strategic Directions Committee Appropriateness Criteria Working Group, American College of Radiology, Society of Cardiovascular Computed Tomography, Society for Cardiovascular Magnetic Resonance, American Society of Nuclear Cardiology, North American Society for Cardiac Imaging, Society for Cardiovascular Angiography and Interventions, and Society of Interventional Radiology. J Am Coll Cardiol. 2006;48(7):1475–97.
2. Kanal E, Barkovich AJ, Bell C, Borgstede JP, Bradley Jr WG, Froelich JW, et al. ACR guidance document on MR safe practices. J Magn Reson Imaging. 2013;37(3):501–30.
3. International Center for Nephrogenic Systemic Fibrosis Registry. [Internet]. [Cited May 8, 2015]. Available from: http://www.icnfdr.org.
4. Marckmann P, Skov L, Rossen K, Dupont A, Damholt MB, Heaf JG, et al. Nephrogenic systemic fibrosis: suspected causative role of gadodiamide used for contrast-enhanced magnetic resonance imaging. J Am Soc Nephrol. 2006;17(9):2359–62.

5. Kallen AJ, Jhung MA, Cheng S, Hess T, Turabelidze G, Abramova L, et al. Gadolinium-containing magnetic resonance imaging contrast and nephrogenic systemic fibrosis: a case-control study. Am J Kidney Dis. 2008;51(6):966–75.
6. ACR Manual on Contrast Media, Version 9, 2013 [Internet] [cited May 8, 2013]. Available from: http://www.acr.org/~/media/ACR/Documents/PDF/QualitySafety/Resources/Contrast%20 Manual/2013_Contrast_Media.pdf.
7. Prince MR, Zhang H, Zou Z, Staron RB, Brill PW. Incidence of immediate gadolinium contrast media reactions. AJR Am J Roentgenol. 2011;196(2):W138–43.
8. Magnetic resonance (Mr) procedure screening form for patients. [Internet] [Cited May 8, 2015]. Available from: http://www.mrisafety.com/SCREENING_FORM/PreScrnF.pdf.
9. Levine GN, Gomes AS, Arai AE, Bluemke DA, Flamm SD, Kanal E, et al. Safety of magnetic resonance imaging in patients with cardiovascular devices: an American Heart Association scientific statement from the Committee on Diagnostic and Interventional Cardiac Catheterization, Council on Clinical Cardiology, and the Council on Cardiovascular Radiology and Intervention: endorsed by the American College of Cardiology Foundation, the North American Society for Cardiac Imaging, and the Society for Cardiovascular Magnetic Resonance. Circulation. 2007;116(24):2878–91.
10. Curtis JW, Lesniak DC, Wible JH, Woodard PK. Cardiac magnetic resonance imaging safety following percutaneous coronary intervention. Int J Cardiovasc Imaging. 2013;29(7):1485–90.
11. Kramer CM, Barkhausen J, Flamm SD, Kim RJ, Nagel E. Standardized cardiovascular magnetic resonance (CMR) protocols 2013 update. J Cardiovasc Magn Reson. 2013;15:91.

Chapter 12
Cardiac MR Protocol Selection

Joseph Soltys

Abstract Cardiac MR (CMR) has tremendous potential for improving cardiac and cardiovascular assessments. Due to high temporal and spatial resolution, CMR is capable of assessing everything from cardiac morphology and function to tissue characterization (viability), perfusion, angiography, and even vascular flow. Image quality however, is highly dependent upon patient compliance and protocol optimization. In addition, it offers alternatives to populations that are sensitive to radiation exposure such as children and women of child bearing age. These tests, though complex, can be mastered with well structured protocols, training and adherence to clinical guidelines.

Keywords Cardiac MR • Morphology • Function • Viability • Perfusion

Background

Cardiac Magnetic Resonance Imaging (CMR) has long been recognized for its potential to provide unique, high quality information for assessing cardiovascular patients. Pioneering work in the 1980s established that MRI could have a role in assessing ischemia and myocardial infarction [1]. Since that time, additional CMR applications have arisen including cardiac morphology [2], cardiac function [3], myocardial viability [4], congenital conditions [5], blood flow [6], and atherosclerotic plaque assessment [7]. However, in order to achieve widespread acceptance and utilization of CMR sites must mutually adopt, implement, and rigorously adhere to protocols and quality control standards.

While the general physics involved remain constant, magnetic field strength considerations, coil design, pulse sequence choice and vendor implementation among other factors confound standardization [8–10]. The Society for Cardiovascular MRI (SCMR), the American College of Radiology (ACR), and the European Society of Cardiology and European Association of Cardiovascular Imaging (EACVI) among

J. Soltys, PhD
MR Physics, Cardiovascular Imaging Technologies, LLC, Kansas City, MO, USA
e-mail: Jsoltys@cvit.com

P.L. Tilkemeier et al. (eds.), *Quality Evaluation in Non-Invasive Cardiovascular Imaging*, DOI 10.1007/978-3-319-28011-0_12

several others have all developed societal guidelines to be used as benchmarks for most CMR laboratories [11, 12].

CMR is a very interactive imaging modality often requiring the scanning technologist to remain attentive and tune sequence parameters to specific patients and, in the case of viability imaging, to the pharmacokinetic washout of the contrast agent. As site specific protocols are developed, they must be descriptive; identifying the pulse sequence to be used, default parameters, and any vendor or application specific instructions so that the scanning technologists know when and how appropriate corrections or additions are to be made. This chapter will address the steps necessary to extend societal guidelines into working clinical protocols.

Basics of Cardiac Magnetic Resonance Imaging (in a Nutshell)

CMR utilizes the process of nuclear resonance to excite hydrogen protons in the tissues of the body. The first step in the process is the introduction of a large and uniform magnetic field (B0) to which the protons will align with or against, precessing at different rates but in equilibrium. B0 field is the large Tesla number describing the system (today 1.5 or 3.0 Tesla systems are common). In order to define a slice plane for imaging within the patient one or more gradient magnetic fields are applied creating linear variations in the B0 field linearly altering the proton precessional frequencies. At the same time the patient is temporarily subjected to radiofrequency (RF) energy designed to elicit a specific response by the protons (pulse sequence). At the end of the pulse sequence the protons are in phase, but will quickly return to the equilibrium state (dephasing) as they release the absorbed RF energy. This released energy is intercepted by a receiver coil and the phase and frequency components are derived via discrete Fourier transform along the spatial encoding gradients which are reconstructed to form the resulting image.

Assessment of Left and Right Ventricular Function

CMR is recognized as a gold standard for the determination of global and local cardiac function by ejection fraction and segmental wall motion and thickening [13], due in part to its high reproducibility [14]. The acquisitions are computer defined and controlled which reduces inter-operator variability and since the imaging field of view is fully three-dimensional CMR does not have the line of sight issues prevalent in modalities such as echocardiography. In a study comparing groups of healthy individuals and congenital conditions measurements of mass, volume, and function, intra-class correlation coefficients of 0.94–0.99 and interoperator coefficients of 0.96–0.99 were observed for the right ventricle [15].

Currently the preferred pulse sequence for functional assessment is an ECG-gated, steady-state free-precession or balanced steady-state free-precession (SSFP and bSSPF) pulse sequence. In a study of 41 patients comparing SSFP and turbo

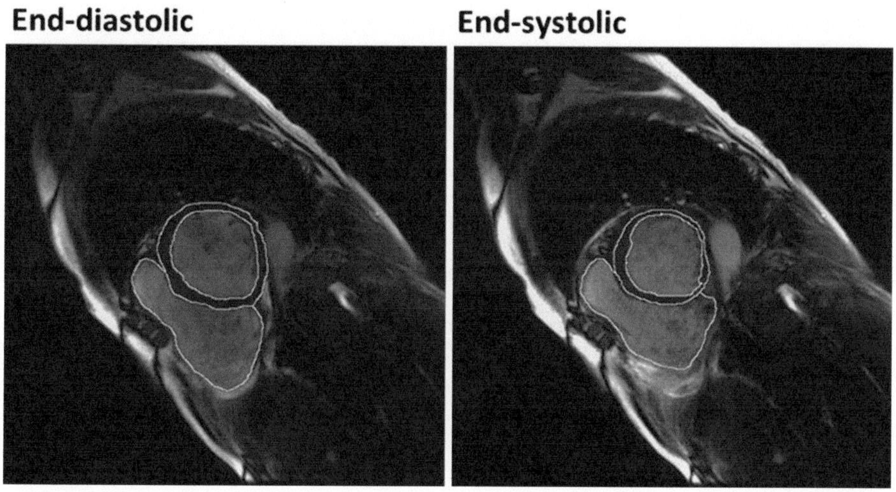

Fig. 12.1 Morphology and function: by measured endocardial volumes (left and right ventricle) and epicardial volumes on each slice obtained from a stack of images through the myocardium, ventricular end-diastolic, end-systolic volumes, stroke volumes, ejection fractions, and mass can all be obtained. There is not much difference in these two images as this person has severe ventricular dysfunction

field echo sequence for ventricular volumes, interoperator variability and success of automatic contour detection, measured volumes were higher with SSFP and automatic contour detection algorithms were more successful [16] (see Fig. 12.1).

The bSSFP sequence is a variant of the gradient echo scheme and is available on all major platforms likely under a vendor specific trade name FIESTA (Fast Imaging Employing Steady State Acquisition) for General Electric; TrueFISP (Fast Imaging with Steady state free Precession) for a Siemens magnet]. The bSSFP sequence provides high signal-to-noise (SNR), excellent contrast between the myocardium and blood pool (based on the T2/T1 ratio of the tissues) and low flow sensitivity ("balanced" gradients) but is very dependent on field homogeneity and thus requires a shim volume over heart [17]. Performing multiple acquisitions along the long axis of the heart allows the resulting images to be stitched together creating a movie demonstrating myocardial contraction throughout the cardiac cycle derives volumes. Segmentation of the endocardium on each slice yields the ventricular volume at the selected location and phase. The segmentation process need only be repeated along the axis for both end diastole and end systole to calculate a global EF, but may be extended to all phases with contours derived (visually, manually, or by various post-processing algorithm) for regional function or if other measures of function are desired. Potential complicating factors for calculations of EF include movements of the mitral valve plane and apex, as well as difficulty with gating from arrhythmias, or from breath-holds. In many cases a long axis localizer view may be utilized, to aid in correction of these motions.

A typical protocol for basic morphological and function of the entire heart is contained in Table 12.1 [11].

Table 12.1 Typical protocol for basic morphological and function of the entire heart [11]

Stage	Purpose	Sequence
Localizer scan	Identify heart position	SSFP/bSSFP
Transaxial stack of entire heart:	Morphology	SSFP/bSSFP or fast spin echo
Short axis localizer	Identify heart position and orientation (short axis, horizontal long axis and vertical long axis)	SSFP/bSSFP
Short axis cine stack of entire heart	Functional assessment: EDV, ESV, RVEF, LVEF	SSFP/bSSFP
Long axis cine slices: 2, 3, and 4 chamber views	Wall motion assessment	SSFP/bSSFP

SSFP steady-state free-precession, *bSSFP* balanced steady-state free-precession, *EDV* end diastolic volume, *ESV* end systolic volume, *RVEF* right ventricular ejection fraction, *LVEF* left ventricular ejection fraction

Protocol for Assessing Cardiac Function

Current protocol for a visual assessment of LV function includes [18]:

1. Simultaneously review cine images of all acquired slices comparing looking for continuity, gating problems, and identify problematic artifacts (if present)
2. Look for ventricular interaction and/or any extracardiac structures as evidence of constriction, shunts, etc.
3. Observe global ventricular function categorizing any wall motion abnormalities (hyperkinetic, normokinetic, hypokinetic, akinetic, or dyskinetic).

Quantitative recommendations include [18]:

1. Calculated/reported parameters:

   (a) Left Ventricle: end-diastolic volume, end-systolic volume, ejection fraction, stroke volume, cardiac output, mass, include body surface area indexed values for each (excluding LVEF)
   (b) Define systole and diastole by smallest and largest LV blood pool volume respectively (in the case of dyssynchrony or severe mitral regurgitation closure of aortic valve defines end-systole).
   (c) Report volumes from LV short axis stack (preferred), alternately rotational long axis views may be used.
   (d) A consistent approach must be used when segmenting papillary muscles from the LV blood pool either excluded (preferred) or included remembering to use appropriate reference values when reporting.
   (e) Include the LV outflow track as part of the LV blood pool volume.
   (f) To determine location of the mitral valve plane use a long-axis reference slice (if correction software available), or on the basal most short axis slice only include blood that is greater than 50 % surrounded by myocardium.

Myocardial Viability

While a great deal can be derived investigating native CMR images, the use of an exogenous contrast agent can heighten CMR's ability to characterize myocardial tissue. The most commonly used contrast agents in CMR are in the same family of gadolinium-based chelates used in central nervous system imaging and magnetic resonance angiography. Each brand available has slightly different pharmacokinetics and magnetic properties, but they all work by influencing the local magnetic field, primarily shortening T1 of the tissues local to the gadolinium molecule.

Before continuing it must be stated that at the time of this writing, the Food and Drug Administration has not approved any gadolinium agent specifically for the investigation of the heart itself, so any cardiac imaging is considered off-label. Suggested links between gadolinium based contrast agents (GBCA) and nephrogenic systemic fibrosis (NSF) have led to changes in both labeling and how these gadolinium based contrast agents (GCBAs) are implemented, especially in patients with impaired renal function [19–22]. Current information can be found from the American College of Radiology and FDA reference documents [23].

Many of the CMR techniques making use of GBCA's are based upon the efforts of Kim et al demonstrating a correlation between gadolinium retained in the ventricular wall and scar tissue [24]. In areas where myocardial tissue has been injured or replaced by fibrotic or scar tissue, the gadolinium molecules take a longer time to transit than through the healthy myocardium and blood pool [25]. When appropriately sequenced with an inversion recovery preparatory pulse, normal tissue recovers more quickly than gadolinium containing tissue [26]. This results in the gadolinium containing tissue appearing as bright, leading to the term "late gadolinium enhancement" (LGE) (see Fig. 12.2; Chap. 11). If the TI is improperly chosen such that the myocardium is not sufficiently nulled, it may appear bright in patches mimicking diffuse LGE or cardiomyopathy. The technologist should choose the TI that best nulls the myocardium [27].

A typical myocardial viability examination will include the previously described morphology and function protocol and also include the following LGE module [11].

1. Pulse sequences:
   (a) 2D segmented inversion recovery GRE or SSFP, Phase-Sensitive Inversion-Recovery (PSIR), and 3D sequences are preferred if patient can perform breath hold otherwise single-shot imaging (SSFP readout) for irregular heart rhythm and/or difficulty breath holding.
2. At least a 10 min delay after GBCA injection (may be shorter if lower dose of GBCA is used). Diastolic imaging is preferred.
3. Repeat cine imaging slice views (short axis and long axis) with similar parameters
4. Use an in-plane resolution (1.4–1.8 mm)
5. Keep duration of acquisition below 200 ms in length (shorter if tachycardia present)

Fig. 12.2 (**a**) Gadolinium is given during adenosine administration (stress perfusion) revealing a defect in the anterior wall, not felt to be artifact on rest perfusion (**b**, lower left corner)

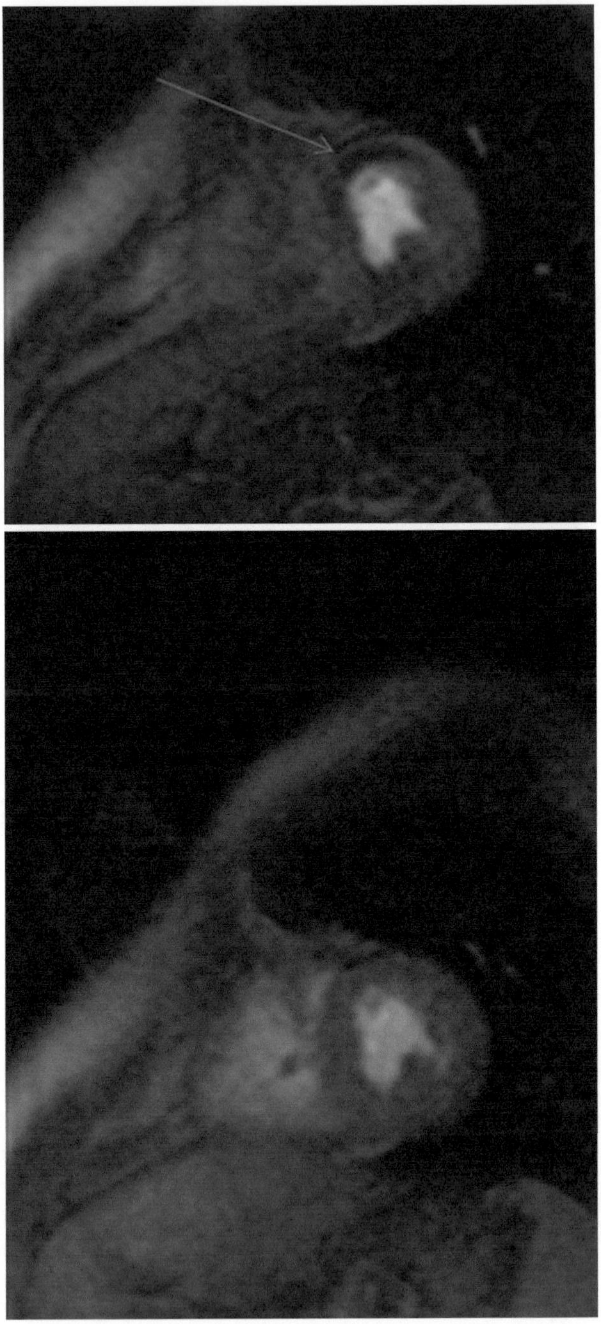

6. Set inversion time to null normal myocardium. Identify with a TI scout if available or repeated single slice acquisitions varying the TI.

Current guidelines for a visual assessment of LGE include [18]:

1. Set the image window and level so that normal myocardium is dark but noise is distinguishable and checking that proper inversion time was used.
2. The presence of LGE may be an area in the myocardium with signal intensity as high as the blood pool (or preferably higher) after ruling out artifacts.
   (a) To rule out artifacts:
      (i) Look for regions of apparent LGE in orthogonal slices (if available)
      (ii) Visually inspect for evidence of artifacts related with the pulse sequence or physiological motion.
3. Determine the location, extent (transmurality), and pattern of the LGE signal (if any) and if it is consistent with CAD or non-CAD disease, using the AHA 17 segment model. Comparison can be made with the morphology and function model cine images to correlate wall motion and thickness with LGE.

Current guidelines for a quantitative assessment are primarily performed to measure extent of LGE for research purposes. The following techniques are recognized but no dedicated statement has been made on their specific use [18]:

1. Manual planimetry
2. The “n”-SD technique
3. The full width half max (FWHM) technique

Like many other exams in cardiac MR, several newer techniques also exist making use of GBCA’s to characterize tissue. Currently, research is being done in the area of T1 mapping (both with and without GBCA’s) linking pathology and tissue characterization with changes in longitudinal recovery of tissues [28].

Myocardial Perfusion

Radionuclide myocardial perfusion imaging (MPI) has greatly benefitted patients with diagnosis, guiding treatment and prognosis of ischemic heart disease [29]. Despite continued progress in reducing the dosage of ionizing radiation to which the patient is exposed, radiation exposure is still a limiting factor of the technology [30]. One of the great advantages of magnetic resonance imaging is the lack of ionizing radiation and higher spatial resolution. CMR perfusion has been demonstrated to report sensitivity and specificity values on par or better to nuclear techniques used today [31, 32]. When perfusion imaging is combined with LGE, the sensitivity, specificity, and accuracy of CMR to detect coronary artery disease has been reported to be 89 %, 87 %, and 88 % respectively [33].

The primary technique for MPI via CMR involves the off label use of the same gadolinium based contrast agents (GBCA) discussed in the previous section (viability). The term "first pass perfusion" (FPP) is often used to reference myocardial perfusion as the images are acquired during an initial bolus of GBCA to provide the greatest amount of image contrast between the native and perfused myocardium. An additional bolus may be administered and a repeat acquisition performed if stress perfusion is to be examined, however less image contrast should be expected on the second acquisition.

How a CMR stress perfusion protocol is acquired depends upon the stressing agent used. The first pass images are more often than not the stress images and are primarily performed after administration of a pharmacological stressing agent. Exercise may also be used but it is nowhere near as widespread as the logistics are only complicated in the MRI suite.

There is considerable variability as to which pulse sequences may be used for perfusion imaging, but current recommendations include the following [11]:

1. Pre-contrast localizer using one of the following sequences making sure slices are as desired.
2. Saturation-recovery imaging with gradient echo-echo planar (GRE-EPI) hybrid, GRE, or SSFP readout. (Inversion recovery was previously used as the preparation pulse for MPI)
3. At least three slices per heart beat using the short-axis view
   (a) Every beat for ischemia for approximately 40–50 beats
   (b) Slice thickness 8 mm
   (c) Parallel imaging, if available
   (d) In-plane resolution (~<3 mm)
   (e) Temporal resolution at most (100–125 ms)
   (f) Give GBCA (0.05–0.1 mmol/kg, 3–7 mL/s) followed by saline flush of at least 30 ml (3–7 mL/s)
   (g) Begin breath-hold before contrast reaches the LV cavity

Stress MPI with CMR are based on the pharmacological agent used:

Adenosine/Regadenoson stress perfusion CMR

1. LV structure and function module (may also be performed between stress and rest perfusion)
2. Adenosine stress perfusion imaging
   (a) (3 min infusion of 140 μg/kg body weight/min, optional up to 210 μg/kg body weight/min).
   (b) First pass perfusion module
   (c) Inject gadolinium during last minute of adenosine

(d) Stop adenosine after imaging for 40–50 heart beats
(e) Monitor ECG and measuring BP at baseline, during infusion, and at least 2 min post-infusion. Alternatively: Regadenoson stress perfusion imaging (bolus injection of 0.4 mg).
(f) First pass perfusion module
(g) Inject gadolinium approximately 2 min after regadenoson
(h) Image for 40–50 heart beats
(i) Monitor ECG measuring BP at baseline and every other minute for at least 6 min after injection.

3. Rest Perfusion (optional if stress images are normal and artifact free)

   (a) Wait at least 10 min for gadolinium to wash out. During this period cine imaging or other evaluation may be performed.
   (b) Repeat perfusion imaging without stressing agent using the same dose of gadolinium (Note: with regadenoson flow may not have returned to baseline after 10 min)

4. Late Gadolinium Enhancement module

   (a) Need to wait at least 5 min after rest perfusion if performed

Dobutamine stress CMR

1. LV structure and function module
2. Dobutamine stimulation

   (a) Start dobutamine at 10 μg/kg body weight/minute increasing by increments of 10 μg/kg body weight/minute every 3 min stop when target heart rate is reached [85 % × (220-age)].
   (b) Add atropine in small incremental doses [0.25 mg fractions (max dose of 2 mg)]
   (c) Repeat three short axis and three long axis cine views during each increment.
   (d) ECG monitoring and measuring BP at each stage.
   (e) Review images (cine) as they are acquired.
   (f) Adjust acquisition parameters (SSFP cine) to align temporal resolution with HR.
   (g) Stop testing at first of new wall motion abnormality, serious side effect(s), or peak heart rate.

Contraindications for Stress Agents

1. Dobutamine

   (a) Severe systemic arterial hypertension (≥220/120 mmHg)
   (b) Unstable angina pectoris
   (c) Significant aortic valve stenosis (Peak aortic valve gradient >50 mmHg or aortic valve area <1 cm^2)
   (d) Complex cardiac arrhythmias including uncontrolled atrial fibrillation

   (e) Hypertrophic obstructive cardiomyopathy
   (f) Myocarditis, endocarditis, pericarditis
   (g) Uncontrolled congestive heart failure

2. Atropine

   (a) Narrow-angle glaucoma
   (b) Myasthenia gravis
   (c) Obstructive uropathy
   (d) Obstructive gastrointestinal disorders

3. Adenosine or Regadenoson

   (a) Second or third degree atrioventricular (AV) block or sinus node dysfunction
   (b) Systolic blood pressure less than 90 mmHg
   (c) Sinus bradycardia (heart rate <40 bpm)
   (d) Active bronchoconstrictive or bronchospastic disease
   (e) Known hypersensitivity to adenosine or regadenoson

Patient preparation and safety is very important when performing any kind of cardiac stress testing. Patients should provide informed consent and are typically required to be off certain medications and not have consumed caffeine (coffee, tea, chocolate, or other food and beverage source) for 12–24 h prior to testing. During the exam the patient should have their blood pressure and electrocardiogram monitored (although the magneto-hydrodynamic effect renders physiological monitoring as unreliable). Furthermore a method of communication should be maintained and all staff involved should be familiar with emergency response procedures.

Structural

Blood Flow

It is possible to quantify the blood flow and velocity through most reasonably sized vessels while attempting to gauge a patients overall condition [34]. This has several useful clinical implications including identification of shunts and detection of valvular disease [35]. While velocity measurements between CMR and echocardiography are generally in good agreement (r=0.87 for mean pressure gradient in aortic stenosis), very recent studies suggest CMR may be better in determining severity of some valvular conditions like mitral regurgitation [36, 37].

The examination of blood flow is accomplished with the introduction of a symmetrical bipolar phase gradient during the phase encoding step of a standard gradient echo sequence. Implementing a phase gradient in this manner allows the discrimination of moving tissues from stationary ones. While the first lobe of the bipolar gradient de-phases the spins of stationary tissues, the second (reverse) lobe de-phases them in the opposite direction (balancing them out) so that there is no net phase difference in the direction of the applied gradient. If an object is moving (e.g. blood) the two gradient lobes will not be experienced equally as the object moves out of range of the reverse lobe before it fully recovers its original phase information, producing a net phase. This net change in phase will be proportional to the velocity of the imaged object and the signal intensity for each voxel can thus be assigned. Fittingly, this type of acquisition is known as phase contrast (PC) imaging.

It should come as no surprise the importance of the parameters defining the bipolar gradient. These characteristics are controlled by the technologist through the maximum velocity encoding threshold (VENC) at the console. The lower the VENC the more sensitive the sequence is to smaller changes in velocity, but if the VENC is lower than the maximum velocity in the vessel then aliasing will occur. In the case of aliasing the flow above the VENC will appear to move in the opposite direction, this is the same phenomenon you witness when looking at the spokes of a wheel speeding up from rest. The desire then is to choose a VENC as close to the maximum velocity expected without going under it. There do exist some post processing solutions to correct aliasing, but it is more commonly accepted that the acquisitions should be repeated.

Beyond the choice of VENC there are a few potential pitfalls to be aware of during phase contrast imaging [38]. First is that the primary assumption in through plane imaging is that the slice is acquired perpendicular to the flow in the vessel. If the perpendicular assumption is invalidated, partial volume errors will accumulate in accordance with how far the imaging plane is from perpendicular [39]. In general the vessel wall and lumen should appear circular in the final reconstructed image (oblong or elliptical likely indicates the angle in one or more planes is off) (Fig. 12.3a–c). Though, in the case of imaging flow through valves, such as a regurgitant jet though the aortic valve, the plane should be perpendicular to the jet itself which may be difficult to determine in some instances or impossible in others (if multiple jets are present in multiple directions). In these cases multiple acquisitions may be required, and properly labeling of your series becomes important. Errors in flow calculations may arise due to background offset (improperly identifying zero velocity) however, in many of the newer scanners this has generally been addressed through improvements in hardware but phantom correction may also be used [40].

Phase contrast imaging for the assessment of blood flow through a vessel is typically performed as part of a larger examination. A typical flow module may include [11]:

1. Additional localizer images for each vessel of interest if oblique or double oblique imaging plane is required.
2. Typical slice thickness (5–8 mm)
3. In plane resolution (at least one tenth of the diameter of vessel)
4. VENC adjusted to expected flow (repeat if aliasing present)
5. Minimum echo time (fast flow/stenoses).
6. Repeat PC acquisition with phantom (optional).

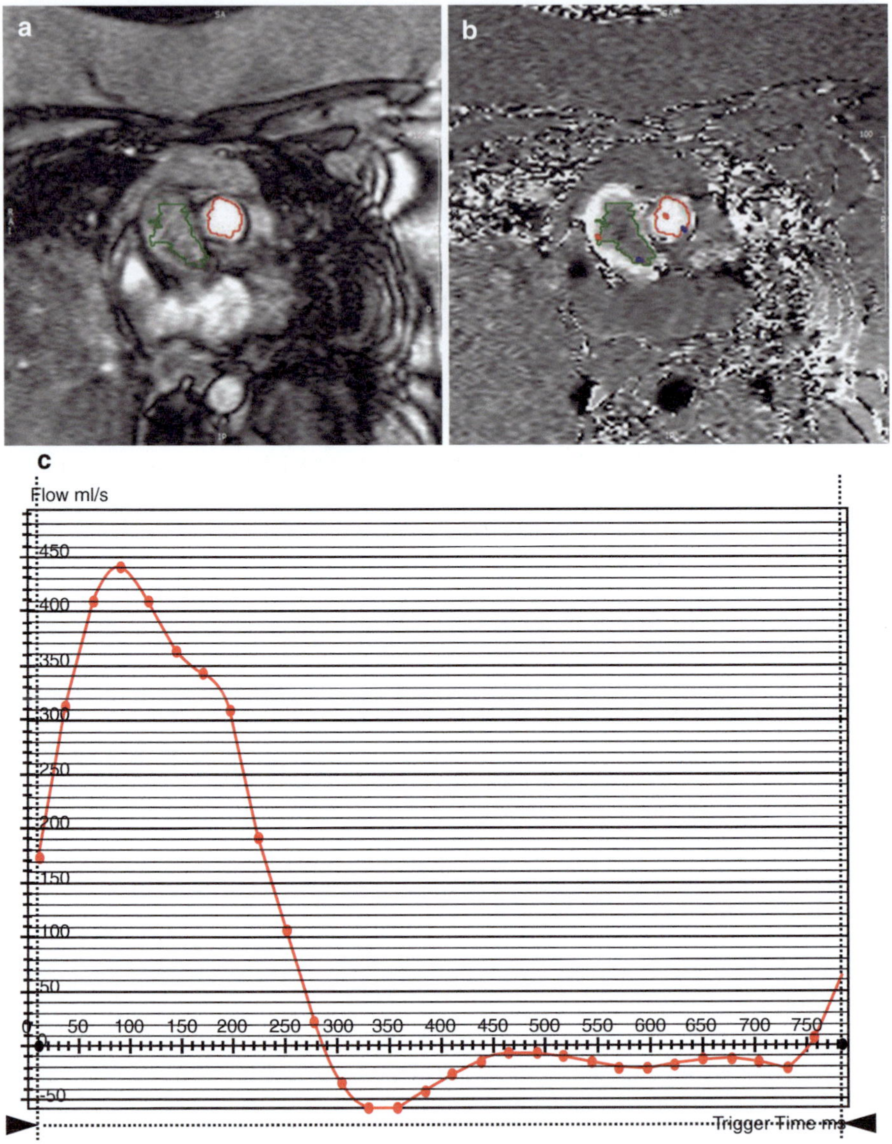

Figure 12.3 (**a**, **b**) Velocity mapping of the PA (*red circle*) is likely more accurate than attempts at assessing flow of the Aorta (*green circle*) due to off axis. (**c**) Sample flow curve generated from a patient with aortic regurgitation

Current guidelines for a visual/quantitative assessment of flows by phase contrast imaging include [18]:

1. For each vessel examined a region of interest (ROI) should be drawn on each phase of the magnitude image along the inside of the lumen wall, then transferring the ROI to the corresponding phase images.
   (a) Values that can be directly calculated:
      (i) Antegrade volume
      (ii) Retrograde volume
      (iii) Peak velocity
      (iv) Mean velocity
   (b) Derived parameters include:
      (i) Net volume [ml|=antegrade volume – retrograde volume
      (ii) Regurgitant fraction [%]=(retrograde volume/antegrade volume)*100
      (iii) Cardiac output (liters/min=(net volume [ml] × heart rate [beats/minute])/1000)
      (iv) Cardiac index (cardiac output/BSA) systemic and by pulmonary branch (if PA branches imaged)
      (v) Regurgitant volume
2. Directly by measuring diastolic flow across the valve of interest and subtracting systolic forward flow
3. Indirectly by measuring stroke volume of cine from functional module and subtracting the forward flow across the associated valve by PC.

As mentioned previously phase contrast imaging is primarily used in the analysis of blood flow through vessels. Flow volume and/or velocity through a particular vessel is most often accomplished with a single bipolar gradient so that phase differences are generated perpendicular to the vessel lumen (through plane imaging), though multiple phase encoding gradients may be applied to measure in-plane and even fully dimensional flow [41]. While the aforementioned (in plane) flow is not widely used in examining blood, the fully dimensional flow has seen impressive progress recently and appears poised to begin moving from research to clinical implementation as the time to both obtain and post process these types of images has dropped.

Conclusions

As an imaging modality, CMR is capable of incorporating protocols to determine cardiac morphology and function, myocardial viability, myocardial perfusion, and blood flow. The protocols discussed here focused primarily on those techniques that are most often employed in standard clinical cardiac MR protocols.

References

1. Goldman MR, et al. Nuclear magnetic resonance imaging: potential cardiac applications. Am J Cardiol. 1980;46(7):1278–83.
2. Fayad ZA, et al. Noninvasive in vivo human coronary artery lumen and wall imaging using black-blood magnetic resonance imaging. Circulation. 2000;102(5):506–10.
3. Rossum V, Albert C, et al. Evaluation of magnetic resonance imaging for determination of left ventricular ejection fraction and comparison with angiography. Am J Cardiol. 1988;62(9): 628–33.
4. Selvanayagam JB, et al. Value of delayed-enhancement cardiovascular magnetic resonance imaging in predicting myocardial viability after surgical revascularization. Circulation. 2004;110(12):1535–41.
5. Knauth AL, et al. Ventricular size and function assessed by cardiac MRI predict major adverse clinical outcomes late after tetralogy of Fallot repair. Heart. 2008;94(2):211–6.
6. Kilner PJ, Gatehouse PD, Firmin DN. Flow measurement by magnetic resonance: a unique asset worth optimising. J Cardiovasc Magn Reson. 2007;9(4):723–8.
7. Jaffer FA, et al. Age and sex distribution of subclinical aortic atherosclerosis a magnetic resonance imaging examination of the Framingham Heart Study. Arterioscler Thromb Vasc Biol. 2002;22(5):849–54.
8. Wieben O, Francois C, Reeder SB. Cardiac MRI of ischemic heart disease at 3T: potential and challenges. Eur J Radiol. 2008;65(1):15–28.
9. Rolf MP, et al. Sequence optimization to reduce velocity offsets in cardiovascular magnetic resonance volume flow quantification-a multi-vendor study. J Cardiovasc Magn Reson. 2011; 13(1):18.
10. Earls JP, et al. Cardiac MRI: recent progress and continued challenges. J Magn Reson Imaging. 2002;16(2):111–27.
11. Kramer CM, et al. Standardized cardiovascular magnetic resonance (CMR) protocols 2013 update. J Cardiovasc Magn Reson. 2013;15(1):1.
12. Woodard PK, et al. ACR practice guideline for the performance and interpretation of cardiac magnetic resonance imaging (MRI). J Am Coll Radiol. 2006;3(9):665–76.
13. Bellenger NG, et al. Comparison of left ventricular ejection fraction and volumes in heart failure by echocardiography, radionuclide ventriculography and cardiovascular magnetic resonance. Are they interchangeable? Eur Heart J. 2000;21(16):1387–96.
14. Grothues F, et al. Comparison of interstudy reproducibility of cardiovascular magnetic resonance with two-dimensional echocardiography in normal subjects and in patients with heart failure or left ventricular hypertrophy. Am J Cardiol. 2002;90(1):29–34.
15. Mooij CF, et al. Reproducibility of MRI measurements of right ventricular size and function in patients with normal and dilated ventricles. J Magn Reson Imaging. 2008;28(1):67–73.
16. Plein S, et al. Steady-state free precession magnetic resonance imaging of the heart: comparison with segmented k-space gradient-echo imaging. J Magn Reson Imaging. 2001;14(3):230–6.
17. Scheffler K, Lehnhardt S. Principles and applications of balanced SSFP techniques. Eur Radiol. 2003;13(11):2409–18.
18. Schulz-Menger J, et al. Standardized image interpretation and post processing in cardiovascular magnetic resonance: Society for Cardiovascular Magnetic Resonance (SCMR) board of trustees task force on standardized post processing. J Cardiovasc Magn Reson. 2013;15(1):35.
19. Kuo PH, et al. Gadolinium-based MR contrast agents and nephrogenic systemic fibrosis 1. Radiology. 2007;242(3):647–9.
20. Bellin M-F. MR contrast agents, the old and the new. Eur J Radiol. 2006;60(3):314–23.
21. Lin S-P, Brown JJ. MR contrast agents: physical and pharmacologic basics. J Magn Reson Imaging. 2007;25(5):884–99.
22. Nacif MS, et al. Gadolinium-enhanced cardiovascular magnetic resonance: administered dose in relationship to United States Food and Drug Administration (FDA) guidelines. J Cardiovasc Magn Reson. 2012;14:18.

23. Cohan RH, Dillman JR, Hartman RP. American College of Radiology Manual on Contrast Media Version 9 ACR Manual on Contrast Media, American College of Radiology. 2013. *Webpage:* http://www.acr.org/~/media/ACR/Documents/PDF/QualitySafety/Resources/Contrast.
24. Kim RJ, et al. The use of contrast-enhanced magnetic resonance imaging to identify reversible myocardial dysfunction. N Engl J Med. 2000;343(20):1445–53.
25. Wagner A, et al. Effects of time, dose, and inversion time for acute myocardial infarct size measurements based on magnetic resonance imaging-delayed contrast enhancement. J Am Coll Cardiol. 2006;47(10):2027–33.
26. Kellman P, Arai AE. Cardiac imaging techniques for physicians: late enhancement. J Magn Reson Imaging. 2012;36(3):529–42.
27. Kim RJ, Shah DJ, Judd RM. How we perform delayed enhancement imaging: HOW I DO…#. J Cardiovasc Magn Reson. 2003;5(3):505–14.
28. Messroghli DR, et al. Modified Look-Locker Inversion recovery (MOLLI) for high-resolution T1 mapping of the heart. Magn Reson Med. 2004;52(1):141–6.
29. Hachamovitch R, et al. Incremental prognostic value of myocardial perfusion single photon emission computed tomography for the prediction of cardiac death differential stratification for risk of cardiac death and myocardial infarction. Circulation. 1998;97(6):535–43.
30. Thompson RC, Cullom SJ. Issues regarding radiation dosage of cardiac nuclear and radiography procedures. J Nucl Cardiol. 2006;13(1):19–23.
31. Wagner A, et al. Contrast-enhanced MRI and routine Single Photon Emission Computed Tomography (SPECT) perfusion imaging for detection of subendocardial myocardial infarcts: an imaging study. Lancet. 2003;361(9355):374–9.
32. Schwitter J, et al. MR-IMPACT: comparison of perfusion-cardiac magnetic resonance with single-photon emission computed tomography for the detection of coronary artery disease in a multicentre, multivendor, randomized trial. Eur Heart J. 2008;29(4):480–9.
33. Klem I, et al. Improved detection of coronary artery disease by stress perfusion cardiovascular magnetic resonance with the use of delayed enhancement infarction imaging. J Am Coll Cardiol. 2006;47(8):1630–8.
34. Pelc NJ, et al. Phase contrast cine magnetic resonance imaging. Magn Reson Q. 1991;7(4):229–54.
35. Cawley PJ, Maki JH, Otto CM. Cardiovascular magnetic resonance imaging for valvular heart disease technique and validation. Circulation. 2009;119(3):468–78.
36. Caruthers SD, et al. Practical value of cardiac magnetic resonance imaging for clinical quantification of aortic valve stenosis comparison with echocardiography. Circulation. 2003;108(18):2236–43.
37. Uretsky S, et al. Discordance between echocardiography and MRI in the assessment of mitral regurgitation severity: a prospective multicenter trial. J Am Coll Cardiol. 2015;65(11): 1078–88.
38. Gatehouse PD, et al. Applications of phase-contrast flow and velocity imaging in cardiovascular MRI. Eur Radiol. 2005;15(10):2172–84.
39. Tang C, Blatter DD, Parker DL. Accuracy of phase-contrast flow measurements in the presence of partial-volume effects. J Magn Reson Imaging. 1993;3(2):377–85.
40. Chernobelsky A, et al. Baseline correction of phase contrast images improves quantification of blood flow in the great vessels. J Cardiovasc Magn Reson. 2007;9(4):681–5.
41. Markl M, et al. Time-resolved three-dimensional phase-contrast MRI. J Magn Reson Imaging. 2003;17(4):499–506.

Chapter 13
Cardiac MR Quality Control

Joseph Soltys

Abstract Every image produced with cardiac MR (CMR) has some amount of artifact in it. These artifacts arise from the physics of MR itself, the assumptions and choices made when sampling, and/or hardware that is not properly working. In order to ensure quality images, it is therefore imperative to follow quality guidelines, such as those presented by the American College of Radiology. These guidelines monitor total system performance so that hardware associated artifacts are not problematic. Technologists and physicians still need to be aware of common non hardware related CMR artifacts and why they are occurring, as they may mimic pathology. A well-trained and experienced technologist able to recognize these artifacts can take corrective action to mitigate them, and the reading physician must also be aware in cases where it is not so obvious or corrective actions are of limited or little help.

Keywords Cardiac MR • Artifact • Ghosting • Aliasing • Quality control

Quality Control: The Magnet

Quality control is paramount to the successful operation and management of a modern clinical MRI suite. Each individual component must be considered (both separately and in conjunction with the others) to ensure diagnostic images are produced. These components include: the main magnet itself including the gradient coils, imaging specific surface coils, the patient handling system ("table"), patient monitoring systems, cooling systems, the computer and controls systems, and the viewing and post processing systems. There is also a human system that interacts with the hardware: the operating staff, patient, and protocols. Only when all of these parts are operate in synchrony can the full range of benefits of MR imaging be achieved. Failure of just a single component can lead to poor or non-diagnostic images at best and/or serious injury at worst.

J. Soltys, PhD
MR Physics, Cardiovascular Imaging Technologies, LLC, Kansas City, MO, USA
e-mail: Jsoltys@cvit.com

P.L. Tilkemeier et al. (eds.), *Quality Evaluation in Non-Invasive Cardiovascular Imaging*, DOI 10.1007/978-3-319-28011-0_13

Fortunately, quality control in MRI need not be a difficult thing. Primarily it boils down to adherence to proper maintenance schedules, regular performance testing, and detailed record keeping. While there is nothing novel about any of these ideas, when they are properly implemented, problematic trends in performance trends can be identified early and corrected, safeguarding both the patient and diagnostic accuracy of the images. Tracking regular preventative maintenance as part of the quality checks is another good idea as it allows any unexpected changes in scanner behavior to be attributed to any system updates that may have occurred.

Historically speaking, MRI quality control has evolved as "best practices" defined by accrediting bodies and the clinical/scientific societies rather than through regulatory pressures, as in modalities that use ionizing radiation. Federal regulations do exist regarding MRI, but are primarily the concern of manufacturers [1, 2]. The American College of Radiology (ACR) accreditation standards define a minimum expected level of MR performance [3]. The testing protocol is focused on well-defined standard pulse sequences designed such that the performance of different style (e.g. standard bore, wide bore, and open bore) and main field strength scanners can readily be assessed [4]. The applicability and level of detail described (what to test, when to test, how to test, and who should perform testing) makes the ACR protocol a useful model for an MRI QC program. Indeed, adherence to ACR phantom testing has been demonstrated to improve the time to resolve scanner problems [5].

Annual testing is a comprehensive assessment of all hardware used during clinical MRI sessions and must be performed by a qualified medical physicist or MR scientist for accreditation. The physicist/scientist qualifications are quite extensive and include a graduate degree in a physical science involving MRI and 3 years of documented experience in a clinical MR environment. For most sites seeking accreditation, it is likely the simplest course of action is to contract with one of the many reputable MRI service companies that regularly perform certification testing and are familiar with the requirements (testing and reporting). All documentation generated over the course of the review must also be maintained by the MRI center.

Per the ACR guidelines, the annual performance review must both include and document the following (ACR Field Guide):

1. Magnetic field homogeneity
2. Slice position accuracy
3. Slice thickness accuracy
4. Performance testing for ALL coils used clinically
   (a) Physical inspection
   (b) Transmitter gain/attenuator verification
   (c) Image signal-to-noise ratio (SNR)
   (d) Image artifact assessment
   (e) Image intensity uniformity
   (f) Year-to-year variations for all of the above should be recorded
5. Geometric accuracy (gradient calibration)

6. High-contrast spatial resolution
7. Low-contrast detectability
8. Acquisition workstation monitor performance
9. Inspection of the physical and mechanical integrity of the system
10. Evaluation of the technologist QC program
11. Assessment of MRI safety program

General monitoring is more limited in scope and can reasonably be performed by a sufficiently trained MRI technologist on either a weekly or daily (preferred) basis. Any technologist performing MRI clinically and likewise performing QC testing must meet at least one of the following certification requirements [6]:

1. Certified by the American Registry of Radiologic Technologists (ARRT), the American Registry of MRI Technologists (ARMRIT), or the Canadian Association of Medical Radiation Technologists (CAMRT) as an MRI technologist (RTMR).
2. Certified by the ARRT and/or have appropriate state licensure and 6 months supervised clinical experience in MRI scanning.
3. An Associate Degree in an allied health field or a bachelor's degree and certification in another clinical imaging field and have 6 month of supervised clinical MRI scanning.

Short term testing should be performed in accordance with the plan developed for your particular site, recorded (including sign-offs), and compared with the manufacturer's guidelines or an established baseline of performance. Any discrepancies outside of the acceptance window or abnormal trends in the performance should immediately trigger a corrective response. Scanning can continue as long as the safety risk to the patient is determined not to be elevated by any of the findings and that images to be acquired are expected to be diagnostic in quality.

The daily (preferred) or weekly quality monitoring should include testing and measurement of the following parameters (ACR Field Guide):

1. Setup and positioning accuracy (including a mechanical inspection of the equipment)
2. Central frequency
3. Transmitter gain or attenuation
4. Geometric accuracy along each of the three major axes
5. High-contrast spatial resolution
6. Low-contrast detectability
7. Image artifact assessment
8. Film printer fidelity when used for primary interpretation
9. Acquisition workstation monitor quality
10. Visual checklist

Meticulous record keeping and regular review of the short term monitoring allows a site to be proactive in remedying hardware problems as they arise. Small changes in performance may not be readily apparent to a continuously scanning technologist, but a well-kept record provides an objective point of comparison so changes can be made before serious artifacts appear in your images that may result in considerable downtime. In the end, proper adherence a quality control regimen requires discipline but the site that is able to demonstrate such diligence will ultimately be in position to reap the rewards of accreditation, less downtime, and quality imaging with MR. In the next few sections we review some of the most common artifacts encountered during a cardiac MR protocol.

Artifact

Despite all of the advancements in hardware and software, CMR still suffers from a relatively slow data acquisition process, which is often the source of image artifacts. The problem arises because the physiological systems we want to image (especially the heart) are inherently dynamic. Physiological movement artifacts can appear as ghosting, and blurring and/or aliasing. The seasoned practitioner of MRI will be quick to inform you that physiological motion is not the only source of artifact with this modality as the basic physics of magnetic resonance allows for their occurrence as well.

In reality, every image produced by MRI has some level of artifact; the determination that must be made is whether or not the artifact observed interferes with the clinical interpretation. In some cases this is problematic as the artifact can hide or mimic pathology (and one needs to look for clues to understand what is occurring) while in other cases we may intentionally introduce artifact to aid interpretation. Generally speaking MRI artifacts can be classified into one of the following groups: magnetic resonance physics, sampling and encoding artifacts and hardware related.

In order to better understand how the artifacts encountered in MRI come to be, it is necessary to understand the origin of the MRI signal, the acquisition process, and how the acquired signal is resolved into the final image. The following sections will include a very brief overview of each part of the MR process and how it is related to some of the most commonly encountered artifacts during a routine cardiac MRI exam. It is assumed that the reader has at least some familiarity with the topics discussed and the interested reader is encouraged to review the CMR chapters in this book and investigate any of the excellent review articles on these topics for more detail.

Nuclear Magnetic Resonance

The scientific basis of modern MRI lies in the phenomena of nuclear magnetic resonance, which for the sake of simplicity we will limit to the hydrogen atom (to which the vast majority of clinical MR units are tuned) [7, 8]. The nucleus of each hydrogen atom, (a single proton) has an intrinsic property called "spin" and a small magnetic moment. In 1946 building upon Nobel winner Isidor Rabi's work, two independent researchers (Edward Purcell and Felix Bloch) demonstrated that nuclei in a strong magnetic field absorbed and released electromagnetic energy according to the Larmor equation and that this could be used to determine the processional frequency of the protons of a sample [9, 10].

The MRI generates a large main magnetic field (B0), uniformly running through the center of the bore of a typical magnet. When an object containing hydrogen (e.g. the patient) is placed inside the main field, the protons will orient along the B0 field in either a high or low energy state producing a slight net magnetization in the direction of the main field (M_Z). At the same time each of the protons will process at a frequency related to the overall strength of the main field (according to the Larmor Equation) but at a random phase so that the net magnetization perpendicular to the main field is zero (M_{xy}). At this point our system is at equilibrium and it is these two components of magnetization (M_Z and M_{xy}) that are manipulated to generate a final image.

Applying a pulse of radio frequency (RF) energy will cause additional protons to temporarily jump into the high-energy state creating a new net magnetization state. After the excitation the protons relax to their equilibrium state, releasing the absorbed energy in an exponentially decaying process called the free induction decay (FID). It is this released energy that we will use to generate our final image. If one were to record the FID signal and perform a Fourier analysis we would see a single peak corresponding to all of the hydrogen contained in the imaged slice of the patient at the Larmor frequency. Useful information, but in order to create an image we need to resolve this information into two planes using a localization process.

In order to create an image in the plane of our selected slice the processional frequencies need to be spatially encoded. We will identify two orthogonal axes in our slice plane and denote one for frequency encoding and the other for phase encoding. In frequency encoding a linear gradient is applied at the time of signal acquisition. This gradient causes protons to process at different frequencies according to their location along the gradient. The phase encode gradient is applied between the initial RF pulse and the generated echo but linearly de-phases the spins along the gradient. In order to resolve all of the phase and frequency combinations all phase encoding steps identified in the image matrix must be accounted for in our sampling. So the entire process of RF excitation, spatial encoding, and sampling process must be repeated until this process is satisfied. Once completed, the raw image data can be Fourier transformed from the frequency domain (K-Space) into our familiar image space for clinical interpretation.

The Basic Data Acquisition Process

The backbone of MRI is the large main magnetic field (B0) generated by the super-cooled magnets. Typical field strengths in use currently are 1.5 and 3.0 Tesla machines (which are considered high field). What is desired and the assumption that is made is that the main field running through imaging location in the center of the bore is uniform (the center of the bore in the most common magnet configuration). When an object containing hydrogen (e.g. the patient) is placed inside the main field, the protons orient along the B0 field in either a high (against the field) or low (with the field) energy state producing a slight net magnetization in the direction of the main field (M_Z). At the same time each of the protons will process at a frequency related to the overall strength of the main field (according to the Larmor Equation) but at a random phase so that the net magnetization perpendicular to the main field is zero (M_{xy}). At this point our system is at equilibrium and it is these two components of magnetization (M_Z and M_{xy}) that will be manipulated to generate data for the final image.

Applying a pulse of radio frequency (RF) energy will cause additional protons to temporarily jump into the high-energy state creating a new net magnetization state. Radio-Frequency energy is in the resonant range for Hydrogen atoms at the magnetic field strengths currently in use. Much like tuning a radio to a specific channel, the clinical MR unit is "tuned" to hydrogen (MRI units can be tuned to other molecules). After the excitation the protons return to their equilibrium state, releasing the absorbed energy in a process called free induction decay (FID). If one were to record the FID signal and perform a Fourier analysis we would see a single frequency peak corresponding to all of the hydrogen contained in the imaged slice of the patient at the Larmor frequency.

In order to create an image, the processional frequency of the hydrogen in our sample needs to be spatially encoded in two dimensions. We will identify two orthogonal axes in our slice plane and denote one for frequency encoding and the other for phase encoding. Frequency encoding is accomplished by applying a linear gradient across the image plane at the time of signal acquisition (also known as the readout gradient). This gradient causes protons to process at different frequencies according to their location along the gradient. The phase encode gradient is temporarily applied after the initial RF pulse but before the frequency gradient causing the spins to linearly de-phase along the gradient. The result of these two gradients is that each location now has a unique combination of phase and frequency. However, not all phase encoding locations be collected at once and in order to resolve all of the phase and frequency combinations all phase encoding steps identified in the image matrix must be accounted for in our sampling. So the entire process of RF excitation, spatial encoding, and sampling process must be repeated until this process is satisfied. Once it is completely collected, the raw image data can finally be Fourier transformed from the frequency domain (K-Space) into our familiar image space for clinical interpretation. Unlike other imaging modalities however, the resulting pixel intensity is not based on an absolute value but rather a relative value based on the observed amplitudes. As you will see, the previous information has been greatly simplified, but adequately demonstrates many of the steps and assumptions made with MR acquisition.

Physics Artifacts

Despite the excitement and promise of CMR, there are some inherent limitations in the underlying physics that must be understood. Artifacts arising from MR physics are always present in the final image to some extent, the challenge is to manage them to a level that does not interfere with diagnosis [11].

Chemical Shift Artifact

In the preceding section, it was mentioned that without the localizing gradients, all of the hydrogen in the sample would process at a single frequency (the Larmor frequency) but this is not wholly accurate. In reality the hydrogen contained within the human body is primarily found in either water or fat based tissues. In the relatively compact water the hydrogen is bonded with a single oxygen molecule while in the much larger fat molecule the majority of hydrogen is bonded with a carbon molecule. The surrounding electron clouds affect the B0 field so that the relatively small water molecule has a much smaller effect than the larger fat molecule. The result is that just as our frequency encoding gradient can cause precession at different frequencies, so too can the chemical structure of the tissue in which the hydrogen is contained. This difference in processional frequency is called a chemical shift and can occur between any two different types of tissue, but we will focus on fat and water. Fortunately the chemical shift between fat and water is constant at 3.5 ppm which converts to a difference of about 220 Hz at 1.5 T and increases linearly with field strength used (about 440 Hz at 3.0 T) [12].

A chemical shift artifact occurs when the water or fat signal is encoded in the wrong frequency location in the final image [13]. This results in a bright signal on one side of the object and a dark signal on the other, known as a Type 1 chemical shift and will occur in either gradient or spin echo sequences. The chemical shift can be reduced by using an appropriate bandwidth (they are inversely related) and/or compared with other views to resolve proper tissue composition [14]. A Type 2 chemical shift or "India Ink Artifact" occurs on gradient echo sequences in voxels containing both fat and water (such as the boundary between muscle and fat (Fig. 13.1). Here, the object in question may appear as though it is outlines with a thick black line. In this particular sequence both the fat and water molecules start off processing in phase, but will quickly de-phase and the resulting image is collected at an echo time (TE) when the fat and water signals effectively cancel each other. The image containing the type 2 chemical shift is said to be "out of phase", the sequence can be adjusted so that the TE is increased and the collection occurs when the fat and water signals eventually come back "in-phase" and the dark outline is gone. Whether an image is acquired in-phase or out-of-phase is the preference of the physician (some like the outline for segmentation while others do not).

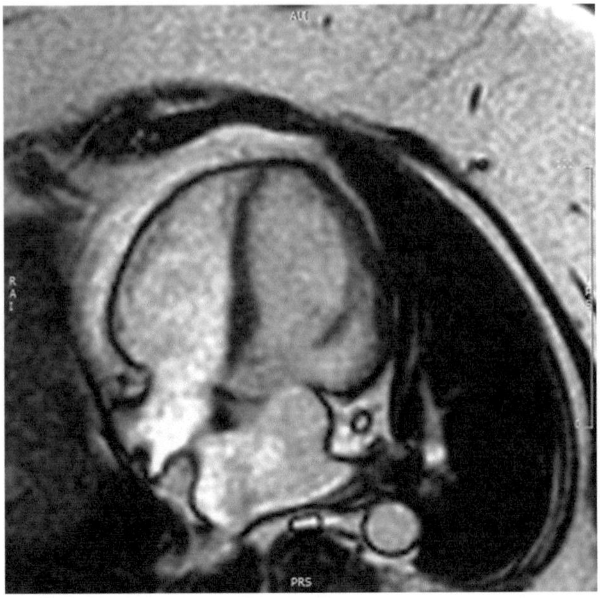

Fig. 13.1 Myocardial fat/water chemical shift interface seen in the lipomatous hypertrophy of the atrial septum and highlighting the coronary sinus within the epicardial fat

Magnetic Susceptibility

Different materials will be temporarily affected by magnetic fields to different extents. This property is known as magnetic susceptibility. Just like the nuclear spins mentioned early, materials can either align against the magnetic field causing it to disperse (diamagnetic) or with the field concentrating it to varying degrees (paramagnetic, super paramagnetic, or ferromagnetic). These small local changes in the B0 field result in changes in processional frequency and de-phasing (especially around tissue boundaries) resulting in loss of signal and geometric distortion. In the presence of sternal wires or other implants, susceptibility will show as an area of signal loss that can extend beyond the area of the implant itself as the ferromagnetic properties of the implant absorb some of the RF energy from the nearby tissues (Fig. 13.2). There is no way to remove these artifacts if they are present, but the extent of the effect can be mitigated by reducing the TE or decreasing the pixel size (increasing resolution) [15]. Magnetic susceptibility is also worse in gradient echo sequences so changing to a spin echo, where appropriate, may provide a solution.

Partial Volume Averaging

As we have seen with the chemical shift artifact, problems can arise when multiple tissues are sampled in the same voxel. In reality, we always have a group of voxels along tissue boundaries that contain a mix of different tissue types. In general the problem occurs when the voxel size is too large (in plane resolution and slice thickness) for the anatomy being imaged. If partial volume effects are too large attempts at quantitative CMR (ejection fraction) will be inaccurate [16] (Fig. 13.3a). In the heart partial volume artifacts can be problematic when investigating fine details in the ventricle and likely contribute to the dark rim artifact observed in myocardial perfusion imaging with MR (Fig. 13.3b).

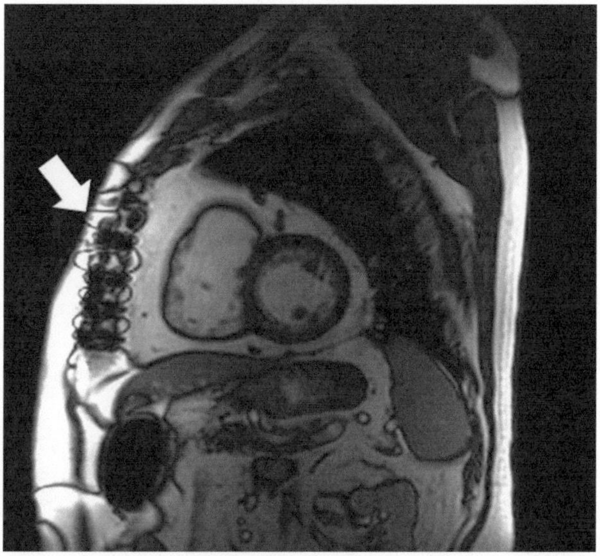

Fig. 13.2 Sternal wire artifact. Short axis balanced steady state free precession acquisition (bSSFP) of a patient with sternal wires. Note the apparent drop in signal in the vicinity of the implant (*arrow*)

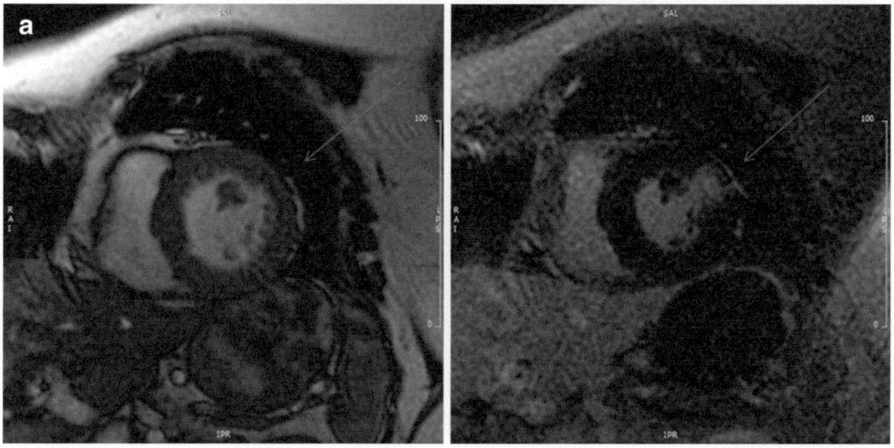

Fig. 13.3 (**a**) Volume averaging: on the right, poor delineation between the blood pool that still retains gadolinium compared with a focal area of late gadolinium enhancement in the anterolateral wall, when compared with the steady state free precession on the *left*. (**b**) Gibbs ringing. Also note the series of *light and dark lined* surrounding each of the dark objects typical of Gibbs ringing artifact seen on both the stress (*above*) and rest images (*below*)

Fig. 13.3 (continued)

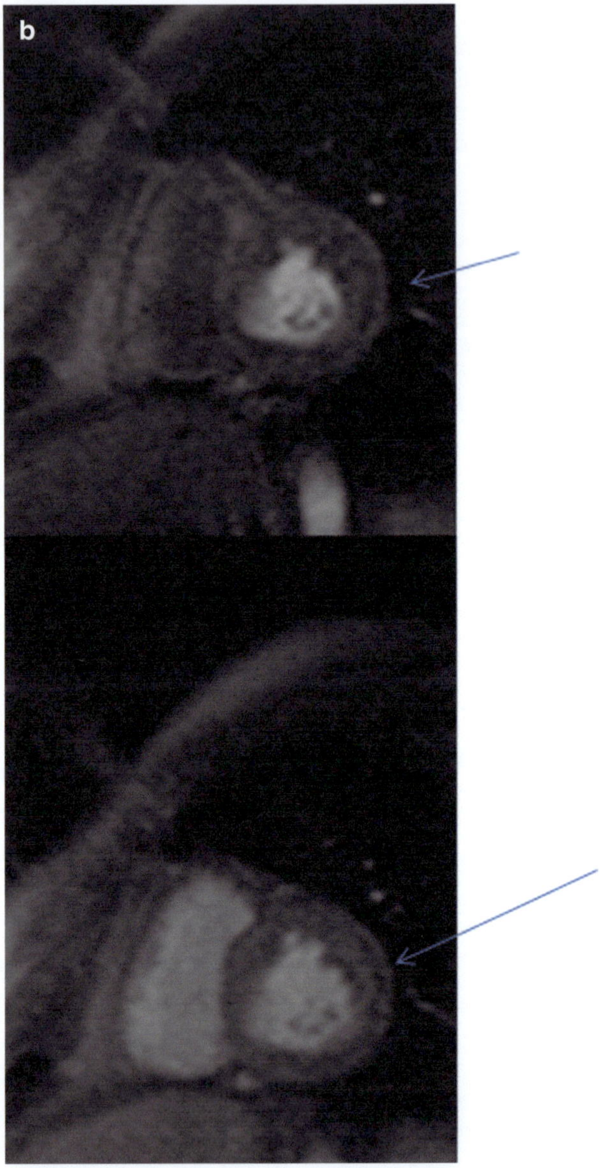

Motion Artifacts

From our review of the basic data acquisition process we can see why any kind of motion would be problematic. Recall that in MRI that there are two steps necessary to localize the NMR signal. By necessity the frequency encoding is repeated multiple times (each time marking a phase encoding step) until the number of acquisitions required completing the image matrix is completed. The frequency points are collected very close to each other temporally, but the phase steps are relatively much further apart (all frequency points are collected at each step in the phase gradient). So anything within the target field of view that moves has the potential to be spatially misplaced. All of the following motion artifacts occur for the same underlying reasons, but properly identifying them will help you find the correct solution.

Ghosting

The most identifiable artifact in cardiac applications is a "ghost" image of an object superimposed over the field of view. The classic example happens when the patient breathes during a study, creating copies of the chest wall propagated across the image (Fig. 13.4a). This arises due to multiple circumstances, but is primarily either due to the patient's own conditioning or fatigue at the length of the protocol. Comparing the acquisition process to the relative movement of the chest wall due to breathing is small during to the time frequency encoding takes and much larger during the phase direction. The "ghosting" will therefore propagate in the phase encoding direction.

Fortunately, there are a number of steps that can be taken to remedy respiratory ghosting, though all require a repeat scan. First though, it should be determined if

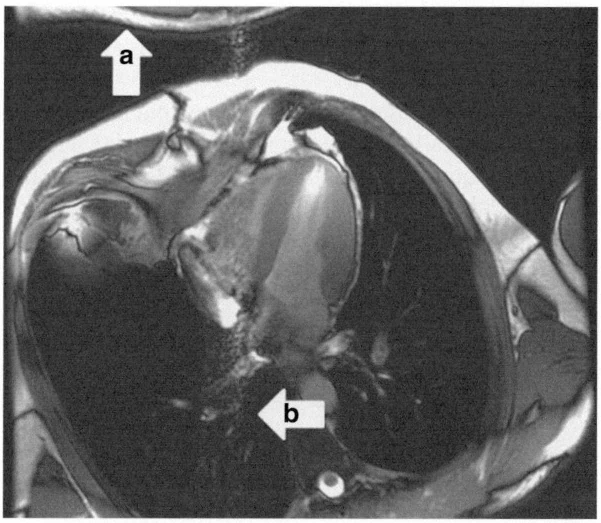

Fig. 13.4 Motion artifacts (*A*) Aliasing with fold-over pulse flow artifacts (*B*) Long axis (four chamber) balance steady state free precession acquisition (bSSFP) with apparent artifacts. Note that the back wall of the thorax is "wrapped" to the *top* of the image (*A*). Also, there is a vertical region of general blurring due to the pulsatile nature of the blood flow in the aorta (*B*)

the ghost image actually interferes with any of the cardiac structures of interest. If not, the protocol can be continued. Some of the simplest remedies to try include: shortening the acquisition by adjusting parameters related to timing or using other accelerated imaging techniques (parallel imaging), swapping phase and frequency encoding directions (to "move" the ghosts away from anatomy of interest), or if available on your machine placing spatial saturation bands on the chest walls (assumes no signal = no ghost). Alternatives include alternating between end-inspiration with end-expiration (with breath-"not"-held). If a patient in unable to comply with a breath-hold at all then a respiratory navigated imaging technique could be used [17].

Cardiac Motion/Blurring

Since the heart is constantly beating, and motion in MRI causes artifact, how then are we able to obtain such beautiful detailed images without massive amounts of ghosting? The answer is that we use cardiac gating by monitoring the electrical activity of the heart with electrocardiogram (ECG) or vectorcardiogram (VCG) [18]. We can then collect data prospectively during the relatively quiet diastolic portion of the cardiac cycle or retrospectively using the gating signal to resolve where data belongs temporally. Essentially, the gating process is used to identify the peak R-wave from which all acquisition timing parameters are derived. Errors in gating occur when the electrodes are improperly placed or damaged and appear as a general blurring of the cardiac structures along the phase encoding direction (Fig. 13.4b). The only solution is to replace the electrodes making sure the ECG/VCG trace is of acceptable quality.

Another form of this error may occur when the patient has a condition where the heart rate changes substantially between beats (arrhythmia). Here, the heart may rapidly move after and acquisition has already started. In this case there is a general blurring of the ventricular wall during different phases of the cardiac cycle making segmentation difficult when trying to evaluate ventricular volumes. Likewise, singular slices may look well defined, however when multiple slices are viewed at the same time, they may "beat" out of phase. In this case a repeat acquisition for the out of phase slices or the entire stack may be necessary, whether enabling "arrhythmia rejection" essentially a built in delay after detection of the R wave or in some cases pharmacological intervention may be necessary.

Pulsatile Flow

Besides the heart and respiratory motion, the blood pulsing through the arteries and veins and can create its own type of ghosting artifact [19]. Since the blood is continuously flowing during the acquisition process, the blood in the imaging at any particular time will not be oriented by the phase encoding gradients and will thus present at random locations along the phase encoding gradient. In some instances these blood vessel “ghosts” can interfere with a particular structure of interest (Fig. 13.4). If an image is affected by phase induced blood flow ghosts they cannot be removed and a repeat acquisition will be necessary swapping the phase and frequency encoding directions or (if available) by applying a saturation band parallel to and along the side of the slice that blood is flowing into. In this way the incoming blood will be saturated and not contribute to the signal intensity upon readout.

Sampling/Encoding Artifacts

Some artifacts can be reasonably dealt with by changing acquisition parameters; these are known as sampling type artifacts. However, being able to mitigate such artifacts requires an understanding which parameters may need to be altered and/or which imaging options are available on your system. Some of the sampling errors most likely encountered during a routing cardiac MR that have not yet been discussed are described below.

Wraparound/Aliasing (Frequency)

The magnetic field extends beyond the field of view defined by the technologist at the console. The frequency encoding gradient actually extends across the entire diameter of the bore. As such, anything inside of the bore will have its processional frequency altered. For spins outside the field of view, they still experience the RF excitation and can contribute to the received signal. What happens is the frequencies outside the FOV will be aliased back into the image by what is called the “wrap-around” or fold-over artifact [20]. In cardiac imaging, if the folded over anatomy does not interfere with any of the cardiac structures then the image is acceptable. Otherwise the technologist may try swapping the direction of phase and frequency encoding or on many systems there is an option for oversampling in the frequency direction which allows for the image to be “unfolded”.

Truncation Artifacts

MRI uses Fourier transforms to generate images from the raw RF signals received. Since all MRI acquisitions are digital, the discretized form of the fast Fourier transform is used to create the end image.. Since the values used are discrete approximations of limited resolution there will be instances where the approximation is difficult to model. In particular along high contrast regions (bright pixels adjacent to dark pixels) there can appear alternating light and dark bands known as Gibb's ringing or a truncation artifact that are the visual result of this approximation (Fig. 13.3b) [21]. This can be remedied by repeating the scan with smaller sized voxels (particularly by increasing the number of phase encoding steps).

Hardware Artifacts

Rapid gradient switching, high magnetic field strengths, heating, and repeated use are all contributing factors to normal wear and tear on the components of a typical clinical MRI unit. In the eventuality that one of these components malfunctions there will be evidence in the end images. Unfortunately, there is little that the technologist can do to remedy hardware problems so following a quality program, like outlined in the previous chapter, can help a site avoid costly downtime. Sometimes however, artifacts related to hardware will show up without warning and need to be recognized as there is no remedy that can be made for these errors without repairs, below is a discussion of some common artifacts to look for.

Field Inhomogeneity (B0 and/or B1)

The first assumption made in MRI is that the magnetic fields used are uniform. This is most likely to be true at the isocenter of the magnetic field with fluctuations becoming more prominent the further from center an observation is made. Inhomogeneity in the magnetic field can cause spins to de-phase more rapidly resulting in signal dropout and geometric distortions in the resulting image. This is similar to what occurs with saturation artifacts, but if the main field is not very homogenous or the shim volumes are unable to make the necessary corrections, then it can become extremely difficult to acquire quality images. Inhomogeneity can be mitigated to some extent by applying a proper gradient shim volume and several correction algorithms have also been proposed to deal with this occurrence [22, 23].

Radio-Frequency Noise Artifacts

As we have seen MRI both transmits and receives RF signals to generate an image. If the scanning environment is not carefully controlled, RF energy from sources external to the MRI can make their way into the final images. These can show up as the "zipper" artifact and a reduction in the overall SNR of the image [24]. The "zipper" artifact appears as a line of static through the image. Spike noise will appear as a light and dark banding across multiple lines. In general the source will be some compromise of the faraday cage of the MRI suite (the door left open, some electronic device maybe for patient monitoring used within the suite with unshielded cabling, or even the lighting used).

Gradient Malfunction Artifacts

Gradients are constantly switching and can sometimes malfunction. When this occurs the resulting image may have severe geometric distortions. Likewise, signal intensity may also drop off along the periphery of the image indicative of eddy currents due to the rapid gradient switching.

Surface Coil Error Artifacts

CMR makes extensive use of surface coils to better accentuate the features of the heart. The typical surface coil is actually made up of multiple individual coils that can be configured to speed up imaging by each recording a part of the dial image. If even a single coil element fails or the signals from each element are not properly combined the result can be a large drop in signal corresponding to the region imaged by the defective element [25]. The only solution is to replace or repair the coil.

Inadequate Study

CMR may be relatively slow and artifact prone, but there are only a handful of cases where an inadequate study may not be repeated. Indeed, one of the great strengths of MRI is that the image planes and acquisition parameters are simple to replicate. Since the setup for an acquisition is stored in the scanner console it can be copied and repeated as often as needed (provided there are no machine faults or loss of table localization). It is worth restating that exams should only be repeated when absolutely necessary as additional scans lengthen the protocol time and may adversely affect image quality. In instances where quantitative data is required, it is beneficial to have a post processing workstation available in the control room so that feedback can be provided while the patient is still in the scanner.

One of the few instances where a scan cannot be repeated involves the use of pharmacological agents. For safety reasons previously discussed, gadolinium-based contrast agents can only be administered in a fashion where the amount and rate are both controlled and limited. Similarly, pharmacological stressing agents (adenosine, regadenoson, or dobutamine) restrict the available acquisition window to the clinically accepted timeframe around administration as defined by safety guidelines.

In the case a contrast enhanced study is inadequate (such as a contrast enhanced MRA, or a viability exam), the first course of action is to decide if there is enough information in the images already collected. If this is not the case then complimentary images should be examined. In the case of viability, myocardial tagging has been demonstrated to correspond well with areas of infarction [26]. However, if a post processing solution is not available a qualitative assessment can still be performed.

In the case of an inadequate first pass perfusion study, the reason for the poor exam should be examined. In some instances a patient may have had caffeine in some form without reporting it to the staff and so the pharmacological agent was unable to adequately increase the heart rate. In this case it is necessary for the clinician to decide whether the patient must be rescheduled for another cardiac MRI or if an alternative test as dictated by the appropriateness criteria is appropriate.

Patient Preparation

This is extensively discussed in Chap. 11. Patient preparation is extremely important when performing cardiac MRI and should begin well before the patient checks-in for the examination [27]. Once the patient has been scheduled to receive a cardiac MRI they should also receive information on what to expect during their procedure (directions on where to go and if any food such as caffeine should be avoided and for how long prior to the exam). This could be something as simple as an informational packet, a link to your facility's webpage, or directions to any of the excellent patient education sites listed at the end of this section. Further, some studies have reported a decrease in patients who underwent relaxation techniques prior to imaging. In many cases, patients prepared with knowledge of what is to come and how to cope are better able to comply with instructions once in the scanner.

As a point of emphasis, the patient's history should be reviewed prior to arrival for any MRI contraindications or allergies/adverse reactions to any pharmaceutical agents that may be used. There is really no reason to have any surprises when a patient that has an extensive medical history shows up to the MRI suite only to first find out during the safety screening that they have a medical device implanted. A lot of scanning time can be lost in the following moments trying to determine if the implant is MR compatible or safe at the field strength to be used. Even if it is deemed safe to continue, artifacts may now render the previously defined protocol useless. In the case of insufficient renal function or allergy to GBCA, a study may have to be non-contrast potentially limiting its overall utility. All of this not only adds to the burden of the technologist, but also adds unnecessary anxiety to the patient, and remember patient compliance is critical in cardiac MRI! Things like this are expected to happen from time to time, but if you find it happening regularly, your site's scheduling procedures should be reviewed.

Provided the necessary safety screening and patient education have taken place in a satisfactory manner the patient can now be physically prepared for placement in the scanner following all safety protocols. Per the safety chapter it is preferable that all patients wear a gown and remove any metallic clothing items (metal may show up in places you least expect so be sure to use a wand or other ferrous metal detector prior to patient placement). Any intravenous lines (MR safe) should be in place prior to placement on the exam table. In systems that include it, an MR safe respiratory bellows will be placed around the patient's abdomen to track patient breathing patterns.

For cardiac MRI some form of physiologic monitoring is necessary for timing of the images, and this is typically accomplished with surface electrodes. This requires preparation of the skin surface where the electrodes will be placed. Hair must be removed and the surface must be clean and dry. An MRI safe conductive gel is then applied to the electrode to help conduct the signal from the heart's electrical activity. Electrodes are then placed to monitor the patient's heartbeat in either an electrocardiogram (ECG) or vector cardiogram (VCG) configuration (this can vary depending on manufacturer). Once the electrodes are in place, your system will provide a waveform that varies with the patient's heart beat. Proper fixation of the electrodes will result in a waveform of sufficient voltage amplitude (consult manufacturer's specifications) and identification of the R-wave for gating purposes. If either is insufficient new electrodes should be repositioned until a satisfactory waveform achieved. Achieving a proper waveform can be particularly difficult in the case of a female patient (due to breast tissue) or obese patients.

Originally ECG was used extensively, but it is subject to the magneto-hemodynamic effect of blood flowing through the aortic arch which can increase the amplitude of the T-wave which would be falsely read as an additional QRS used to define systole leading to development and acceptance of VCG [28]. This is very important because timing for all image acquisition is based off of this information, and such an error would effectively cut the time for image acquisition effectively in half or lead to additional artifacts in the collected images. The VCG configuration addresses this by resolving the electrical vectors in three dimensions. Recent developments to simplify patient monitoring setup have included acoustic monitoring that not only listen for the valves closing but can also track respiratory motion [29]. This system proposes to essentially reduce patient monitoring setup to the placement of a stethoscope placed on the chest and under the cardiac coil.

It is necessary to note that the types of monitoring mentioned are insufficient to assess the patient's condition, and are used solely for timing the collection of image data. Additionally, pulse oximeter monitoring may be used, but it not as robust as the VCG or ECG techniques.

Once the monitoring device is in place the appropriate imaging coil may now be placed. Cardiac applications typically make use of a surface phased array coil of various numbers of elements. To avoid overheating/burning the patient the coil will typically be placed on top of a towel or two. Positioning of the coil is important as signal strength decreases exponentially in an inverse relationship with the size of the coil. In order to ensure that sufficient signal is available the sagittal localizer images should be reviewed. The hyper intense signal observed on the anterior and posterior chest walls should fully encase the cardiac anatomy of interest and should be of level from front to back. If the signal does not fully cover the anatomy of interest the patient should be removed from the bore, the coil should be repositioned in the necessary direction, and the localizer repeated and reviewed until adequate covered is obtained. Once satisfied, the patient setup can be considered complete.

Summary

Quality control starts with scheduling the patient with adequate preparation, but also preparing the magnet for the patient beforehand. Artifacts are inevitable in CMR imaging, but they can be eliminated, mitigated, or at times, enhanced to aid in your examination.

References

1. Federal Food Drug and Cosmetics Act, Chapter V, Subchapter C – electronic product radiation control.
2. Title 21 Code of Federal Regulations, Subchapter J – radiological health, Parts 1000–1005.
3. Woodard PK, et al. ACR practice guideline for the performance and interpretation of cardiac magnetic resonance imaging (MRI). J Am Coll Radiol. 2006;3(9):665–76.
4. American College of Radiology. Site scanning instructions for use of the MR phantom for the ACR MRI accreditation program. 2002.
5. Chen C-C, et al. Quality assurance of clinical MRI scanners using ACR MRI phantom: preliminary results. J Digit Imaging. 2004;17(4):279–84.
6. American College of Radiology, ACR practice parameter for continuing Medical Education (CME). 2014.
7. Ridgway JP. Cardiovascular magnetic resonance physics for clinicians: part I. J Cardiovasc Magn Reson. 2010;12(1):71.
8. Biglands JD, Radjenovic A, Ridgway JP. Cardiovascular magnetic resonance physics for clinicians: part II. J Cardiovasc Magn Reson. 2012;14:66.
9. Bloch F, Hanson W, Packard M. Nuclear infraction. Phys Rev. 1946;69:127.
10. Purcell E, Torrey H, Pound R. Resonance absorption by nuclear magnetic moments in a solid. Phys Rev. 1946;69:37–8.
11. Zhuo J, Gullapalli RP. MR artifacts, safety, and quality control 1. Radiographics. 2006;26(1):275–97.
12. Merkle EM, Dale BM. Abdominal MRI at 3.0T: the basics revisited. Am J Roentgenol. 2006;186(6):1524–32.
13. Dietrich O, Reiser MF, Schoenberg SO. Artifacts in 3-T MRI: physical background and reduction strategies. Eur J Radiol. 2008;65(1):29–35.
14. Bitar R, et al. MR pulse sequences: what every radiologist wants to know but is afraid to ask 1. Radiographics. 2006;26(2):513–37.
15. Morelli JN, et al. An image-based approach to understanding the physics of MR artifacts. Radiographics. 2011;31(3):849–66.
16. van der Geest RJ, Reiber JHC. Quantification in cardiac MRI. J Magn Reson Imaging. 1999;10(5):602–8.
17. Haacke EM, Lenz GW. Improving MR image quality in the presence of motion by using rephasing gradients. Am J Roentgenol. 1987;148(6):1251–8.

18. Chia JM, et al. Performance of QRS detection for cardiac magnetic resonance imaging with a novel vectorcardiographic triggering method. J Magn Reson Imaging. 2000;12(5):678–88.
19. Lotz J, et al. Cardiovascular flow measurement with phase-contrast MR imaging: basic facts and implementation 1. Radiographics. 2002;22(3):651–71.
20. Stadler A, et al. Artifacts in body MR imaging: their appearance and how to eliminate them. Eur Radiol. 2007;17(5):1242–55.
21. Pusey E, et al. Magnetic resonance imaging artifacts: mechanism and clinical significance. Radiographics. 1986;6(5):891–911.
22. Irarrazabal P, et al. Inhomogeneity correction using an estimated linear field map. Magn Reson Med. 1996;35(2):278–82.
23. Feinberg DA, Oshio K. Gradient-echo shifting in fast MRI techniques (ERASE imaging) for correction of field inhomogeneity errors and chemical shift. J Magn Reson. 1969;97(1):177–83.
24. Bernstein MA, Huston J, Ward HA. Imaging artifacts at 3.0 T. J Magn Reson Imaging. 2006;24(4):735–46.
25. Murakami JW, Hayes CE, Weinberger E. Intensity correction of phased-array surface coil images. Magn Reson Med. 1996;35(4):585–90.
26. Kim YJ, et al. Delayed enhancement in hypertrophic cardiomyopathy: comparison with myocardial tagging MRI. J Magn Reson Imaging. 2008;27(5):1054–60.
27. Kramer CM, et al. Standardized cardiovascular magnetic resonance (CMR) protocols 2013 update. J Cardiovasc Magn Reson. 2013;15(1):1.
28. Fischer SE, Wickline SA, Lorenz CH. Novel real-time R-wave detection algorithm based on the vectorcardiogram for accurate gated magnetic resonance acquisitions. Magn Reson Med. 1999;42(2):361–70.
29. Frauenrath T, et al. Acoustic cardiac triggering: a practical solution for synchronization and gating of cardiovascular magnetic resonance at 7 Tesla. J Cardiovasc Magn Reson. 2010;12(1):67.

Chapter 14
MRI Report

Ibrahim M. Saeed

Abstract Cardiac magnetic resonance imaging is a complicated process involving many experts in order to obtain required images. As a result of this complicated process a report reflecting the acquisition parameters and physician interpretation is a key product. Key elements of the report have been defined by the American College of Radiology and the Inter-Societal Accreditation Commission. These include five major areas: Demographics, relevant clinical information and indication, procedure and materials, findings and impression. Additionally, the report should be signed and dated and communicated in a timely manner to enable best care.

Keywords Cardiac magnetic resonance • Reporting elements • Reporting standards • Timeliness

Introduction

Multiple imaging societies have published a joint health policy statement [1] on the imaging report, which includes several principles, such as clinical relevance, completeness, clarity, consistency, reproducibility, practicality, and adequacy for billing. The structured report should have a balance of ease of use, rigor and flexibility. Consideration was also given to both commonality to the process and content, but also an opportunity for innovation and proprietary development.

An issue for cardiac MRI (CMR) is that, while most other imaging modalities are designed for syntactic and semantic interoperability (that is exchange of data between electronic medical record systems and other receivers of data), compatibility and multimodality comparability is somewhat challenging in the setting of CMR. Although one could compare an MRI with the hemodynamic information of

I.M. Saeed, MD, FACC, FAAP
Saint Luke's Mid America Heart Institute Cardiovascular Consultants,
University of Missouri, Kansas City, MO, USA
e-mail: isaeed@saint-lukes.org; imsaeed@gmail.com

P.L. Tilkemeier et al. (eds.), *Quality Evaluation in Non-Invasive Cardiovascular Imaging*, DOI 10.1007/978-3-319-28011-0_14

an echocardiogram, or the anatomical description of a CT, or even the metabolic data described by a nuclear cardiology report; no other modality provides information about tissue characterization as does CMR. Therefore, while one could, as an example, extend the terminology of viability of transmural presence of late gadolinium enhancement in an effort to compare with a viability PET study, it would not have the ability to compare these fields for lipomatous hypertrophy of the atrial septum, edema or microvascular obstruction following a myocardial infarction, an inversion recovery time suggestive of cardiac amyloidosis, or a darkened liver with a low T2* time suggestive of hemochromatosis. There are so many sequences such as those focusing on edema, ischemia, fat, infarction, inflammation, iron, expansion of the extracellular volume, fibrosis, and others that continue to be developed, and that are vendor dependent, that it can be challenging to be consistent.

Effective communication is a critical component of diagnostic imaging and quality patient care. As part of this, the report should promote optimal patient care and support the ordering health care provider in that regard in a timely manner. Furthermore, interpretation of images necessitates cooperation amongst many stakeholders (and therefore relevant sections), including those for administrators, clinicians, and interpreting physicians. Review with previously available clinical information is critical.

Key Elements

The American College of Radiology (ACR) has established practice parameters for communication of diagnostic findings [2]. Similarly, there are specific requirements that the Intersocietal Accreditation Commission [3]. These are combined and summarized below, but the IAC also suggests in its guidelines that an experienced technologist should be able to reproduce the exam based on the description provided:

1. Standardized reporting format. A computer-generated template is recommended by the ACR.
2. Demographics
   (a) Facility where the study was performed
   (b) Patient identifier or name.
   (c) Ordering health care provider, or if self-referred
   (d) Name or type of examination
      (i) This often involves relevant CPT codes.
   (e) Date of examination (and time if relevant, and more than one per day).
   (f) Technologist who performed the exam
   (g) Recommended additional demographic data elements
      (i) Date of dictation
      (ii) Date and time of transcription

(iii) Patient's date of birth (or age)
(iv) Patient's gender.

3. Relevant clinical information that serves as indication for the test
4. Body

   (a) Procedures and Materials

      (i) Sequences performed and imaging planes
      (ii) Type and amount of contrast media used or other medications
      (iii) Catheters or devices involved
      (iv) Patient reactions or complications.

   (b) Findings that use appropriate anatomic, pathologic, or radiologic terminology

      (i) These should be Cardiac MRI specific (see below)
      (ii) All of the MRI examination images must be reviewed by the interpreting member of the medical staff or the Medical Director.
      (iii) Pertinent positives and negatives

   (c) Limitations including identifying factors that may compromise the exam's sensitivity and specificity.
   (d) Address the clinical issue
   (e) Comparison with prior studies and reports.

5. Impression (or Conclusion)

   (a) Should be a specific section
   (b) If a specific diagnosis is possible, then given; otherwise a differential diagnosis if appropriate.
   (c) Follow up or additional diagnostic studies to clarify or confirm the impression should be suggested if appropriate
   (d) Significant patient reactions.

Cardiac MRI Specific

Although the above suggestions are relevant for all radiologic studies, the ACR also released specific suggestions for the interpretation of CMR in 2014 [4]. It acknowledged several indications for CMR and highlighted below are those indications that are recommended for assessment of specific parameters:

1. Acquired heart disease

   (a) Dynamic cardiac anatomy and left ventricular (LV) function

      (i) Using the standard 17-segment model [5] for LV wall motion assessment
      (ii) Quantifications of LV volumes and ejection fraction.
      (iii) At least qualitative assessment of the right ventricle.

(iv) Chamber-sizes are recommended to be indexed for body surface, gender, and age and with corresponding Z-scores when relevant, and compared with referenced norms.

(b) Assessment of cardiomyopathies, myocardial fibrosis, and infarction

(i) Including pattern and distribution of late gadolinium enhancement if relevant

(c) Assessment of ischemia with pharmacologic agents

(i) Including related EKG and hemodynamic findings.
(ii) Stress agents used.

(d) Characterization of masses
(e) Characterization of the pericardium
(f) Valvular disease

(i) Stenosis including quantification of peak systolic velocity combined with the modified Bernoulli equation [6] and/or planimetry
(ii) Regurgitant volumes and fractions.

(g) Coronary artery disease, in particular if any proximal stenoses or aneurysms or detected, or the patency of bypass grafts.
(h) Pulmonary vein assessment, including anatomy.

2. In the setting of congenital heart disease, Shunts (atrial or septal defects), quantification of their size (the ratio of pulmonary-to-systemic-flow, or Qp:Qs); and overall complex anomalies including pericardial anomalies (such as absence or partial defects); valve disease; and/or extracardiac vascular anomalies.

Timeliness and Other Principles

There are several other principles that are included in this definitive document:

- It should be proofread with limitations on abbreviations or acronyms.
- It should be verified (manually or electronically) and signed by the Medical Director or a member of the medical staff. Date of the interpreting physician's signature.
- The physician's final interpretation, whether paper, electronic, or voice, must be available within two working days of the examination date.
- The final, verified, signed report should be transmitted to the referring physician within four working days, unless awaiting additional clinical information. These include any relevant images when requested.
- The permanent record should be archived and retrievable for future reference.

Communication

As stated above, the final, verified, signed report should be transmitted to the referring physician within four working days, unless awaiting additional clinical information. These include any relevant images when requested.

If there are other communications than the final report, preliminary findings need to be documented specifically as the preliminary report. Any variations with the final report need to also be documented. Non-routine communications, such as those with a need for immediate or urgent intervention, discrepant findings that may adversely affect patient health, or those findings that do not require immediate intervention but may result in an adverse patient outcome over time should be documented.

References

1. Douglas PS, Hendel RC, Cummings JE, Dent JM, Hodgson JM, Hoffmann U, et al. ACCF/ACR/AHA/ASE/ASNC/HRS/NASCI/RSNA/SAIP/SCAI/SCCT/SCMR 2008 health policy statement on structured reporting in cardiovascular imaging. J Am Coll Cardiol. 2009;53(1):76–90.
2. Practice parameter for communication of diagnostic imaging findings [database on the Internet]. www.acr.org. Revised 2014. Available from: http://www.acr.org/~/media/C5D1443C9EA4424AA12477D1AD1D927D.pdf.
3. The IAC standards and guidelines for MRI accreditation [database on the Internet] (2014) Available from: http://www.intersocietal.org/mri/standards/IACMRIStandardsJuly2014.pdf.
4. ACR–NASCI–SPR practice parameter for the performance and interpretation of cardiac magnetic resonance imaging (MRI) [database on the Internet] Amended 2014 [cited 2014]. Available from: http://www.acr.org/~/media/61ECDDA970F34D58AD79A8657EAE1BFA.pdf.
5. Cerqueira MD, Weissman NJ, Dilsizian V, Jacobs AK, Kaul S, Laskey WK, et al. Standardized myocardial segmentation and nomenclature for tomographic imaging of the heart. A statement for healthcare professionals from the Cardiac Imaging Committee of the Council on Clinical Cardiology of the American Heart Association. Circulation. 2002;105(4):539–42.
6. Caruthers SD, Lin SJ, Brown P, Watkins MP, Williams TA, Lehr KA, et al. Practical value of cardiac magnetic resonance imaging for clinical quantification of aortic valve stenosis: comparison with echocardiography. Circulation. 2003;108(18):2236–43.

Chapter 15
MRI: Laboratory Accreditation and Quality Improvement Program

Ibrahim M. Saeed

Abstract Given the complex nature of cardiac magnetic resonance imaging it is important to have in place a robust quality improvement program that is a partnership between the physician and the technologist. Laboratory accreditation will be reviewed as a mechanism for building a high quality laboratory. Key components of this program will be reviewed including physician recognition of artifacts, scheduling, technologist training, review of imaging data and interpreter quality control. It is important to recognize those events which should never occur during a cardiac magnetic resonance imaging study. General and specific safety recommendations will be reviewed.

Keywords Quality improvement • Laboratory accreditation • Imaging artifact • Interpreter quality control • "never" events

Laboratory Accreditation

Accreditation of cardiac magnetic resonance (CMR) laboratories by one of three CMS approved accrediting bodies, the American College of Radiology (ACR), the Intersocietal Accreditation Commission (IAC) or the Joint Commission, is an important recognition of the quality of the entire imaging process. Given that CMR is considered an advanced imaging modality, accreditation is required for reimbursement by Medicare as a result of the Medicare Improvements for Patients and Providers Act of 2008. Each organization has unique aspects of their accreditation program that may make one a better 'fit' than another with regard to a laboratory and its specific characteristics, e.g. hospital based, free standing, or multi-modality.

The ACR model is more often utilized by laboratories that have multiple imaging modalities that are being accredited simultaneously. The Joint Commission pathway

I.M. Saeed, MD, FACC, FAAP
Saint Luke's Mid America Heart Institute Cardiovascular Consultants,
University of Missouri, Kansas City, MO, USA
e-mail: isaeed@saint-lukes.org

P.L. Tilkemeier et al. (eds.), *Quality Evaluation in Non-Invasive Cardiovascular Imaging*, DOI 10.1007/978-3-319-28011-0_15

is commonly used by laboratories that are undergoing routine accreditation visits by the Joint Commission, hospital based facilities for example. The IAC pathway can be utilized by all laboratories and includes a broad assessment of a laboratory's performance from three perspectives: staff qualifications, patient testing and a quality improvement program.

Specifics of the ACR program have been included in Chap. 13. The ACR program has specific requirements to assess image quality and equipment performance using a proprietary phantom, any appropriately designed phantom will suffice as part of a local QC program (ACR reference). Other groups, like The Intersocietal Accreditation Commission (IAC) [1] or the Joint Commission [2], provide similar guidelines, but do not specifically define how the testing is to be performed, only what must be included as part of the QC testing. The ACR model specifically defines both an annual examination (long term monitoring) and a daily/weekly (short term) monitoring schedule.

In distinction to the accreditation of laboratories, physicians can achieve individual certification documenting their skills from the Society of Cardiovascular Magnetic Resonance (SCMR). The process requires board certification in an appropriate cardiovascular subspecialty, initial and ongoing participation in coursework relative to CMR, performing the required number of interpretations and participation in ongoing quality management /improvement programs in the laboratory. Details can be located on the SCMR website, www.scmr.org.

Identifying What Steps Need to Be Evaluated for Quality

Performing a cardiac MR (CMR) study is highly complex and involves multiple steps including, scheduling, patient preparation, sequence optimization, image acquisition, processing and reporting. However, critical to success is the ability to repeat the process again and again, in an efficient manner. To ensure success, follow-up information regarding all aspects of CMR is necessary, including the impact on patient management and outcome. Furthermore, complications and inadequate/inaccurate studies require careful review. The directors (technical and medical) would ideally have a process in place where each of these steps is continually reviewed.

Scheduling is critical to success. Selection of a device, such as a 1.5 T or a 3 T magnet is important as well as when an extended scan is required-both mandate forethought and planning. Schedulers also must prepare the patient, and also serve as the front line for MR safety by reviewing one of the established contraindication checklists. For any concerns or questions, they often communicate with the MR technologists or the directors.

Physician education is important to the success of a CMR program. The interpreting and supervising physicians as well as the medical director for the laboratory must have all of the required training elements to insure appropriate oversight of the individual patient studies and the overall functioning of the laboratory. This includes the required assessment of the technical quality, patient safety, patient selection and appropriate protocol selection, image review and inter/intra observer interpreter variability and other elements of an ongoing quality assurance program. The physician(s) must participate in ongoing education to insure they are aware of and have implemented the latest techniques to insure the highest quality patient studies possible.

Technologists are critical to the success of a CMR program. While often highly trained, they should also seek guidance from the director to help guide the sequence parameters, which is a significant investment in time from the physician and group practice or hospital. Furthermore, for each indication a **sequence protocol** is reviewed by the medical director or interpreting physician beforehand for appropriateness, with any suggestions to alter the established protocol, such as valvular heart disease or congenital issues. In the meantime, depending on the sequence, the protocol may be "locked" with minor adjustments, so as to maintain efficiency. Finally, regular constructive feedback is given. Technologists must regularly attend educational conferences and maintain appropriate certification.

An MR examination typically generates a large amount of **imaging data**. Most practices have an archival system such as PACS. There are several post-processing solutions that allow the user to calculate the ejection fraction, quantify flow or tissue characterization, 3D rotation for multiplanar reformatting or maximum intensity projections, or viewing a region of interest in orthogonal planes. The ability to recall, reprocess and reinterpret studies after initial acquisition is an important part of the imaging process as the post-acquisition/processing review of a study can often occur on an independent workstation.

Interpreter quality control can be difficult, particularly at a smaller institution where not many CMR readers exist. Multi-modality conferences may help to ensure validation and cross-correlation. This may be done by comparing LVEF measurements between CMR and other modalities and determine why variations may exist, such as whether or not the papillary muscles are included in the assessment. Similarly, comparison of post-gadolinium images with nuclear cardiology techniques is also important. Finally, follow up to see if evaluation of pathology (such as whether viable tissue did or did not recover after revascularization, or if tumor pathology was consistent with interpretation) is critical.

"NEVER-EVENTS" and MR Safety

Introduction

While the use of magnetic resonance does not have any of the inherent risks associated with ionizing radiation, there are still many safety considerations of which to be aware. Of primary concern are the main magnetic field forces, radiofrequency heating, patients with implants or metal working history, and the operating noise from gradient switching [3]. MRI safety requires continued education and constant vigilance because the magnetic field is always present and the array of implanted medical devices in use is constantly changing.

The Main Magnetic Field

The MR suite is first and foremost designed around the strength of the main magnetic field of the unit. While there are no readily recognized adverse biological effects with exposure to the magnetic fields utilized in clinical MRI, environmental factors can become dangerous [4]. Within this field (which rapidly grows in strength with proximity to the bore) even the most benign seeming objects will become subject to force or torque wanting to move or twist. This can lead to them to become dangerous projectiles. The high field strengths typically in use are also strong enough to pull larger sized items like chairs, floor buffers, and gurneys into the bore [5]. The most effective way to prevent this from occurring is to physically restrict access to and control movement around the vicinity of the magnet and implement a rigorous screening process [6, 7].

Once inside the magnet room (Zone 4) make note of the five Gauss line. This line is a three dimensional bubble surrounding the magnet and defining the point at which the static field strength greatly increases and is regularly defined in site planning prior to installation. Items that normally do not behave as magnetic may exhibit magnetic attraction within this area. Often the line will be marked on the floor of the scanning room to explicitly mark the transition point. All screening should take place outside of the magnet room (see below for suggestions) paying special attention to patients with prior medical implants to ensure their safety as they may be at particularly high risk of injury (see section "Medical implants").

RF Heating

The same RF energy used to excite the hydrogen protons will also cause heating (both core and locally) potentially leading to injury if not controlled [8]. Exposure to RF is measured by the specific absorption rate (SAR), an estimate of heating based on the patient's mass measured in Watts per kilogram [9]. These values are typically presented as a running average of exposure over a 6 min or 10 s period. Clinical limits are based upon standards developed by the International Electrotechnical Commission standards (IEC 60601-2-33). The FDA further recommends RF exposure levels limiting core temperature rise of 1 °C and local heating dependent upon body region. Fortunately, the standard operating modes of all modern scanners limit the amount of RF energy a patient may receive. Local heating is typically limited to the skin's surface and can thus be dissipated in part by utilizing the onboard patient cooling systems. There have been instances of injury due to the use of non-compliant patient monitoring leads, looping wires, and clothing, but these can be avoided by strict adherence to proper patient preparation guidelines. Patients with prior medical implants may be at particularly high risk of local heating injury and require special attention (see section "Medical implants").

Medical Implants

Special consideration must be given to patients scheduled to undergo an MRI with prior medical devices [3]. There have been a great many advancements in the design and manufacture of medical devices many of which are able to safely be imaged with MR. Devices may experience any or all of the previously mentioned effects. Static devices may displace under the force and torques generated in the magnetic field, electronic devices may malfunction under the RF excitation, and/or the RF excitation may also cause dangerous local heating. This is further complicated by the fact that a device may be MR compatible at one field strength (1.5 T) but not another (3.0 T) so it is important to always confirm that implanted devices are safe for the magnetic field to be used. An excellent resource, "The List" is found online at www.mrisafety.com and is continuously updated and lists whether devices may be safely imaged at particular field strength.

Noise

The gradient switching systems on a clinical MRI scanner generate a lot of loud noise (up over 115 dB) that can permanently damage hearing and result in injury [10].

This is easily addressed by always making sure that all patients are properly fitted with appropriate hearing protection (headphones, earplugs, or both) prior to beginning the exam. Many of these systems incorporate a way for patients to receive instructions from the technologist and also listen to music or other entertainment during the exam. The patient should also be encouraged to maintain communication with the technologist during the exam and notify if at any time the noise level they experience increases because the earplugs/earphones become too loose.

General MRI Safety Suggestions

1. Control the environment
   (a) Limit access to the control room/magnet room
   (b) Everyone clears pockets and is screened for metal items before every entry into magnet room
   (c) Always screen patients before entering the MRI suite/bore

(d) Implement a magnetic detector curtain on door or wand to screen individuals entering the scanning room for metal.
(e) Screen all items to be used in the MR suite. Label all MRI safe items. DO NOT allow unscreened outside items in. Especially while the patient is in the bore. Assume all unscreened items are magnetic.

2. Patient Safety
   (a) Be aware of SAR limits.
   (b) ALWAYS have hearing protection properly installed on patient.
   (c) ALWAYS have multiple methods for communication with the patient.
      (i) Engage often with the microphone
      (ii) Emergency "squeeze ball"
   (d) NO LOOPS in coil wires or on patients
   (e) NEVER inject a contrast agent without a physician present.
   (f) All patients should use the medical gowns and remove belts, earrings, rings, change in pockets, or any other items that MAY contain metal
      (i) Even underwire in bra or other clothing may pose a hazard in the magnet
   (g) Screen the patient.
      (i) Double check patient medical records
      (ii) Implants must be verified as MR SAFE/MR compatible FOR THE FIELD strength of the magnet being used to image (lookup or verify with manufacturer). When in doubt pull the records and verify. DO NOT simply rely on the patients' memory. "Trust… but verify".
   (h) Take special care when patient is under anesthesia and unable to communicate.
3. Practice Safety
   (a) Have a safety and emergency response plan.
      (i) Use signage to clearly mark emergency response items.
   (b) Practice rapid removal of patient from magnet.
   (c) All necessary safety equipment should be immediately available or on the emergency cart
   (d) Use proper monitoring equipment.

Technical: Equipment

A quality assurance program for technical performance of the equipment is essential to assuring high quality images. A rigorous quality assurance program for the laboratory must be developed and monitored by the technologists, physicians and laboratory administrative leadership routinely. The requirements of such a program are outlined in detail in Chap. 13.

Development of a Quality Assurance Program

The development of a quality assurance program must be part of the initial setup of the laboratory and must be designed to meet the specifics of the equipment, physical facility, staff, and most importantly the patients being tested and imaged. Such a program needs to be part of an accreditation program and undergo periodic review to insure it is meeting the needs of the laboratory. This would include revision as new technology and techniques are developed and clinically implemented, new cameras are added, new staff (technologists or physicians) join the laboratory or any other changes are implemented that could affect the quality of the complex CMR imaging chain.

Conclusion

A high quality CMR laboratory must have a multi-dimensional approach to quality assurance and improvement that is based in an accreditation process. The process must include all aspects of a CMR study: appropriate patient selection; patient preparation; technical quality; qualified personnel; selection of appropriate protocols to address the clinical question; image interpretation quality assurance, including comparison to other modalities; addressing "never" events and mechanisms to assure they do not occur; and generating a timely and high quality report communicating the results succinctly and meaningfully. Performance at this high level will insure the continued growth of CMR as a technology to meet increasing patient needs and demands.

References

1. Intersocietal Accreditation Commission. "The IAC Standards and Guidelines for MRI Accreditation." 2012. Available from: http://www.intersocietal.org/mri/main/mri_standards.htm
2. The Joint Commission. Facts about Ambulatory Care Accreditation. [Internet]. 2014 [cited 2014 December 12]. Available from: http://www.jointcommission.org/assets/1/18/Ambulatorycare_1_112.PDF.
3. Levine G, Gomes A, Arai A, Bluemke D, Flamm S, Kanal E, Martin ET, Smith JM, Wilke N, Shellock F. Safety of magnetic resonance imaging in patients with cardiovascular devices: an American Heart Association Scientific Statement From the Committee on Diagnostic and Interventional Cardiac Catheterization, Council on Clinical Cardiology, and the Council on Cardiovascular Radiology and Intervention: Endorsed by the American College of Cardiology Foundation, the North American Society for Cardiac Imaging, and the Society for Cardiovascular Magnetic Resonance. Circulation. 2007; 2878–91.
4. Schenck JF. Safety of strong, static magnetic fields. J Magn Reson Imag. 2000;12(1):2–19.
5. Chaljub G, et al. Projectile cylinder accidents resulting from the presence of ferromagnetic nitrous oxide or oxygen tanks in the MR suite. Am J Roentgenol. 2001;177(1):27–30.
6. Kanal E, et al. American College of Radiology white paper on MR safety. Am J Roentgenol. 2002;178(6):1335–47.

7. Shellock FG, Spinazzi A. MRI safety update 2008: part 2, screening patients for MRI. Am J Roentgenol. 2008;191(4):1140–9.
8. Dempsey MF, Condon B. Thermal injuries associated with MRI. Clin Radiol. 2001;56(6):457–65.
9. Shellock FG. Radiofrequency energy-induced heating during MR procedures: a review. J Magn Reson Imag. 2000;12(1):30–6.
10. Price DL, De Wilde JP, Papadaki AM, Curran JS, Kitney RI. Investigation of acoustic noise on 15 MRI scanners from 0.2T to 3T. J Magn Reson Imag. 2001;13:288–93. doi:10.1002/1522-2586(200102)13:2<288::AID-JMRI1041>3.0.CO;2-P.

Part IV
PET

Chapter 16
Cardiac PET Imaging: Clinical Applications and Patient Selection

Gary V. Heller, James A. Case, and Abhijit Ghatak

Abstract This chapter describes clinical value of cardiovascular PET imaging. This includes a detailed examination of a variety of applications, including the detection of coronary artery disease, assessment of myocardial viability and the diagnostic value for identification of cardiac sarcoidosis and infection imaging. Patient selection for Cardiovascular PET imaging procedures is also discussed, and appropriate use criteria as it applies to cardiac PET.

Keywords Cardiac PET • Nuclear cardiology • Quality measures • Appropriate use criteria • Clinical applications • Patient selection

Introduction

Over the past several years, many SPECT laboratories have integrated cardiac positron emission tomographic (PET) imaging into their testing armamentarium. The reasons for considering cardiac PET are: better image quality, greater efficiency, lower radiation exposure, and higher diagnostic accuracy over conventional SPECT imaging. There are approximately 250 laboratories throughout the United States currently performing some form of cardiac PET imaging procedures. The number of laboratories using PET cameras has increased steadily in part due to the availability of radiotracers rubidium-82 and NH13-ammonia and the growing body

G.V. Heller, MD, PhD (✉)
Department of Cardiovascular Medicine, Morristown Medical Center, Atlantic Healthcare System, Gagnon Cardiovascular Institute, Morristown, NJ, USA

Research Section, Intersocietal Accreditation Commission, Ellicott City, MD, USA
e-mail: garyvheller@gmail.com

J.A. Case, PhD
Technical Director, Cardiovascular Imaging Technologies, Kansas City, MO, USA

A. Ghatak, MD, MRCP
Southwest Heart PC, 2525 S Telshor Blrd, Las Cruces, NM 88011, USA
e-mail: ghatak.abhijit@gmail.com

P.L. Tilkemeier et al. (eds.), *Quality Evaluation in Non-Invasive Cardiovascular Imaging*, DOI 10.1007/978-3-319-28011-0_16

of literature supporting its use. This chapter will discuss data regarding cardiac PET imaging, particularly focusing upon perfusion but also highlighting other aspects of cardiac PET such as viability assessment and inflammation/infection imaging, patient selection including appropriate use relating to PET and protocols.

Myocardial Perfusion Imaging with PET

Positron emission tomography utilizes a unique particle, the positron, to create the light that is recorded by the imaging system. Positrons are identical in every respect (mass, lepton number, spin) to electrons, with the exception of their charge; electrons being negatively charged and positrons (the electrons anti-particle) being positively charged. When positrons come in contact with electrons, they completely annihilate; converting all of their energy into two 511 keV photons travelling 180° opposite each other [1]. Because of this geometry, the origin of a radioactivity decay can be localized without the use of lead septa. This phenomenon significantly increases the resolution and sensitivity over Single Photon Emission Computed Tomography. The PET scanner accomplishes this with a system of detectors arranged in a 360 ring around the patient. Using a series of very fast detectors (<15 ns), the camera can quickly identify photon pairs that came from the same decay (Fig. 16.1). An additional benefit of PET is that the images can easily be corrected for soft tissue attenuation. Because both the forward and reverse photons are needed to register a true coincidence, the total attenuation is the sum of the forward attenuation plus the reverse attenuation. The total attenuation length for the line of sight is *independent* of where the annihilation event takes place. This fact greatly increases the simplicity of resolving attenuation artifact and as such improves its accuracy and diagnostic certainty. Attenuation correction is used in essentially all cardiac PET studies.

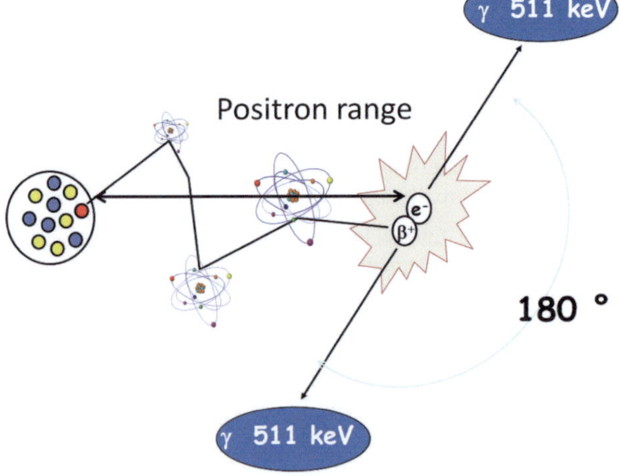

Fig. 16.1 Schematic description of positron emission and annihilation events

Table 16.1 Summary of whole body radiation exposures for common cardiac imaging procedures

Protocol	Modality	Radiation dosage
Dual isotope imaging (Tl-3 mCi, Tc-30 mCi)	SPECT	35 mSv [2]
Thallium stress (3 mCi) reinjection (1 mCi)	SPECT	34 mSv [2]
Low dose (10 mCi)/high dose same day (40 mCi), Rest-stress Tc-99 m	SPECT	12.4 mSv [2]
Stress only Tc-99 m with high sensitivity SPECT camera	SPECT	1.2 mSv [2]
Stress-rest 2 day Tc-99 m	SPECT	18.6 mSv [2]
Rest-Stress Rb-82 in 2D (50 mCi rest, 50 mCi stress)	PET	4.6 mSv [3]
Rest-Stress Rb-82 in 3D(30 mCI rest, 30 mCi stress)	PET	2.8 mSv [3]
Rest-Stress Ammonia (40 mCi)	PET	3.2 mSv [2, 4]
FDG viability (10 mCi)	PET	7 mSv [5]
Cardiac CTA	CT	2–25 mSv [6]
Diagnostic catheterization	Planar x-ray	2.7–8.8 mSv [7]

SPECT single photon emission computed tomography, *PET* positron emission tomography, *CT* computed tomography

Radiation exposure from medical imaging has become an important topic for patient care. Both PET and SPECT tracers expose the patient to some radiation, although minimal and generally approximately that of only several fold that of annual background radiation [2–7]. With the most commonly used protocols for SPECT, radiation dosages can be as high as 20 mSv for a same day Tc-99m study and higher for 2 day and dual isotope protocols. Newer protocols, imaging systems and software techniques for SPECT imaging can substantially reduce the radiation exposure to approximately 6–10 mSv (see Table 16.1). However, the use of cardiac PET imaging and tracers provides typical exposure to as low as 2–6 mSv using Rubidium-82 [3] and for NH^{13} ammonia 4–6 mSv [4].

Diagnostic Accuracy of Cardiac PET Perfusion

Cardiac PET perfusion has been associated with a high diagnostic accuracy for the detection of obstructive coronary artery disease. Several recent meta-analysis have demonstrated superiority of cardiac PET over SPECT imaging [8, 9]. These analyses of the literature demonstrated higher specificity of PET, as well as sensitivity. The specificity improvement most likely was due to a reduction of attenuation artifact and higher image quality without gut and liver impact. However, note, both sensitivity and specificity were higher with PET than SPECT, suggesting the value of PET is more than specificity alone. In a clinical setting, Bateman et al. demonstrated superior diagnostic accuracy in comparable patients between SPECT and PET imaging [10]. In this study, diagnostic accuracy was significantly better in both genders and independent of body mass, although patients with high body mass index did benefit (Fig. 16.2). In this study, the ability to identify multi-vessel CAD

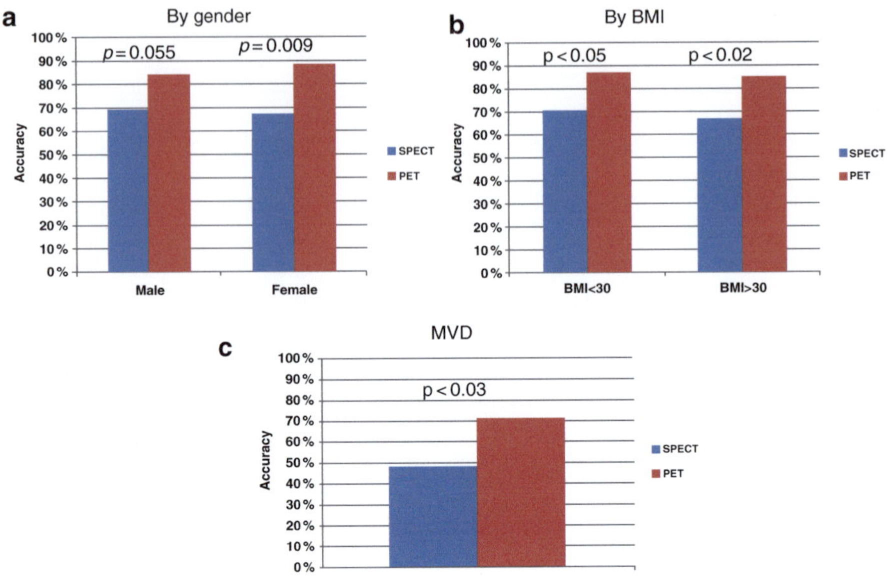

Fig. 16.2 Diagnostic accuracy of cardiac PET vs cardiac SPECT. Diagnostic accuracy is significantly better for PET than SPECT in both genders as well as obese and normal body weight patients. The ability to identify multi-vessel CAD was also significantly better with PET than SPECT [6]

was statistically higher with PET, most likely due to better tracer characteristics and image quality.

Risk stratification with SPECT has been an important contribution to its clinical value. This is based upon the concept that patient management decisions, particularly with regards to medical therapy or coronary intervention can be made on the basis of the size and severity of the SPECT abnormality. Risk stratification data has also been described with cardiac PET perfusion imaging. Cardiac PET identifies patients who are at low, moderate or high risk for future cardiac events. In the largest study to date, Dorbala et al. demonstrated superior risk stratification following cardiac PET studies and classification of patients between low intermediate and high risk for future coronary events [11]. In addition, PET was particularly helpful in female patients [11]. In this studies, risk stratification in women was well-documented at a low radiation exposure (3 mSv on average). This is of considerable importance as women presenting for nuclear imaging trend towards being younger and therefore more vulnerable effects of to radiation exposure.

The improved diagnostic accuracy, image quality and risk stratification may provide an economic advantage over SPECT with regards to invasive procedures following the nuclear procedure. Merhige et al. [12] compared downstream catheterization in patients from his laboratory undergoing SPECT or PET as well as SPECT outcomes from previously published large multicenter study (Fig. 16.3) [13]. Results demonstrated that fewer patients underwent either cardiac catheterization

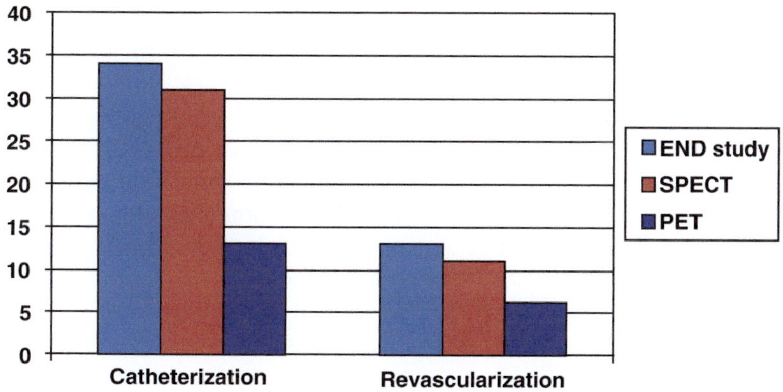

Fig. 16.3 Downstream cardiac catheterization following cardiac SPECT or PET. Data demonstrate significantly fewer catheterizations following PET rather than SPECT. However, the percentage of interventions in those who underwent catheterization was significantly higher after PET than SPECT [8]

with PET than either of the SPECT databases. Of importance, however, the percentage of patients undergoing intervention following cardiac catheterization was significantly higher for PET than SPECT. This suggests a reduction in the unnecessary number of catheterizations based upon false positive SPECT results, with more precise utilization of interventional procedures.

An emerging advantage of cardiac PET perfusion imaging is the ability to measure regional and global myocardial blood flow and flow reserve. Absolute quantification of myocardial blood flow is accomplished by acquiring a dynamic sequence of images beginning prior to the injection of the radiotracer and the following the kinetic uptake process over time. By applying a mathematical model for the uptake process, the blood flow supply can be calculated. The most common model used is the single compartment model as described by Lortie et al. [14], although other models are also used [15] and two compartment models [16]. Comparisons of different software applications implementation of these models demonstrate that a high degree of reproducibility and interchangeability is possible so long as the same imaging protocol and kinetic models are employed [17]. Myocardial blood flow has been assessed with dipyridamole, adenosine, and more recently regadenoson, using both rubidium-82 and ammonia NH-13. Renauld et al. [18] quantified the normal range of blood flow at rest as between 0.33 and 1.3 ml/g/min and 2.36–3.56 ml/g/min in a group of healthy volunteers using dipyridamole. Resting flows also are related to the product of the systolic blood pressure and heart rate, which needs to be keep in mind when evaluating data [19]. There is developing experience with regadenoson indicating similar vasodilator properties [20].

The addition of absolute blood flow measurements has been demonstrated to improve the diagnostic accuracy of PET. When myocardial blood flow is normal in the absence of a perfusion abnormality, it effectively excludes the presence of multivessel CAD [21]. Abnormal, absolute, flow also has been demonstrated to be useful in the identification of balanced ischemia [22], identification of the true extent of multivessel disease [23], and identifying diffusely reduced flow in conditions of microvascular disease [24].

Several studies have demonstrated increased risk stratification capabilities combining perfusion and myocardial blood flow to place patients in more precise risk categories [24–27]. Herzog et al. 2009 identified a significant increase risk of major cardiac events in patients with a normal perfusion scan and abnormal blood flow reserve [28]. This same study also demonstrated a significant increase in risk of death in patients with an abnormal perfusion study with abnormal global flow reserve vs abnormal perfusion study and normal global flow reserve (7.1 % vs 25.7 % respectively, $p<0.05$). Figure 16.3 illustrates an example of normal perfusion and blood flow.

Myocardial Function Using PET Imaging

An advantage of cardiac PET imaging is that ventricular function assessment can be performed at both rest and peak stress, and in the case of vasodilator stress, during active hyperemia. The assessment of ventricular function at rest is similar to other non-invasive strategies such as echocardiography, SPECT imaging, and radionuclide angiography. Correlation between ventricular function assessed by cardiac PET in comparison to these modalities is excellent [29, 30]. Stress ventricular function is performed during active hyperemia with all available vasodilator agents and therefore more closely represents ischemic changes than with SPECT in which data are acquired after cessation of the ischemic event.

Vasodilator stress with dipyridamole and regadenoson have a similar effect on LVEF, increasing the LVEF by 8 % percentage points in normal patients. The presence of a reversible wall motion abnormality has been associated with identification of multivessel disease [31] as well as a worse outcome [31, 32]. The presence of left ventricular dysfunction is also associated with a higher risk of cardiac death particularly in the presence of perfusion abnormalities [33–37].

Myocardial Viability Using FDG PET Imaging

Hibernating myocardium can occur in regions of chronic hypoperfusion where the tissue remains alive but in a low metabolic state [38], reflected as minimal or absent perfusion or akinesis by ventricular function. In the low metabolic state of hibernation, glucose metabolism replaces free fatty acid. A direct assessment of myocardial viability can by performed with PET by determining the regions of the myocardium that are engaged in glucose metabolism specifically with the metabolic tracer F-18-Fluorodeoxyglucose (FDG).

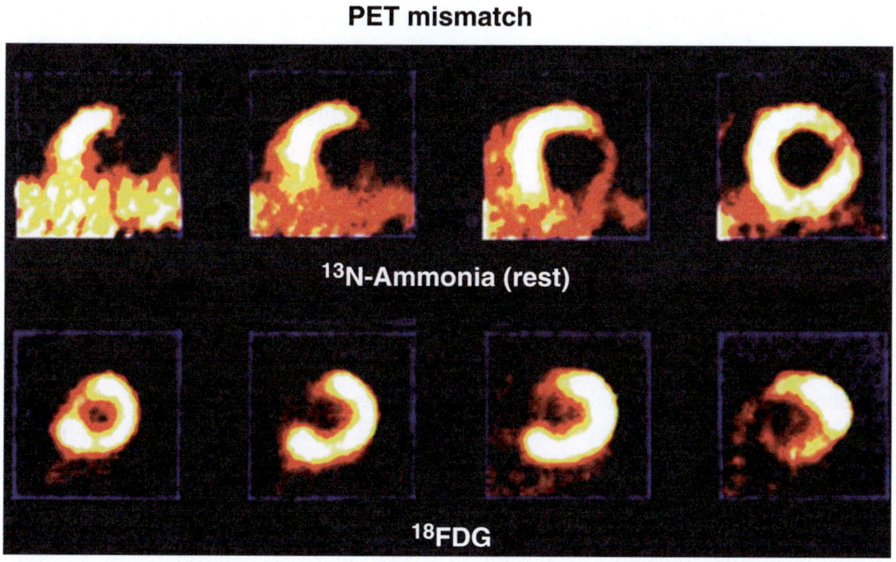

Fig. 16.4 Example of FDG mismatch for myocardial Viability. NH3 ammonia perfusion on the *upper row* shows minimal uptake in the lateral and inferior walls, indicating no viability. The *lower row* demonstrates PE FDG activity in the same areas, consistent with viability in the inferior and lateral distribution

FDG viability imaging is performed by first using a glucose load, either intravenously or orally, to elevate blood sugar levels. The blood sugar levels are then lowered using insulin. Blood sugar must be closely monitored to identify a target blood sugar level for injecting FDG, usually at 150 mg/dL. Typical dosages of FDG are between 10 and 20 mCi, estimated to be 4–5 mSv radiation exposure. Viable myocardium can be identified in regions with little or no perfusion but with clear FDG uptake (FDG mismatch pattern). A matched pattern on cardiac PET, where both perfusion and metabolism are reduced, is consistent with scar (prior infarction), and non-viability.

Several studies have shown that the presence of glucose activity in the area of the hypoperfused myocardium indicates viability and subsequent revascularization results in better patient outcomes [38–40]. An example of a mismatch between perfusion and FDG is shown in Fig. 16.4. In this case, ^{13}N ammonia, a perfusion agent demonstrates little to no activity in the lateral and inferior wall. The FDG study demonstrates glucose activity in the hypoperfused area, an indication for myocardial viability.

Myocardial viability assessment for patients being considered for CABG has been a mainstay in the decision to proceed to surgery. However, this approach recently came under scrutiny from the data of the STICH trial [35]. In this prospective trial, neither thallium-201 nor technetium 99-m viability assessment was shown to be predictive of outcomes. This trial was not one of a prospective randomization based upon imaging results, which may have contributed to the outcomes. It should be noted that FDG imaging was not part of the STICH trial and may have been more effective at identifying hibernating myocardium. Several other prospective studies conducted do demonstrate value of FDG imaging for viability assessment [39–41]. These data as well as the concept of PET FDG imaging suggest this is a very useful tool for assessment of myocardial viability and is currently being used in many centers in both Canada and the United States.

Inflammation/Infection Imaging with PET

Cardiovascular PET imaging has moved into areas unrelated to assessment of patients for CAD. This takes advantage of the properties of FDG as well as potentially other PET tracers. As an example, FDG imaging has been applied to assess the presence of cardiac sarcoidosis activity. Sarcoidosis is a systemic inflammatory disease which affects many organ systems throughout the body. Although systemic sarcoidosis often has a favorable outcome, when the myocardium is involved, the morbidity and mortality rate increases substantially. Cardiac sarcoidosis has been identified in as many as 25 % of all patients with systemic sarcoid and may lead to heart block, ventricular arrhythmias, and eventually heart failure and a worse prognosis [42]. Steroids and other therapies may prevent and even improve the progression of left ventricular dysfunction thus having effective diagnostic methods is essential.

Assessment of cardiac involvement with sarcoidosis is difficult because standardized tests for diagnosis are still developing (echo, PET, MR) and the therapies such as steroids or methotrexate have considerable side effects and may not offer benefit. Further, because of the focal nature of cardiac involvement, diagnosis, including myocardial biopsy has been difficult [42].

PET evaluation of cardiac involvement of sarcoidosis using FDG imaging has been used in the clinical arena for several years [43–45]. Recent data has been accumulating to demonstrate the clinical value sarcoid assessment, risk stratification and therapy monitoring using FDG PET. Blankstein and colleagues in 2014 reported that an abnormal FDG PET study carries a higher risk of cardiac death/ventricular tachycardia than normal and even higher in patients with perfusion abnormalities [46]. The presence of FDG activity in the right ventricle places the patient at a particularly high risk. Figure 16.5 demonstrates a patient with FDG activity in the left ventricle consistent with sarcoid inflammation. Data have been published using sarcoid assessment in identifying patients for implantable cardioverter defibrillator therapy [47, 48]. Recent data suggest that therapies can make a difference in patient outcomes, especially when cardiac FDG uptake is reduced on subsequent imaging [49].

Protocols for evaluation of cardiac sarcoidosis are not standardized. However, a principal is to patient preparation for the assessment of sarcoidosis is to first suppress glucose metabolism. A metabolic change is induced by using a glucose free diet using high fat dietary preparation. This suppresses glucose metabolism in the

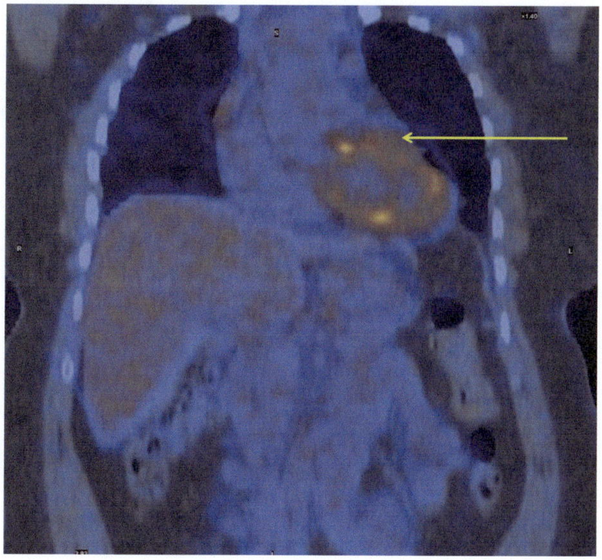

Fig. 16.5 Example of FDG uptake in the myocardium of a patient with systemic sarcoid, indicating active cardiac inflammation

myocardium and, allowing the uptake in the sarcoid lesions to be visualized. Theoretically this uptake relates to active inflammation, not necessarily sarcoid tissue changes.

Additional diagnostic applications of cardiac PET are possible, including the detection of amyloidosis with FDG imaging and resting myocardial perfusion (generally using rubidium or ammonia PET. More recently, FDG PET has also been applied to infections both within and without the heart including the following indications: evaluation of prosthetic valves [50], implanted devices [51] and graft infections [52]. Further studies are needed to fully validate these applications, but several laboratories are currently using these procedures clinically. Further down the line of development is an F-18 neuronal imaging agent, similar in properties to mIBG, but with much higher image quality, a substantial current limitation [53, 54].

Radiation Exposure

Radiation exposure has become an important aspect of all procedures which utilize ionizing radiation, including x-ray, CT and nuclear imaging. Efforts are being made on a national level to encourage reduction of radiation exposure in individual patients by reducing the number of repeat studies, reducing the dose of radiotracers administered and using new technologies to accomplish those goals. An information statement from ASNC has recommended at least 50 % of patients in a given laboratory receive <9 mSv for a routine study [55] and that PET is preferred over standard SPECT for radiation reduction.

The radiation exposure for both available PET flow tracers has been examined and has demonstrated that patient exposure is below that recommended by ASNC [55]. Senthamizhchelvan et al. determined the radiation dose of Rubidium-82 to be 0.9 mSv per 20 mCi [3], for an individual patient radiation exposure for rest/stress Rb-82 ranges of 2–5.4 mSv, depending upon camera systems and tracer dose. Changing from 2D to 3D imaging promises further reductions without loss of image quality; potentially improving systems sensitivity [56, 57]. Radiation exposure for NH3 ammonia is 4–6 mSv, and for FDG studies also 5–7 mSv. Hunter et.al. also compared radiation exposure in an average 75 kg person [58] and found significant radiations dose reductions using Rb-82 PET in their laboratory compared with reported radiation doses for Thallium 201 and Tc-99 m SPECT [2] (see Table 16.1).

Cardiac PET Patient Selection and Protocols

Clinical PET Perfusion Imaging

Selecting the patient for cardiac PET perfusion imaging is emerging based upon several features. Of importance, the Appropriate Use Criteria [59–61] established by the American College of Cardiology and sponsoring organizations state that these criteria can be used for all radionuclide imaging, thereby also including PET. In general, CMS (Centers for Medicare and Medicare Services) approve the use of PET at the discretion of individual physicians. Insurance companies and Radiology Business Manager (RBM) organizations vary considerably in payment for cardiac PET. The most commons approvals are for patients with BMI over 30 (sometimes 40) or an inconclusive SPECT study. Thus, if cardiac PET is available patient selection intead SPECT is important. The accepted reasons for performing PET over SPECT include the following considerations:

1. **Is the patient able to exercise**? Approximately 95 % of cardiac PET perfusion imaging is performed with the agent rubidium-82. The rubidium half-life of 75 s precludes exercise in patients, as the tracer needs to be injected with the patient under the camera. Ammonia-13 use is limited because of a short half-life of 10 min and because it is cyclotron produced. Because of the short half-life, the cyclotron needs to be within very close proximity or on campus, rarely occurring. Exercise with ammonia is possible, but difficult. Thus, if a patient can perform adequate exercise, SPECT imaging is recommended, as it is impractical to perform exercise routinely with PET. Patients who can exercise should not be routinely changed to pharmacologic stress just based on test preference, as there is no literature supporting superiority. This may change when any of the F-18 agents (cyclotron produced, but 2 h half-life) are FDA approved. However, for some patients with adequate exercise capacity, there still may be some value to cardiac PET as described below.

2. **Is the patient going to undergo pharmacologic stress**? In this case patients unable to undergo exercise, PET perfusion imaging offers a fast, efficient test with high diagnostic accuracy and low radiation exposure (2–6 mSv). A recent Information Statement by the American Society of Nuclear Cardiology regarding radiation exposure recommended the use of Cardiac PET when available to offer the lowest radiation exposure to the patient possible [55]. In practices in which both SPECT and PET are available, pharmacologic stress with PET is generally recommended in all such patients.
3. **Inconclusive SPECT study**? This is a commonly accepted indication for PET, regardless of whether the previous SPECT study was performed by exercise or pharmacologic stress. However, the objective may be to avoid these situations by performing PET first in certain patients.
4. **Is the patient Obese**? Cardiac PET uses radiotracers with energy levels approximately fourfold higher than SPECT agents. This offers considerably less attenuation artifact, especially in obese patients as well is much improved image quality. Furthermore, the routine application of attenuation correction in PET reduces the number of inconclusive tests due to soft tissue attenuation. One of the most commonly approved indications for PET is in obese patients, due to superior image quality and accuracy. In most cases, exercise capacity in such patients is limited.
5. **Patients with known CAD**. In patients with known CAD, especially those post procedures (PCI or CABG), the questions are generally very specific for re-stenosis (PCI) or evaluation for new disease vs incomplete revascularization in the case of CABG. Cardiac PET offers better discrimination between single and multi-vessel ischemia [6] and this test is can provide critical direction towards no catheterization or if the latter, CABG vs PCI.
6. **Concern for limiting radiation exposure**. Radiation exposure is an important societal concern, especially in younger patients and especially in women. As such, cardiac PET may be preferred in selected patient groups (Table 16.1).

Appropriate Use Criteria as It Relates to Cardiac PET

The Appropriate Use Criteria (AUC) for cardiac radionuclide imaging (RNI) was first published in 2005 (Hendel et al.) and updated in 2009 [60]. This was followed by further publications including 2014 [61] which was for multimodality imaging and the terms “Appropriate”, “Uncertain” and “Inappropriate” were replaced by “Appropriate”, “May be Appropriate” or “Rarely Appropriate” In these AUC publications PET and SPECT MPI were categorized under the same heading of cardiac RNI. A more detailed description of the AUC and its complete use is reviewed in the SPECT Section, Chap. 20. Below are selected examples which may apply to cardiac PET.

Detection of CAD/Risk Assessment

Symptomatic Patients Includes Those with Chest Pain Syndromes or Angina Equivalent

Stress PET is considered **Appropriate** for the following indications in these patients.

(a) Low pre-test probability of CAD with uninterpretable ECG or unable to exercise.
(b) Intermediate pre-test probability of CAD with interpretable ECG and able to exercise
(c) Intermediate pre-test probability of CAD with uninterpretable ECG or unable to exercise.
(d) High pre-test probability of CAD with interpretable ECG and able to exercise.

High pre-test probability of CAD with uninterpretable ECG or unable to exercise.

For symptomatic patients with Low pre-test probability of CAD with interpretable ECG and able to exercise, the use of stress imaging is considered Rarely Appropriate.

Asymptomatic Patients (Without Symptoms or Ischemic Equivalent)

In general, any testing of asymptomatic patients with either SPECT for PET is considered Rarely Appropriate. PET imaging is not considered Appropriate for these patients irrespective of their overall global coronary heart disease risk (CHD), interpretability of the ECG and ability to exercise. The use of Calcium Scoring is gaining favor, and may be performed with a PET/CT camera.

(a) The following indications are considered **Rarely Appropriate** in asymptomatic patients: Low global CHD risk, regardless of ECG interpretability and ability to exercise.
(b) Intermediate global CHD risk with interpretable ECG and able to exercise.

The following indications are considered **May be Appropriate**:

(a) Intermediate global CHD risk with uninterpretable ECG or unable to exercise.
(b) High global CAD risk with interpretable ECG and able to exercise.
(c) High global CAD risk with uninterpretable ECG or unable to exercise.

In Patients with Other Cardiovascular Conditions

In patients with newly diagnosed systolic or diastolic heart failure patients without prior CAD evaluation cardiac PET Imaging is considered Appropriate. In patients without ischemic equivalent and no prior cardiac evaluation PET imaging is considered Appropriate in evaluation of patients with sustained ventricular tachycardia (VT), ventricular fibrillation, exercise induced VT or non-sustained VT, frequent premature ventricular complexes (PVC), or prior to initiation of antiarrhythmic therapy in patients with high global CAD risk. In patients with infrequent PVCs and new onset atrial fibrillation (AF) use of PET imaging is regarded as May Be Appropriate.

In patients with syncope without ischemic equivalent, cardiac PET imaging is graded as Appropriate in those with intermediate or high global CAD risk and May be Appropriate in those with low global risk.

Prior Testing

Prior Testing Without Intervening Revascularization

A. In patients with abnormal prior testing repeat testing within 90 days is considered "Appropriate" in the following scenarios:

    (a) Abnormal rest ECG findings (potentially ischemic in nature such as LBBB, T-wave inversions) in patients with low global CAD risk.
    (b) Abnormal rest ECG findings (potentially ischemic in nature such as LBBB, T-wave inversions) in patients with intermediate to high global CAD risk.
    (c) Abnormal prior exercise ECG test.
    (d) Obstructive CAD on prior coronary CT study or angiography.
    (e) Abnormal prior cardiac CT calcium score (Agaston score >100)

B. In patients with uncertain results from prior testing, repeat testing within 90 days with equivocal, borderline or discordant prior noninvasive evaluation where obstructive CAD remains a concern performing a PET scan is graded "Appropriate" when the prior test was an exercise ECG test or a coronary CT. In the case in which the prior study was a stress SPECT study, performing a repeat PET scan is considered "May be Appropriate".
C. In Asymptomatic or stable patients follow up testing after 90 days:

    - In patients with abnormal prior exercise ECG, stress imaging, coronary CT or angiogram test repeating a PET scan within 2 years is graded "Rarely Appropriate", and beyond 2 years as "May Be Appropriate".
    - In patients with prior coronary Agatston score of <100 repeating PET scan is considered as Rarely Appropriate. In patients with low to intermediate or high global CAD risk and Agatston score between 100 and 400 and those with a score above 400, repeat scan is graded May be Appropriate.
    - In asymptomatic patients with normal prior exercise ECG, stress imaging, or angiogram (invasive or noninvasive) testing repeat scan is marked Rarely Appropriate in those with low CAD risk and intermediate to high CAD risk with the test done within the last 2 years. If the patient with intermediate to high CAD risk had a normal test ≥2 years ago repeat PET is considered May Be Appropriate.

- In patients with stable symptoms and normal prior exercise ECG, stress imaging, or angiogram (invasive or noninvasive) testing repeat scan is marked Rarely Appropriate in those with low CAD risk and intermediate to high CAD risk with the test done within the last 2 years. If the patient with intermediate to high CAD risk had a normal test ≥2 years ago repeat PET is considered May Be Appropriate.

D. Follow up testing in patients with new or worsening symptoms:

- In patients with normal or abnormal prior exercise ECG testing, non-obstructive or obstructive disease on angiogram (invasive or noninvasive), abnormal CCTA calcium score >100, or normal prior stress imaging, performing a PET scan is graded Appropriate.
- Repeating PET imaging with an already abnormal prior stress imaging is considered May Be Appropriate.

Post Revascularization (PCI or CABG)

- In symptomatic patients performing a PET scan is considered Appropriate.
- In asymptomatic patients performing a scan is considered Appropriate only in the setting of incomplete revascularization when additional revascularization is being considered.
- In asymptomatic patients with prior left main stent, ≥5 years after CABG or ≥2 years after PCI, repeating a PET scan is graded as May be Appropriate.
- In asymptomatic patients <5 years after CABG or <2 years after PCI, repeating a PET scan is graded as Rarely Appropriate.

Tracer Selection for Cardiac PET Perfusion Imaging

Once the patient is determined a candidate for cardiac PET perfusion imaging, protocol selection is based upon the tracer used and the reason for the study. This section will discuss cardiac PET tracers currently available. The three FDA-approved PET radionuclide tracers for clinical cardiac applications are Rubidium-82(82Rb), N-13 Ammonia (^{13}NH3) and Fluorine-18 Fluorodeoxyglucose (18 F-FDG). ^{82}Rb and ^{13}NH3 are used as perfusion agents while 18 F-FDG has been used as viability tracer and more recently for identification of inflammation/infection. FDG is not useful as a stress perfusion agent.

Rubidium-82

The most commonly used PET perfusion tracer is Rubidium-82. Its mechanism of uptake is a cation and a K^+analog, similar to thallium-201 [62–65]. It has a first-pass extraction of 65 % (less than Ammonia but substantially higher than current SPECT technetium tracers) [66–68] and utilizes energy for myocardial uptake via Na/K--ATPase pump [63, 64]. ^{82}Rb has a half-life of 75 seconds. Because the patient has very little tracer activity at the end of the test, radiation exposure to the staff and public can be minimized. One of the major advantages of ^{82}Rb over $^{13}NH_3$ is that ^{82}Rb is produced in a commercially available generator by decay from ^{82}Sr without the need for a cyclotron. The parent ^{82}Sr has a half-life of 25.5 days; thus, the same generator is used for 4–6 weeks for ^{82}Rb production, and can be delivered on-site. Protocols for ^{82}Rb are very efficient and in situations in which a PET/CT camera is available, a rest/stress study can be completed in less than 30 min. Protocols using dedicated PET cameras with line source attenuation correction can be completed within 45 min.

NH3-Ammonia

^{13}NH3 ammonia was the first cardiac PET tracer developed and subsequently approved for clinical use by the FDA. It is cyclotron-produced, and because of the short half-life, 10 min, the production site must be very close to or on location of the clinical site. The necessity for an on-site cyclotron has limited ammonia use clinically. Recently, "desk-top" cyclotrons have been developed to be placed in the same facility as the stress laboratory and may make this agent more practical for use, but as of present has not been implemented. Part of the interest in this agent is that ^{13}N-ammonia has an excellent first-pass extraction of 80 % exhibiting a linear relationship with myocardial blood flow up to very high flow rates [68]. It provides high quality images with excellent spatial resolution with a clear blood-to-myocardial delineation. A disadvantage of ammonia is decreased retention in the lateral wall compared to the rest of the myocardium, which is yet to be explained [68, 69]. This tracer suffers from significant liver and lung uptake particularly in patients with heart congestion leading to artifacts [70]. Despite these limitations, image quality is excellent in experienced laboratories.

F-18 Perfusion Imaging

^{18}F-flurpiridaz is a perfusion tracer under Phase III investigation in the United States. As with other F-18 agents, it has a longer half-life of 110 min (compared to rubidium or ammonia) allowing regional production possible and unit delivery to clinical sites. This longer half-life also makes this agent compatible with exercise stress testing potentially expanding the role of cardiac PET imaging in such patients who have good exercise capacity, currently not considered appropriate. This agent has excellent spatial resolution owing to its short positron range and it has almost a linear uptake proportional to the blood flow; potential leading to higher sensitivity to smaller defects and accurate flow quantification [71–73].

Another potential candidate for a perfusion PET agent is BFPET. BFPET is a PET perfusion imaging agent undergoing preliminary Phase II evaluation [74]. Further development is need to establish its efficacy, but Phase I data does indicate reasonable myocardial uptake [75].

Stress Modality for Cardiac PET Imaging

Pharmacological stress is the most commonly employed stress modality for current PET perfusion studies utilizing ^{82}Rb and ^{13}NH3. This can be performed using vasodilator stress (regadenoson, dipyridamole or adenosine) or inotropic stress (dobutamine). Rubidium-82. In general, patients who can exercise sufficiently for testing purposes are more often referred for SPECT imaging.

Exercise PET MPI, both treadmill [76] and supine bicycle [77, 78] is feasible for ^{13}NH3 and has been shown to induce larger and more severe stress and ischemic perfusion defects as compared to dipyridamole [78] stress in patient achieving adequate exercise level. However the successful performance of the exercise stress ^{13}NH3 PET requires significant coordination of the cyclotron laboratory and the imaging team. Currently, F-18 Flurpiridaz which is in Phase 3 has more favorable pharmacodynamics characteristics including longer half -life to make exercise testing a viable option in the future.

PET Contraindications

Contraindications to Cardiac PET are the same as other stress protocols, such as ability to safely perform exercise and specific conditions for pharmacologic stress agents such as regadenoson, adenosine, dobutamine and dipyridamole. Claustrophobia may be an issue in some patients. s. Cardiac PET cameras require entry by the patient into the “bore” which varies in depth depending on the camera With some patients claustrophobia may be an issue. The staff should discuss this with the patients prior to the entry into the laboratory. Some patients respond successfully to medications, but then need to provide alternate forms of transportation as these medications render driving unsafe.

References

1. Richards KA, Heller GV. Cardiac positron emission tomography. Nuclear Cardiology: Practical Applications. 2nd ed. McGraw Hill. 2010. p. 149–59.
2. Strauss HW, Miller DD, Wittry MD, Cerqueira MD, Garcia EV, Iskandrian AS, Schelbert HR, Wackers FJ, Balon HR, Lang O, Machac J. Procedure guideline for myocardial perfusion imaging. J Nucl Med Technol. 2008;36(3):155–61.
3. Senthamizhchelvan S, Bravo PE, Esaias C, et al. Human biodistribution and radiation dosimetry of 82Rb. J Nucl Med. 2010;51:1592–9.
4. Package insert for N-13 ammonia, January 5, 2011. The Feinstein institute for medical research, Manhasset.
5. ICRP Publication 106, Annex C biokinetic models and dose tables. Ann ICRP. 2008;38(1–2): 51–162.
6. Abbara S, Arbab-Zadeh A, Callister TQ, Milind Y, Desai MY, Mamuya W, Thomson L, Weigold G. SCCT guidelines for performance of coronary computed tomographic angiography:

a report of the society of cardiovascular computed tomography guidelines committee. J Cardiovasc Comput Tomogr. 2009;3:190–204.
7. Delichas MG, Psarrakos K, Molyvda-Athanassopoulou E, Giannoglou G, Hatziioannou K, Papanastassiou E. Radiation doses to patients undergoing coronary angiography and percutaneous transluminal coronary angioplasty. Radiat Prot Dosim. 2003;103:149–54.
8. Parker MW, Iskandar A, Limone B, et al. Diagnostic accuracy of cardiac positron emission tomography versus single photon emission computed tomography for coronary artery disease; a bivariate meta-analysis. Circ Cardiovasc Imaging. 2012;5:700–7.
9. McArdle BA, Dowsley TF, deKemp RA. Does Rubidium-82 have superior Accuracy to SPECT perfusion imaging for the diagnosis of obstructive coronary disease? A systematic review and meta-analysis. J Am Coll Cardiol. 2012;60:1828–37.
10. Bateman T, Heller GV, McGhie I, et al. Diagnostic accuracy of rest/stress ECG-gated rubidium-82 myocardial perfusion PET: comparison with ECG-gated Tc-99m-sestamibi SPECT. J Nucl Cardiol. 2006;12:24–33.
11. Dorbala S, Di Carli MF, Beanlands RS, et al. Prognostic value of stress myocardial perfusion positron emission tomography: results from a multicenter observational registry. J Am Coll Cardiol. 2013;15(61):176–84.
12. Merhige ME, Breen WJ, Shelton V, et al. Impact of myocardial perfusion imaging with PET and (82)Rb on downstream invasive procedure utilization, costs, and outcomes in coronary disease management. J Nucl Med. 2007;48:1069–76.
13. Hachamovitch R, Nutter B, Hlatky MA, et al. Patient management after noninvasive cardiac imaging results from SPARC (Study of myocardial perfusion and coronary anatomy imaging roles in coronary artery disease). J Am Coll Cardiol. 2012;31(59):462–74.
14. Lortie M, Beanlands RS, Yoshinaga K, Klein R, DaSilva JN, deKemp RA. Quantification of myocardial blood flow with 82Rb dynamic PET imaging. Eur J Nucl Med Mol Imaging. 2007;34:1765–74.
15. Yoshida K, Mullani N, Gould KL. Coronary flow and flow reserve by PET simplified for clinical applications using rubidium-82 or nitrogen-13-Ammonia. J Nucl Med. 1996;37:1701–12.
16. Herrero P, Markham J, Shelton ME, Bergmann SR, Herrero. Implementation and evaluation of a two-compartment model for quantification of myocardial perfusion with rubidium-82 and positron emission tomography. Circ Res. 1992;70(3):496.
17. Nesterov SV, et al. Quantification of myocardial blood flow in absolute terms using ^{82}Rb PET imaging: the RUBY-10 study. J Am Coll Cardiol Img. 2014;7:1119–27.
18. Renaud JM, DaSilva JN, Beanlands RS, DeKemp RA. Characterizing the normal range of myocardial blood flow with ^{82}rubidium and ^{13}N-ammonia PET imaging. J Nucl Cardiol. 2013;20(4):578–91.
19. Czernin J1, Müller P, Chan S, Brunken RC, Porenta G, Krivokapich J, Chen K, Chan A, Phelps ME, Schelbert HR. Influence of age and hemodynamics on myocardial blood flow and flow reserve. Circulation. 1993;88(1):62.
20. Goudarzi B. Comparison of the myocardial blood flow response to regadenoson and dipyridamole: a quantitative analysis in patients referred for clinical 82Rb myocardial perfusion PET. Eur J Nucl Med Mol Imaging. 2011;38(10):1908–16.
21. Naya M, Murthy VL, Taqueti VR, et al. Preserved coronary flow reserve effectively excludes high-risk coronary artery disease on angiography. J Nucl Med Off Publ Soc Nucl Med. 2014;55(2):248–55.
22. Ziadi MC1, Dekemp RA, Williams K, Guo A, Renaud JM, Chow BJ, Klein R, Ruddy TD, Aung M, Garrard L, Beanlands RS. Does quantification of myocardial flow reserve using rubidium-82 positron emission tomography facilitate detection of multivessel coronary artery disease? J Nucl Cardiol. 2012;19(4):670–80.
23. Kajander SA, Joutsiniemi E, Saraste M, et al. Clinical value of absolute quantification of myocardial perfusion with 15O-water in coronary artery disease. Circ Cardiovasc Imaging. 2011;4:678–84.
24. Yoshinaga K, Katoh C, Noriyasu K, et al. Reduction of coronary flow reserve in areas with and without ischemia on stress perfusion imaging in patients with coronary artery disease: a study using oxygen 15 labeled water PET. J Nucl Cardiol. 2003;10:275–83.

25. Ziadi MC, Dekemp RA, Williams KA, et al. Impaired myocardial flow reserve on rubidium-82 positron emission tomography imaging predicts adverse outcomes in patients assessed for myocardial ischemia. J Am Coll Cardiol. 2011;9(58):740–8.
26. Murthy VL, Naya M, Foster CR, et al. Improved cardiac risk assessment with noninvasive measures of coronary flow reserve. Circulation. 2011;124:2215–24.
27. Dorbala S, Vangala D, Sampson U, et al. Value of vasodilator left ventricular ejection fraction reserve in evaluating the magnitude of myocardium at risk and the extent of angiographic coronary artery disease: a 82Rb PET/CT study. J Nucl Med. 2007;48:349–58.
28. Herzog BA, Husmann L, Valenta I, et al. Long-term prognostic value of 13N-ammonia myocardial perfusion positron emission tomography: added value of coronary flow reserve. J Am Coll Cardiol. 2009;54(2):150–6.
29. Brunken RC, Chen MS, Lohmann KA, Howe WC, Bruckbauer T, Kaczur T, Bynel B, DiFilippo. LVEF measurements from cardiac PET/CT images obtained using CT based attenuation correction. J Nucl Cardiol. 2004;11(4):S13.
30. Slart RH, Bax JJ, de Jong RM, de Boer J, Lamb HJ, Mook PH, Willemsen AT, Vaalburg W, van Veldhuisen DJ, Jager PL. Comparison of gated PET with MRI for evaluation of left ventricular function in patients with coronary artery disease. J Nucl Med. 2004;45(2):176–82.
31. Dorbala S, Hachamovitch R, Curillova Z, et al. Incremental prognostic value of gated Rb-82 positron emission tomography myocardial perfusion imaging over clinical variables and rest LVEF. JACC Cardiovasc Imaging. 2009;2:846–54.
32. Lertsburapa K, Ahlberg AW, Bateman TM, et al. Independent and incremental prognostic value of left ventricular ejection fraction determined by stress gated rubidium 82 PET imaging in patients with known or suspected coronary artery disease. J Nucl Cardiol. 2008;15:745–53.
33. Auerbach MA, Schöder H, Hoh C, et al. Prevalence of myocardial viability as detected by positron emission tomography in patients with ischemic cardiomyopathy. Circulation. 1999;99:2921–6.
34. Allman KC, Shaw LJ, Hachamovitch R, et al. Myocardial viability testing and impact of revascularization on prognosis in patients with coronary artery disease and left ventricular dysfunction: a meta-analysis. J Am Coll Cardiol. 2002;39:1151–8.
35. Bonow RO, Maurer G, Lee KL, et al. Myocardial viability and survival in ischemic left ventricular dysfunction. N Engl J Med. 2011;364:1617–25.
36. Tarakji KG, Brunken R, McCarthy PM, Al-Chekakie MO, Abdel-Latif A, Pothier CE, Blackstone EH, Lauer MS. Myocardial viability testing and the effect of early intervention in patients with advanced left ventricular systolic dysfunction. Circulation. 2006;113:230–7.
37. Tillisch J, Brunken R, Marshall R, et al. Reversibility of cardiac wall-motion abnormalities predicted by positron tomography. N Engl J Med. 1986;314:884–8.
38. Egert S, Nguyen N, Brosius III FC, et al. Effects of wortmannin on insulin- and ischemia-induced stimulation of GLUT4 translocation and FDG uptake in perfused rat hearts. Cardiovasc Res. 1997;35:283–93.
39. Beanlands RSB, Nichol G, Huszti E, et al. F-18-fluorodeoxyglucose positron emission tomography imaging-assisted management of patients with severe left ventricular dysfunction and suspected coronary disease. A randomized controlled trial (PARR-2). J Am Coll Cardiol. 2007;50(20):2002–12.
40. Maddahi J. Factors influencing predictive value of FDG imaging for evaluating myocardial viaibility. J Nucl Cardiol. 2004;11(5):524–6.
41. Beller GA. More evidence for the survival benefit of coronary revascularization versus medical therapy in patients with ischemic cardiomyopathy and hibernating myocardium. Circ Cardiovasc Imaging. 2013;6:355–7.
42. Silverman KJ, Hutchins GM, et al. Cardiac sarcoid: a clinico-pathologic study of 84 unselected patients with systemic sarcoidosis. Circulation. 1978;58:1204–11.
43. Ishmaru S, Tsujino I, Takei T, et al. Focal uptake on 18F-fluoro-2 deoxyglucose positron emission tomography images indicates cardiac involvement of sarcoidosis. Eur Heart J. 2005;26: 1538–43.

44. Yamagishi H, Shirai N, Takagi M. Identification of Cardiac Sarcoidosis with (13)N-NH(3)/(18)F-FDG PET. J Nucl Med. 2003;44:1030–6.
45. Kida K, Yoncyama K, Kohayashi Y, Takano M, Akashi YJ, Miyake F. Late gadolinium enhancement on cardiac magnetic resonance images diagnostic standard and guidelines for sarcoidosis (in Japanese). Jpn J Sarcoidosis Granulomatous Disord. 2007;27:89–102.
46. Blankstein R, Osborne M, Naya M, et al. Cardiac positron emission tomography enhances prognostic assessments of patients with suspected cardiac sarcoidosis. J Am Coll Cardiol. 2014;63:329–36.
47. Schuller JL, Zipse M, Crawford T, et al. Implantable cardioverter defibrillator therapy in patients with cardiac sarcoidosis. J Cardiovasc Electrophysiol. 2012;23:925–9.
48. Betensky BP, Tschabrunn CM, Zado ES, et al. Long-term follow-up of patients with cardiac sarcoidosis and implantable cardioverter defibrillators. Heart Rhythm. 2012;9:884–91.
49. Osborne MT, Hulten EA, Singh A, et al. Reduction in 18F-fluorodeoxyglucose uptake on serial cardiac positron emission tomography is associated with improved left ventricular ejection fraction in patients with cardiac sarcoidosis. J Nucl Cardiol. 2014;21:166–74.
50. Saby L, Laas O, Habib G, et al. Positron emission tomography/computed tomography for diagnosis of prosthetic valve endocarditis: increased valvular 18F-fluorodeoxyglucose uptake as a novel major criterion. J Am Coll Cardiol. 2013;61:2374–82.
51. Sarrazin JF, Philippon F, Tessier M, et al. Usefulness of fluorine-18 positron emission tomography/computed tomography for identification of cardiovascular implantable electronic device infections. J Am Coll Cardiol. 2012;59:1616–25.
52. Saleem BR, Pol RA, Slart RH, et al. 18F-Fluorodeoxyglucose positron emission tomography/CT scanning in diagnosing vascular prosthetic graft infection. Biomed Res Int. 2014;2014:471971.
53. Jacobson AF, Senior R, Cerqueira MD. Myocardial iodine-123 meta-iodobenzylguanidine imaging and cardiac events in heart failure. Results of the prospective ADMIRE-HF (AdreView Myocardial Imaging for Risk Evaluation in Heart Failure) study. J Am Coll Cardiol. 2010;55:2212–21.
54. Sinusas AJ, Lazewatsky J2, Brunetti J, et al. Biodistribution and radiation dosimetry of LMI1195: first-in-human study of a novel 18F-labeled tracer for imaging myocardial innervation. J Nucl Med. 2014;55:1445–51.
55. Cerqueira MD, Allman KC, Ficaro EP, et al. Recommendations for reducing radiation exposure in myocardial perfusion imaging. J Nucl Cardiol. 2010;17:709–18.
56. Cherry SR, Dahlborn M, Hoffman EJ. 3D PET using a conventional multislice tomography without septa. J Comput Assist Tomogr. 1991;15(4):655–68.
57. Watson C, Newport D, Casey M, DeKemp R, Beanlands R, Schmand M. Evaluation of simulation-based scatter correction for 3-D PET cardiac imaging. IEEE Nucl Sci Symp Conf Rec. 1997;44:90–7.
58. Hunter C, Ziadi MC, Etele J, Hill J, et al. Rest and stress dosimetry for Rubidium-82 using new effective dose estimates based on dynamic PET/CT imaging in humans. J Nucl Med. 2010;26:40D–2.
59. Henzlova MJ, Cerqueira, MD, Hansen CL, et al. ASNC imaging guidelines for Nuclear cardiology procedures stress protocols and tracers. J Nucl Cardiol. 2009;16:164–94.
60. Hendel RC, Berman DS, Di Carli MF, et al. ACCF/ASNC/ACR/AHA/ASE/SCCT/SCMR/SNM 2009 Appropriate use criteria for Cardiac Radionuclide Imaging: a Report of the American College of Cardiology Foundation Appropriate Use Criteria Task Force, the American Society of Nuclear Cardiology, the American College of Radiology, the American Heart Association, the American Society of Echocardiography, the Society of Cardiovascular Computed Tomography, the Society for Cardiovascular Magnetic Resonance, and the Society of Nuclear Medicine. J Am Coll Cardiol. 2009;53:2201–29.
61. Wolk MJ, Bailey SR, Doherty JU, et al. American College of Cardiology Foundation Appropriate use Criteria Task ACCF/AHA/ASE/ASNC/HFSA/HRS/SCAI/SCCT/SCMR/STS 2013 multimodality appropriate use criteria for the detection and risk assessment of stable

ischemic heart disease: a report of the American College of Cardiology Foundation Appropriate Use Criteria Task Force, American Heart Association, American Society of Echocardiography, American Society of Nuclear Cardiology, Heart Failure Society of America, Heart Rhythm Society, Society for Cardiovascular Angiography and Interventions, Society of Cardiovascular Computed Tomography, Society for Cardiovascular Magnetic Resonance, and Society of Thoracic Surgeons. J Am Coll Cardiol. 2014;63:380–06.

62. Garcia EV, Galt JR, Faber TL, et al. Principles of nuclear cardiology imaging. In: Dilsizian V, Jagat N, editors. Atlas of nuclear cardiology. 4th ed. New York: Springer Science; 2013. p. 1–53.
63. Love WD, Burch GE. A comparison of potassium 42, rubidium 86, and cesium 134 as tracers of potassium in the study of cation metabolism of human erythrocytes in-vitro. J Lab Clin Med. 1953;41:351–62.
64. Love WD, Romney RB, Burch GE. A comparison of the distribution of potassium and exchangeable rubidium in the organs of the dog, using rubidium. Circ Res. 1954;2:112–22.
65. Selwyn AP, Allan RM, L'Abbate A, et al. Relation between regional myocardial uptake of rubidium-82 and perfusion: absolute reduction of cation uptake in ischemia. Am J Cardiol. 1982;50:112–21.
66. Meerdink DJ, Leppo JA. Experimental studies of the physiologic properties of technetium-99m agents: myocardial transport of perfusion imaging agents. Am J Cardiol. 1990;66:9E–15.
67. Leppo JA, Meerdink DJ. Comparison of the myocardial uptake of a technetium-labeled isonitrile analogue and thallium. Circ Res. 1989;65:632–9.
68. Nienaber CA, Ratib O, Gambhir SS, et al. A quantitative index of regional blood flow in canine myocardium derived noninvasively with N-13 ammonia and dynamic positron emission tomography. J Am Coll Cardiol. 1991;17:260–9.
69. Beanlands RS, Muzik O, Hutchins GD, et al. Heterogeneity of regional nitrogen 13-labeled ammonia tracer distribution in the normal human heart: comparison with rubidium 82 and copper 62-labeled PTSM. J Nucl Cardiol. 1994;1:225–35.
70. Tamaki N, Ruddy TD, Dekamp R, et al. Myocardial perfusion. In: Wahl RL, Buchanan JW, editors. Principles and practice of positron emission tomography. Philadelphia: Lippincott, Williams & Wilkins; 2002. p. 320–33.
71. Huisman MC, Higuchi T, Reder S, et al. Initial characterization of an 18F-labeled myocardial perfusion tracer. J Nucl Med. 2008;49:630–6.
72. Nekolla SG, Reder S, Saraste A, et al. Evaluation of the novel myocardial perfusion positron-emission tomography tracer 18F-BMS-747158-02: comparison to 13N-ammonia and validation with microspheres in a pig model. Circulation. 2009;119:2333–42.
73. Yu M, Guaraldi MT, Mistry M, et al. BMS-747158-02: a novel PET myocardial perfusion imaging agent. J Nucl Cardiol. 2007;14:789–98.
74. Shoup TM, Elmaleh DR, Brownell AL, Zhu A, Guerrero JL, Fischman AJ. Evaluation of (4-[18F]Fluorophenyl)triphenylphosphonium ion. A potential myocardial blood flow agent for PET. Mol Imaging Biol. 2011;13(3):511–7.
75. Elmaleh D, Kardan A, Barrow S, Dragotakes A, Correia J, Weiss S, Goumnerov B, Kundakovic L, Gewirtz H, Fischman A. A phase I study evaluating dosimetry and myocardial pharmacokinetic behavior of BFPET, a new F-18 labeled tracer for myocardial perfusion imaging. J Nucl Med. 2009;50 Suppl 2:420.
76. Chow BJ, Beanlands RS, Lee A, et al. Treadmill exercise produces larger perfusion defects than dipyridamole stress N-13 ammonia positron emission tomography. J Am Coll Cardiol. 2006;47:411–6.
77. Tamaki N, Yonekura Y, Senda M, et al. Myocardial positron computed tomography with 13N-ammonia at rest and during exercise. Eur J Nucl Med Mol Imaging. 1985;11:246–51.
78. Krivokapich J, Smith GT, Huang SC, et al. 13N ammonia myocardial imaging at rest and with exercise in normal volunteers. Quantification of absolute myocardial perfusion with dynamic positron emission tomography. Circulation. 1989;80(5):1328–37.

Chapter 17
Cardiac PET Quality Control for Imaging, Patient Preparation and Reporting

James A. Case and Gary V. Heller

Abstract Cardiac positron emission tomographic imaging offers significant improvements in image quality over other nuclear approaches. These improvements can only be achieved with strict adherence to imaging protocols and quality control procedures. This begins with an understanding of the physics of PET, PET systems and the clinical differences of cardiac PET from other approaches. These core concepts can then be integrated into a process for reducing image artifacts, reducing radiation exposure and improving the patient care.

Keywords PET • Quality control • Myocardial perfusion imaging • Myocardial blood flow

Physics of PET Imaging: History of Cardiac PET

Positron Emission Tomography (PET), relies on the annihilation of a positively charged particle (an anti-electron or positron) with a conventional electron to produce two high energy gamma rays traveling 180° from each other. The prediction of the existence of positrons was first proposed by Paul Dirac in 1928 [1], and ultimately discovered in 1932 by Carl D. Anderson [2]. Positrons, though stable in vacuum, annihilate almost immediately when they come in contact with electrons; producing a complete conversion of the mass of the two particles (511 keV/c^2) into energy. This unique property of positrons, the complete conversion of the positron-electron pair into two photons of identical energies (511 keV), was recognized as

J.A. Case, PhD
Technical Director, Cardiovascular Imaging Technologies, Kansas City, MO, USA
e-mail: jcase@cvit.com

G.V. Heller, MD, PhD (✉)
Department of Cardiovascular Medicine, Morristown Medical Center, Atlantic Healthcare System, Gagnon Cardiovascular Institute, Morristown, NJ, USA

Research Section, Intersocietal Accreditation Commission, Ellicott City, MD, USA
e-mail: garyvheller@gmail.com

P.L. Tilkemeier et al. (eds.), *Quality Evaluation in Non-Invasive Cardiovascular Imaging*, DOI 10.1007/978-3-319-28011-0_17

potentially revolutionary for medical imaging. The first application of positron annihilation medical imaging was first explored in by Brownell et.al. 1953 for imaging brain tumors [3]. This technique was later expanded to tomographic imaging in 1971 [4].

Myocardial perfusion PET with ^{13}N ammonia was one of the first practical implementations of PET in the myocardium [5–7]. ^{13}N ammonia produces high quality myocardial perfusion images with favorable responses to changes in blood flow. The short half-life of ^{13}N requires a nearby cyclotron for production, thereby limiting the number of sites that can use it. A more practical approach is to employs a generator to produce the radionuclide. ^{82}Rb was studied in 1986 as a generator produced potassium analog for the detection of myocardial infarction [8–10]. Using a ^{82}Sr generator ($t_{1/2}$ – 28 days), a user could be provided with an on-site generator every 4 weeks.

Metabolic cardiac imaging continues to be of interest. ^{18}F labeled deoxyglucose (FDG) has long been used for imaging myocardial viability [11, 12] and has been also used for imaging of ischemic activation [13] and sarcoid imaging [14]. Additionally, metabolic agents have been explored for fatty acid metabolism and cardiac denervation [15, 16].

Positron Decay and Annihilation

The cascade of events of an annihilation event begins with an unstable parent atom. As the parent decays, a proton is converted into a neutron-positron-neutrino by product. The positron is then emitted at a high energy into the surrounding material.

In vacuum, this positron would be stable, similar to the electron. Like conventional beta emission, the positron first must thermalize in the medium prior to annihilation. Once at rest it will "pick-off" an electron from the surrounding material and annihilate, creating two 511 keV photons traveling 180° opposite from each other. The two photons travel exactly 180° from each other in the center of momentum frame, but not in the lab frame. The thermal motion of the positronium will create a small, but measurable relativistic shift in the angles the two photons when measured in the lab frame.

This thermalization length of the positron causes the annihilation event to drift from the parent radionuclide, reducing the overall resolution of the image. For ^{18}F, the maximum energy of the emerging positron is 633 keV, leading to a thermalization length is 0.239 cm [17, 18]. However for ^{82}Rb, the maximum energy of the positron is 3.148 MeV, leading to a maximum thermalization length of 1.561 cm.

Though many atoms, such as ^{18}F and ^{13}N decay to a stable nuclear state, some atoms, such as ^{82}Rb, can decay to an unstable nuclear state. For these atoms, the decay to an unstable state results in the emission of a nuclear gamma ray (a "prompt gamma") in addition to the two photons produced by the positron annihilation. In the case of ^{82}Rb, 13 % of all decays result in a prompt gamma ray (776 keV) [19]. These gamma rays can influence the scatter correction algorithms of the imaging system producing significant artifacts [20, 21].

PET Imaging Systems

Detector Systems

The detection of the two photons emitted from a positron annihilation event requires a system that can measure the energy and position of both of the 511 keV photons. In particular, the system must determine if any two photons received by the scanner are a true pair of annihilation photons (trues) or simply the chance coincidence of two un-related photon events.

Most PET scanners consist of a system of concentric rings of multiple detector blocks around a central axis. Each of these detectors consists of a scintillator crystal and a small array of photo-multiplier tubes (see Fig. 17.1). The physical properties of the scintillator crystal determine much of the performance of the PET scanner. Ideally, a scintillator crystal has a high stopping power (to reduce the depth the gamma rays penetrate before being recorded), high light output per event (needed to differentiate photon energies), and a rapid light curve decay (to minimize the time needed to record the photon event and have the crystal ready to receive the next event. Several common scintillator crystal properties are summarized in Table 17.1 [22, 23].

Response time of the system describes how effective a system can differentiate random events from true coincidence. To accomplish this, a coincidence timing window of <10 ns is needed to differentiate true pairs from random coincidence event. As challenging as that may appear, most modern PET scanners have coincidence windows of <5 ns, making it possible to not only differentiate the difference between randoms and trues, but utilize the differences in the arrival times of the two annihilation photons to localize the annihilation event along the line of site [24].

The intrinsic sensitivity of PET is typically much higher than SPECT due to the fact that localization of the annihilation event does not require the use of collimation. Despite this fact, a large number of PET imaging systems use a system of septa to reduce scatter and randoms. These septa significantly reduce the sensitivity of the imaging system, potentially increasing system sensitivity by a factor of two to five times [25]. Extraction of the septa can greatly improve system sensitivity and improve image quality (discussed later in this chapter).

Attenuation Correction

In contrast with SPECT, attenuation correction is almost always applied in the processing of cardiac PET [26]. The geometry of PET makes it possible to estimate attenuation without knowing the depth of the annihilation event in the patient. Unlike SPECT, the attenuation of a true event is the sum of the attenuation both 511 keV photons; specifically the total attenuation along the line of response

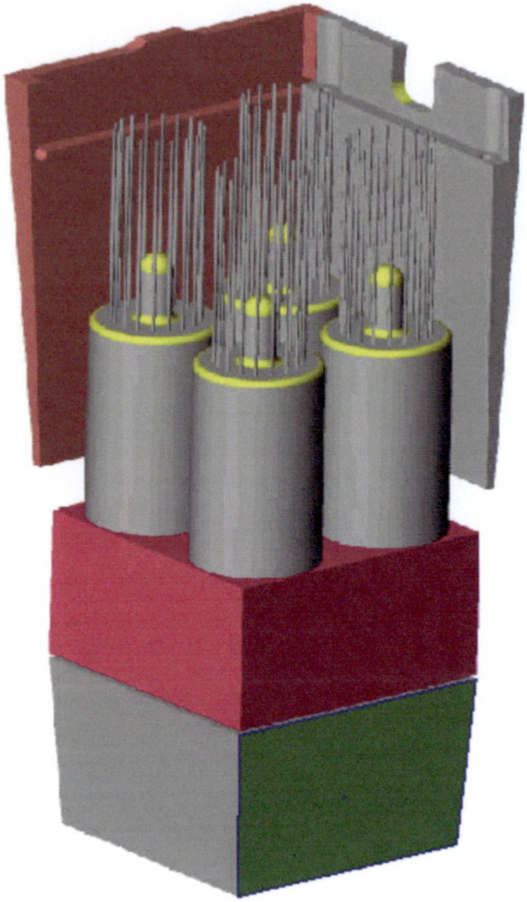

Fig. 17.1 Single detector of a PET scanner typically consists of a scintillator block and four photomultiplier tubes. The PET scanner consists of a concentric rings of these detector blocks in a 360° ring

Table 17.1 Listing of physical properties of common PET scintillator crystals

	LSO	GSO	BGO	NaI
Density (g/cc)	7.4	6.7	71.	3.6
Effective (Z)	66	59	75	51
Mean free path (cm)	1.16	1.43	1.05	2.88
Decay constant (ns)	40	60	300	230
Relative light yield	75	25	20	100

(see Fig. 17.2). Therefore, the correction that is applied is independent of where the annihilation event took place along a line of response.

The attenuation estimate can either be made using an external positron source or x-ray based computed tomography. Though, in principle either of these approaches can be used, their unique properties require different approaches to quality control.

Line source attenuation correction, "dedicated PET", typically utilizes an external Ge-68 line source rotating around the patient to create a patient specific map of

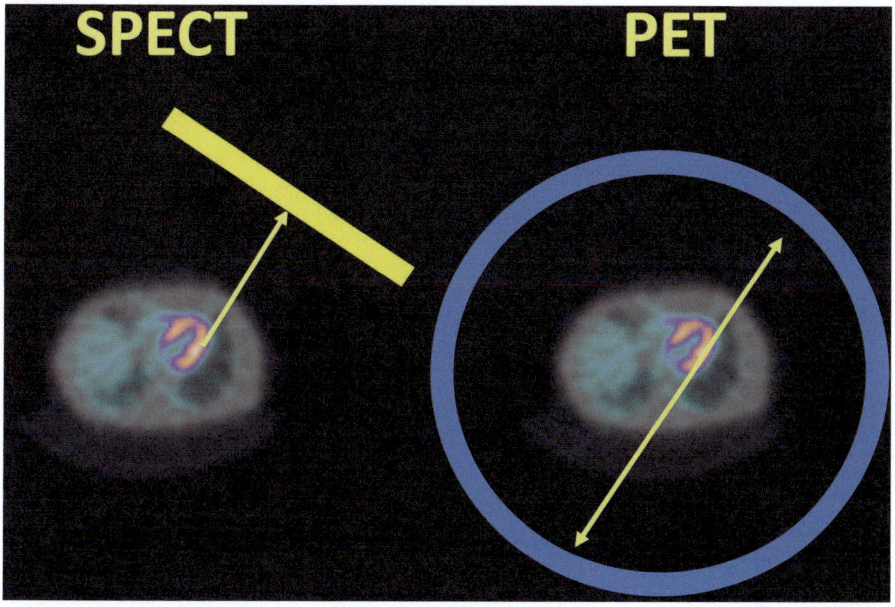

Fig. 17.2 The amount of attenuation in SPECT (*top*) is depend on the depth of the source radiation. The amount of attenuation in PET (*bottom*) is only dependent on the total attenuation along a line of site, making attenuation correction mathematically much more reliable

the attenuation. Because the source photons are positrons, there is no need to translate the attenuation coefficients from the transmission energy to the emission energy. Another advantage of dedicated PET is the attenuation map is acquired while the patient is free breathing. This reduces misregistration and breathing artifacts when compared to PET/CT [27, 28]. Finally, the radiation dosage from a dedicated PET scanner is typically less than an x-ray based CT (though dosage reducing strategies can be employed to minimize x-ray radiation dosage). One possible limitation of dedicated PET is some systems require long transmission acquisition scans (4–8 min). Newer reconstruction methods reduce the number of counts required, reducing the acquisition time to 60–90 s [29].

Another approach for obtaining the transmission study is to use a X-ray based CT attenuation correction using a hybrid PET/CT camera [30]. These cameras are equipped with a PET scanner and CT scanner fused to one another. When performing PET/CT, one should consider:

1. Minimization of the CT dosage attenuation correction. This may mean reducing the mAs and/or kVp of the acquisition. Newer acquisition protocols also allow for modulation of the tube current to reduce patient dosage [31].
2. Using an appropriate scanner pitch based on the manufacture's recommendation to optimize patient dosage, minimize patient breath-hold times and minimize misregistration artifacts. Coordination with the PET/CT scanner manufacturer is essential to establishing the optimal pitch.

3. Though implanted metal devices is not necessarily a contra-indication for PET/CT the user must confirm the appropriate corrections are present in the transmission reconstruction algorithm to remove these artifacts [32, 33].
4. Most PET/CT systems require some method of controlling the patient breathing. It is essential the user not only understand the breathing algorithm that is to be employed (free-breathing, in expiration, shallow free breathing, etc.) but train the patient on the correct breathing before the scan begins [33–36].

Randoms, Scatter Correction and Prompt Gamma

PET imaging also can be influence by photon scatter, random coincidences between unrelated photons (randoms), and contamination from nuclear gamma rays (prompt gamma contamination). Photon scatter in PET is caused by the scattering of the emitted photons off of electrons in the patients. This scattered radiation degrades image quality by reducing image contrast and distorting the final image. Scatter contamination in PET primarily reduces the overall contrast in the image, and to a lesser degree distorting the appearance of the image. When a photon is scatter in PET, it loses its correlation to the original annihilation event and its pair, causing the photon pair event to be recorded far from the annihilation event (see Fig. 17.3).

One of the challenges of 3D imaging is the increased photon scatter component requires accurate scatter compensation [37]. The most common approach utilizes a model based approach to estimate the scatter component [37–39]. These methods

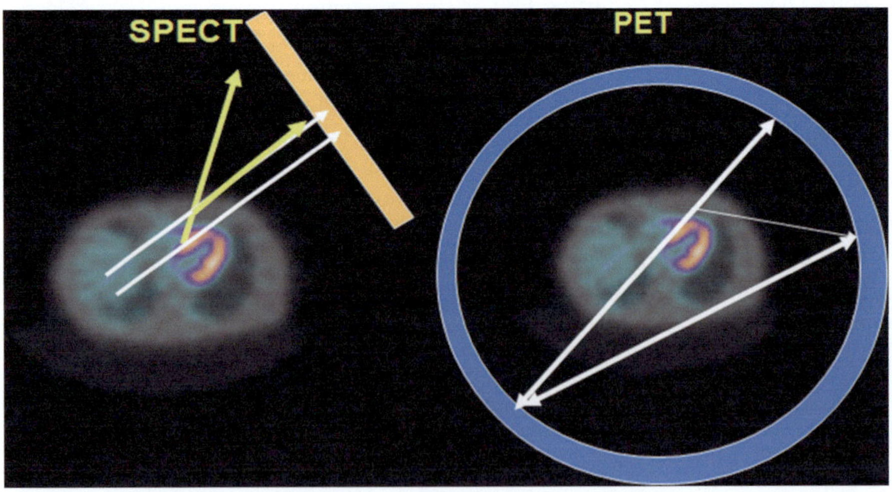

Fig. 17.3 When photons are scattered in SPECT (*top*), the recorded location of the scattered photon often near the location of the unscattered events. In PET (*bottom*), the location of a pair event is the combination of the scatter and unscattered photon event. Because of this, the scatter events have little correlation with the source distribution

perform well for ^{13}N and ^{18}F studies, however, they must be modified to account for the additional, 776 keV prompt gamma in 13 % of ^{82}Rb decay events [40]. When these photons are not accounted for, the over-correction for scatter can reduce specificity from 90 % to 22 % [20].

Random events (randoms), are a result of un-related photon events being recorded within the timing acceptance window of the system. Random events degrade image contrast, however because random photons are from unrelated annihilation events they largely only reduce overall image contrast. Hence, most randoms correction algorithm are implemented by subtracting a constant from the entire image [41].

Image Reconstruction

Because attenuation correction is applied prior to reconstruction, either filtered back projection (FBP) or iterative reconstruction can be used for creating three dimensional tomograms. Most modern reconstruction algorithms for PET utilize an iterative, ordered subsets/expectation maximization algorithm [42].

Iterative reconstruction algorithms use a step wise updating algorithm to "search" for a source distribution that could produce the projection data observed. It relies on a model (the projector), of the transport of photons through the patient to the camera. In principle, this projector can be used to model any physical process in the photon transport, thus giving it considerably more flexibility than the FBP algorithm.

Imaging Protocols

The American Society of Nuclear Cardiology has developed imaging guidelines for the development of cardiac PET imaging protocols and should be consulted when developing clinical protocols [43]. Almost all cardiac PET perfusion studies are performed using vasodilator stress (though dobutamine may also be used). Patients should refrain from used of any product containing caffeine and other substances that could interfere with the vasodilator. For specific requirements, practitioners should refer the package insert of the vasodilator [44].

For most studies, this single infusion site can be used for both the vasodilator and the ^{82}Rb. A notable exception is when adenosine is used as the vasodilator. Because of the short half-life of adenosine, it is impractical to switch between the low flow rate adenosine to the high flow rate ^{82}Rb without bolusing the adenosine into the heart or interrupting the flow of adenosine. Stress testing using ^{13}N-ammonia is considerably less restrictive than Rb-82, allowing for vasodilator and exercise testing.

Prior to the study, technologists will need to apply ECG patches for both the 12 lead cardiac monitoring system and 3 lead ECG triggering system for the scanner. Once patients have been prepared, they are positioned supine in the scanner system.

Because attenuation correction is applied in all cardiac PET studies, it is possible to image patients with an arm down, however, it is important that the arm is immobilized and is free from the infusion activity.

The first stage of imaging is the transmission study, either acquired using CT or line source. For PET/CT systems, a low dosage chest planar image for positioning followed by a low dosage chest CT for attenuation correction will then be acquired of the mediastinal region. For dedicated PET systems, a line source transmission study is acquired for both positioning and attenuation correction. The transmission studies must be repeated if patient positioning is not correct.

The resting perfusion study typically follows the transmission study. Delivery of the ^{82}Rb using a generator cart requires strict adherence to the manufacturer's recommendations for dose delivery, QC and general operations. Persons using a ^{82}Rb generator should obtain training from the manufacturer prior to using the generator cart. Because of the very short half-life of RB-82 (75 s), it is important to begin emission collection quickly after this injection. However, due to considerable blood pooling, a brief delay of 90–120 s is important. Studies that incorporate measurement of myocardial blood flow however, require that the dynamic flow acquisition study be started prior to the infusion [45–47].

These imaging studies can be acquired either using a list mode (inclusion of all photon pair events) or a frame mode. In principle, these two modes will yield similar results, however list mode acquisitions do offer some additional flexibility to create multiple studies from a single data acquisition. Practically, frame mode and list mode acquisitions do not appear to be different either quantitatively or visually [48, 49].

Dipyridamole as the stress agent has been extensively studied for use with cardiac PET. In a study comparing matched adenosine SPECT and dipyridamole PET, Bateman et al. [50] demonstrated improved sensitivity and specificity for the global detection of CAD. Experience with regadenson stress is less robust, but most recent publications indicate similar imaging properties when compared to dipyridamole [51, 52]. Many PET laboratories are now using regadenoson. Idealized imaging protocols are summarized in Fig. 17.4.

PET Image Artifacts

Misregistration

Misregistration of the transmission and emission datasets is the one of the most significant sources of image artifacts in cardiac PET. This artifact is a result of the sequential acquisition of the emission and transmission datasets. When a patient moves between the transmission and emission scans, the attenuation map is improperly applied to the emission data: over corrected some regions, while under-correcting others. The resulting artifacts can lead to lwo diagnostic certainty and reduced diagnostic accuracy.

In a study of 1,177 patients, Loghin et al. [27] reported that 21 % of all resting cardiac PET studies had detectable misregistration artifacts, and in a separate study it was observed as little as 1 cm can introduce a 10 % drop in lateral wall counts [53]. Gould et al. [28] examined the effect on misregistration on image interpretation and demonstrated as many as 40 % of all PET/CT studies would have a change in diagnosis after misregistration correction was applied. Imaging guidelines recommended that all cardiac PET studies be routinely examined for misregistration and corrected whenever possible (see Fig. 17.4).

By far the most common technique for misregistration correction is a rigid shift of the transmission and emission data sets [54]. The user can interactively visualize

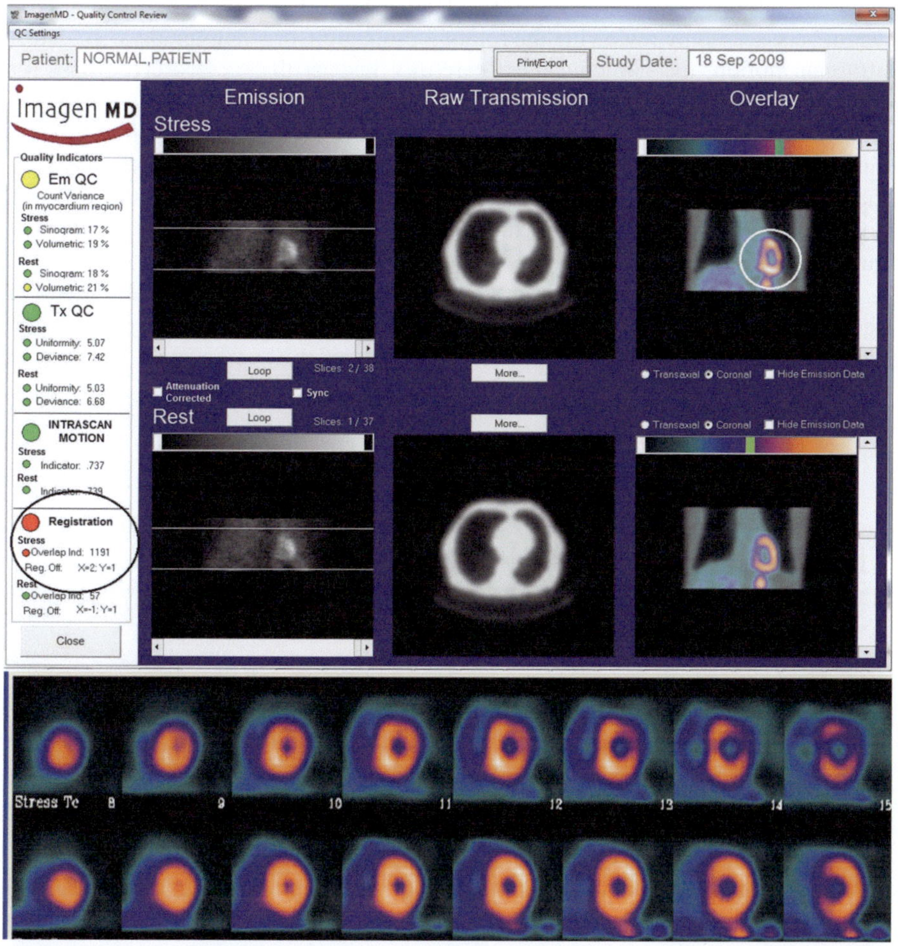

Fig. 17.4 PET data should routinely be inspected for misregistration by using an overlay of the transmission and emission data (*top*). Misregistration artifact are often impossible to distinguish from actual perfusion defects (*bottom*) When misregistration is detected, misregistration compensation must be applied before image interpretation

an overlay of the transmission and emission data and move one of the datasets relative to the other until a satisfactory positioning is obtained. An alternative approach is to fill the attenuation map with soft tissue values where the heart is overlaying the lung field [55].

Intrascan Motion

Another potential source of interpretive uncertainty is motion restricted to the emission scan alone, or intrascan motion. This can be a result of respiration, coughing, talking or patient motion [56]. Unlike SPECT imaging, intrascan motion cannot be assessed by reviewing the rotating projection, or sinogram data. To detect intrascan motion, the clinician must carefully inspect the reconstructed data for losses in image fidelity. It is also helpful for the technologist, nurse or others to note when they see a patient obviously moving during the acquisition. For those patients with a single movement the instrascan motion artifact will appear as two matching image defects, 180° apart (Fig. 17.5). This can be complicated if a patient moves more than once, as the resulting myocardial image can appear more uniformly blurred and/or misshapen.

At this time, there are no commercially available intrascan motion correction algorithms, however there are several investigators exploring approaches that incorporate dynamic list-mode data [57]. Because of this, care should be taken to

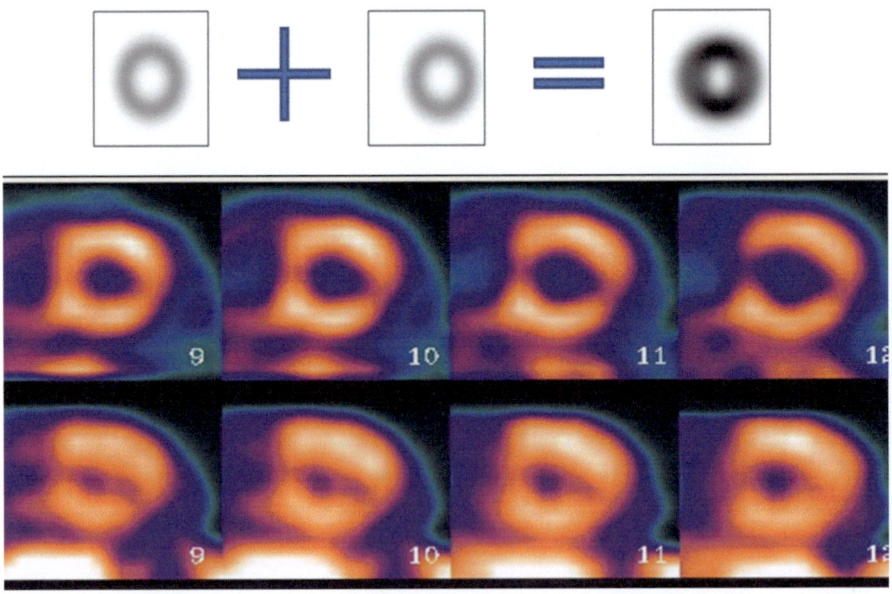

Fig. 17.5 Intrascan motion (motion exclusive to the emission study) reduces overall image fidelity. It often can be identified as matching artifacts in the short axis cuts, separated but 180°

insure patients are still and awake throughout the study. Unfortunately, repeating the study may be the only option to resolve this issue.

PET/CT Specific Artifacts

Cardiac PET studies can be corrected for attenuation either using line source or a CT based transmission study using a relatively short acquisition time, <2 min. As discussed earlier, the two major sources of potential artifacts in PET/CT are: improper patient breath holds during the CT and metallic implants.

There are three common techniques for the breath hold for CT attenuation correction: cine CT/Free breathing, end-expiration breath hold, shallow free breathing: In principle, all of these techniques can obtain good quality transmission scans, however some scanners may be incapable of performing the desired CT scan. The cine CT/free breathing performs multiple CT scans over the same point to obtain an average diaphragm position. Tube current is also reduced to minimize radiation. This creates an averaging effect similar to dedicated PET [34]. This technique is very straight forward to apply for compatible scanners because it requires little effort on the part of the patient to acquire this type of CT map. The drawback is that leaving the patient in the scanner for up to 1 min could potentially deliver an unacceptably high radiation dosage, unless a very low tube current is possible (<8 mAs). It may also be necessary to employ a CT reconstruction algorithm that is specific to the Cine CT/Free Breath protocol. Users should consult with their PET/CT vendor to confirm that their scanners can deliver correct X-ray tube settings and reconstruction to perform this protocol.

For the end-expiration breath hold technique, the patient is instructed to hold their breath after breathing out to achieve a best positioning of the diaphragm. This method differs from end-inspiration breatholding, which distort the shape of the lungs and lowers the diaphragm [35, 36]. This technique relies on training the patient prior to the study on how to hold their breath during the end-expiration pause of the breath cycle. During normal breathing, the diaphragm spends most of its time in a light expiration phase, with short cycles between inspiration and expiration movement. This protocol attempts to extend the time of the expiration pause to allow for the CT scan. For most multi-slice systems ($\geq$16 slices) the duration of the breath hold is <10 s. However, breath holds for two and four slice systems can exceed 20 s, making them prohibitively long for many cardiac patients.

For the shallow free breath technique, the patient is allowed to breathe throughout the CT scan; however they are instructed to take small breaths [36]. The shallow free breath protocol can be employed on most systems. The protocol encourages the patient to maintain a light breathing respiratory cycle to minimize diaphragm motion. This technique can produce good quality transmission maps; however, if the patient cannot maintain shallow breathing or if they take a breath at the wrong time, the resulting transmission map can be un-usable. If the shallow free breath protocol is used, the technologist must review the transmission study immediately after the CT scan and repeat the CT scan if necessary.

Metal Artifacts

Patients with implanted metal devices, surgical clips, wires, etc. can be challenging to image with PET/CT because of the high efficiency of metals to absorb x-rays. Presence of these metal objects near the heart can introduce artifacts in upwards of 50 % of patients [32]. However, the presence of metallic objects in the field of view of the heart should not be considered necessarily a contraindication to cardiac PET/CT imaging, when appropriate corrections are applied.

Several approaches have been proposed for removing the influence of metallic objects from the CT attenuation maps [29, 58]. One approach to correcting for this is a simple replacement or segmentation of the transmission maps of water attenuation values in regions with known metallic artifacts is sufficient to correct CT attenuation maps that are influenced by metal. Another algorithm utilizes a thresholding and reprojection reconstruction technique which offers a more quantitative approach to remove the influence of metallic objects [33].

Quality Control of Absolute Blood Flow Measurements

Absolute blood flow measurements using myocardial perfusion PET are rapidly gaining acceptance because of their ability to assess normality and identify disease in challenging patients [59, 60]. These techniques rely on a dynamic acquisition of the tracer kinetics and a model for tracer transport from the blood into the cell.

To calculate the absolute blood flow, it is necessary to obtain a dynamic series of measurements of the blood pool concentration of the injected activity and the myocardial uptake. This can be obtained as either a dynamic framed data set or a list-mode study. Unlike perfusion PET, these dynamic acquisitions must be started before the infusion of the PET tracer. The first dynamic frame is free of any counts from the radiotracer. Beginning the acquisition late can lead to an underestimation of the blood pool concentration and thereby and overestimation of the myocardial blood flow. To avoid these quantitation errors, the dynamic data must be inspected to verify the following:

1. Minimal counts in the first frame.
2. Early blood pool stage clearly visualized
3. Sufficient counts in the frames containing the uptake information.
4. Adequate blood pool clearance in the later stages of the dynamic study.

Reconstruction of the dynamic studies requires utilizing a reconstruction algorithm that maintains the absolute concentration or at the very least the relative relationship between reconstructed counts and activity.

Accurate measurement of the myocardial uptake can be challenging due to the effect of spillover from the blood pool into the myocardium and blurring. A partial volume correction must be applied to obtain an accurate estimate of the myocardial uptake [61]. These partial volume corrections are very sensitive to the filtering of the image and therefore filtering must always be done in accordance with the recommendation of the quantitation software used.

In addition to the accurate location of the myocardial boundary, it is essential that the blood pool ROI is appropriately centered over the target structure (either the left atrium or left ventricle). Inaccurate positioning of the blood pool ROI can cause inaccuracies and potentially mask true disease (Fig. 17.6).

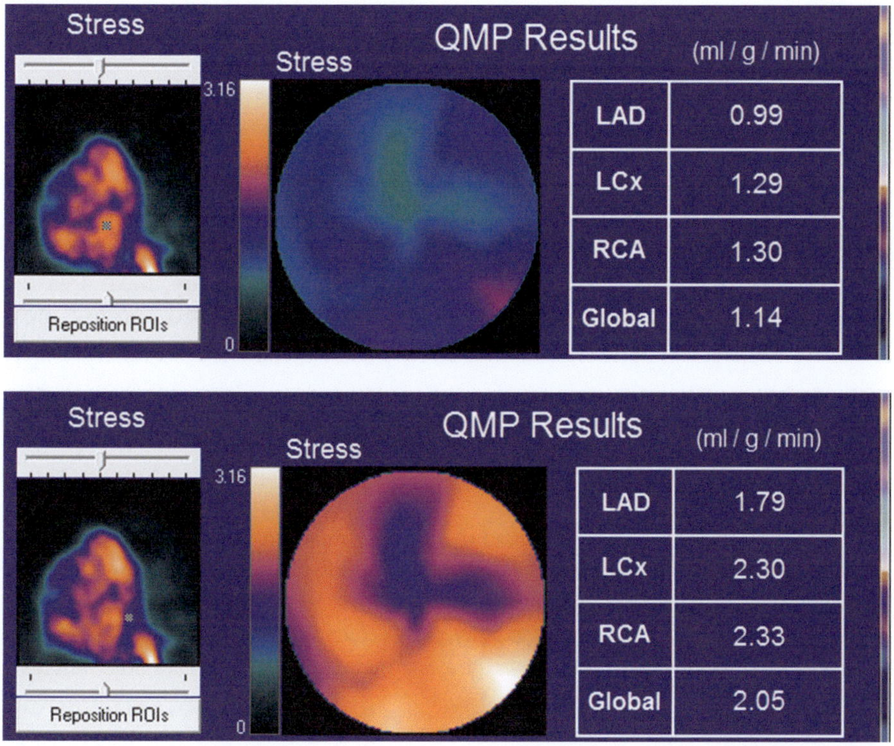

Fig. 17.6 The determination of absolute blood flow is one of the most important, unique measurements that can be made in cardiac PET. However, improper identification of the blood pool region of interest can lead to highly inaccurate blood flow measurements. In the top image, a patient with extensive atherosclerosis and radically reduced blood flow can appear completely normal if the blood pool region of interest is not centered on the blood pool

Image Interpretation

Despite the best efforts of technologists and clinicians, sub-optimal quality images do occur and it is essential that the clinician understand how to recognize artifacts. Simply reviewing the reconstructed tomograms is insufficient to for image assessment. Prior to image interpretation, each image should be inspected for:

1. Quality of emission datasets
2. Quality of transmission datasets
3. Misregistration between the transmission and emission datasets
4. Motion exclusive to either the transmission or emission datasets (intrascan motion)
5. Secondary (non-cardiac) findings in either the emission or transmission data sets

Emission Datasets Assessment

Emission datasets should be reviewed for camera artifacts and count sufficiency. This assessment is performed by reviewing either the sinogram data or a raw (non-attenuation corrected), rotating projection of the trues data. When reviewing the raw rotating projection data, patient motion cannot be assessed. The raw projection data should be set in motion and inspected for: (1) overall count density, (2) horizontal lines likely due to a bad normalization, (3) dark block object(s) rotating with projection likely due to a detector malfunction, and (4) secondary, focal areas of uptake. Possible attenuation artifact do not need to be assessed because most attenuation artifacts will be removed with attenuation correction is applied.

Transmission Dataset Assessment

The transmission datasets are inspected using a transmission volume viewer that will allow the user to scroll through the entire transmission volume. The transmission volume should be inspected for: (1) Truncation of the patient volume, (2) "hot" or "cold" bands in the image, likely due to low counts, and (3) clearly delimitated lung boundaries. PET/CT images should also be reviewed for any metal artifacts or breath hold failures.

Misregistration Artifact Recognition

The identification of misregistration is done using an overlay of the emission and transmission datasets. Clinicians reviewing the overlay should first confirm that no part of the emission image of the myocardium is visible overlaying the transmission image of the lungs. The review should be made in a coronal and/or transaxial view, scrolling through the entire volume, reviewing the entire volume.

The identification of excessive left lateral shift in the emission data can be visualized in the transaxial images as a dropout in counts in the emission image at the interface between the heart and the lung field. Right-lateral shift can be visualized as an artifact boosting of lateral wall counts, extending posteriorly sometime forming a "hook" around the left lung. Positive vertical misregistration is identified as an anterior drop it counts at the interface between the heart and lung. Negative vertical misregistration is identified as a "shelf" of excessive counts in the inferior wall.

Intrascan Motion

Another potential source of interpretive uncertainty is intrascan motion from respiration, coughing, talking or patient motion [56]. This motion is different than misregistration because all of the motion is confined to the emission data set. Unlike SPECT imaging, intrascan motion cannot be seen by reviewing the rotating projection, or sinogram data. To detect intrascan motion, the clinician must carefully inspect the reconstructed data for losses in image fidelity. For those patients with a single movement the instrascan motion artifact will appear as two matching image defects, 180° apart (Fig. 17.5). This can be complicated if a patient moves more than once, the resulting in a more uniformly blurred image. It is also helpful it the technologist/nurse carefully observes the patient during the rest and stress acquisition and notes whether motion has occurred.

Correction for intrascan motion is not currently possible with PET. As a result, if intrascan motion artifacts are too severe, studies may need to be repeated. Technologists should be observant during the study acquisition. If the patient moves during rest, it may be possible to repeat the resting study immediately after the first resting scan. This option is not possible following the stress acquisition. Thus, cautioning the patient during patient preparation is critical to avoid as much motion as possible (see next section).

Patient Preparation

Generally, patient preparation for a cardiac PET perfusion study is similar to SPECT study. That is, the patient must be informed of the risks of either pharmacologic stress in the case of rubidium-82 laboratories and either pharmacologic stress or exercise stress in laboratories who use ^{13}N ammonia. In addition, there are some specific issues for optimal patient preparation:

1. Radiation exposure: Radiation exposure is a concern for many patients and referring physicians. Nuclear laboratory staff must be prepared to explain in sufficient detail the radiation risks of cardiac PET procedures, in relative terms and absolute:

(a) Rubidium-82: The radiation exposure for Rubidium-82 is 0.9 nSv/20 mCi [62]. The average dose is 40–60 mCi at rest and stress for 2D imaging (3.6–5.4 mSv) and for 3D imaging 20–40 mCi at both rest and stress (1.8–3.6 mSv).
(b) Ammonia-13. The radiation exposure is estimated at 4–6 mSv for two injections of 20 mCi (rest and stress) [63].
(c) Context: These radiation doses are approximately two to threefold lower than the standard single isotope SPECT study (10–15 mCi at rest, 30–45 mCi at rest, 9–15 mSv estimated, [64]. These PET radiation levels also meet the ASNC recommended levels for patients undergoing nuclear cardiology imaging [65]. Finally these levels are at or below the annual radiation exposure of the average American (6.2 mSv).

2. Explaining the PET Procedure:
Common causes of suboptimal PET imaging relate to the patient cooperation during the procedure. Thus, the patient must be informed of certain aspects of the procedure before proceeding:

(a) Camera: PET cameras can to be large, especially if associated with CT with a smaller gantry opening. The gantry is circular and tubular and as a result, some patients may experience claustrophobia. The patient should be informed about the nature of the scan and if they will be required to have more than just their head within the gantry opening.

(b) Protocol positioning. The field of view of PET systems is typically smaller than SPECT systems. As a result patient positioning is critical. For PET/CT, this can be easily accomplished with a quick topographic scan prior to PET imaging. With dedicated systems, the can require using the transmission scan as a positioning scan. Technologists should be trained on using the transmission scan for positioning. If a patient must be repositioned, the transmission scan must always be repeated.

(c) Pharmacologic stress; Stress testing in cardiac PET is almost always performed using pharmacological stress. Patients must be informed of the potential side-effects prior to placing the patient in the camera. They must be informed that despite the patient's discomfort, it is essential the patient remain still throughout the entire stress test.

The Cardiac PET Report

A crucial aspect of laboratory quality control is the report which is submitted to the referring physician. Excellent laboratory practices in all other aspects such as camera quality, artifact recognition, and patient preparation can fail if the report is inadequate, incorrect or incomplete.

Table 17.2 Required reporting elements: IAC nuclear cardiology [66]

1	Demographics of faculty including address, phone number
2	Referring healthcare provider name
3	Clinical indications/history
4	Timeliness: date of study performed and finalized
5	Description of procedure
6	Non-radioactive drug administration including dosages
7	Exact radioactive tracer dose for rest/stress
8	Use of standard nomenclature
9	Defect quantification
10	Wall motion finding
11	Integrated stress and nuclear report
12	Succinct impression
13	Signature of interpreting physician
14	Date of report finalization

There have been several important documents describing critical elements in the cardiac SPECT report (see Table 17.2). Necessary elements of the Nuclear Cardiology Report has been standardized report template by the Intersocietal Accreditation Commission (IAC) Nuclear Division requirements [66]. The report should encompass:

1. Indication: The reason for the test, should be consistent with reimbursement coding language. These indications will be replaced by Appropriate Use Criteria.
2. Clinical history: Previous history of CAD, risk factors, previous procedures, new or current symptoms, and other relevant information.
3. Procedure details:

   (a) Stress test stressor, amount administered, administration technique, clinical vital signs (HR, BP), clinical and ECG response to stress test)
   (b) Imaging test: tracer and dosage used, administration details, imaging system description, other details.

4. Findings:

   (a) Quality of study and QC challenges.
   (b) Ventricular enlargement (yes/no or quantitative), lung activity.
   (c) Tracer distribution: overall and location of any defects. Estimate of severity of defects.
   (d) Gated study: LVEF, regional wall motion and thickening.
   (e) Transient Ischemic Cavity Dilation (TID). This is much more common with Cardiac PET perfusion than SPECT, and should be included in every report, in the defect quantification section.
   (f) Reversible wall motion abnormalities: It is very common to capture both rest and stress data during the acquisition of cardiac PET perfusion data. As a

result, both rest and stress wall motion should be assessed on a global and regional basis. Reporting on both are important because reversible wall motion abnormalities and changes in ejection fraction are much more common with PET than SPECT and should be reported [67, 68].

(g) Absolute myocardial blood flow: The ability to measure global and regional myocardial blood flow at stress and rest conditions as well as differences (termed coronary flow reserve) has been shown to have both diagnostic and prognostic significance from multiple publications [66]. Data are now emerging that this information should be reported. Bateman, Gould and DiCarli have proposed a categorization of how to report the findings for the first time and suggest the following categories: (a) normal flow augmentation (b) abnormal flow augmentation and (c) no flow augmentation [66, 69, 70].

5. Impressions:

   (a) Overall impression: abnormal/normal/ischemic
   (b) Defect location, extent and severity
   (c) Overall ventricular function and regional functional abnormalities, if present.
   (d) Changes from prior studies.
   (e) The report should be completed in a timely fashion (IAC mandates 1–2 days)

Summary

Cardiac PET imaging can produce significantly higher quality images of the myocardium when compared to SPECT. However to achieve this, technologist and clinicians must implement robust quality control procedures to insure that data is acquired property and necessary corrections are applied. When applied properly, the resulting images have greatly reduced artifacts, and improved contrast and resolution. Patient preparation is critical to avoid artifacts that may impact on diagnostic accuracy. Reports should contain all of the recommended IAC Nuclear elements as well as aspects unique to cardiac PET.

References

1. Dirac PAM. The quantum theory of the electron. Proc R Soc Lond A. 1928;1:610–24.
2. Anderson CD. The positive electron. Phys Rev. 1933;43(6):491–4.
3. Brownell GL, Sweet WH. Localization of brain tumors with positron emitters. Nucleonics. 1953;11:40–5.
4. Brownell GL, Burnham CA, Hoop B and Bohning DE. Quantitative dynamic studies using short-lived radioisotopes and positron detection. In: Proceedings of the symposium on dynamic studies with radioisotopes in medicine, Rotterdam. August 31 – September 4, 1970. IAEA. Vienna. 1971. p. 161–72.

5. Schelbert HR, Phelps ME, Hoffman EJ, Huang SC, Selin CE, Kuhl DE. Regional myocardial perfusion assessed with N-13 labeled ammonia and positron emission computerized axial tomography. Am J Cardiol. 1979;43:209–18.
6. Schelbert HR, Phelps ME, Huang SC, et al. N-13 ammonia as an indicator of myocardial blood flow. Circulation. 1981;63:1259–72.
7. Hutchins GD, Schwaiger M, Rosenspire KC, Krivokapich J, Schelbert H, Kuhl DE. Noninvasive quantification of regional blood flow in the human heart using N-13 ammonia and dynamic positron emission tomographic imaging. J Am Coll Cardiol. 1990;15:1032–42.
8. Gould KL. Clinical cardiac PET using generator-produced Rb-82: a review. Cardiovasc Intervent Radiol. 1989;12(5):245–51.
9. Goldstein R, Mullani N, Wong W, Hartz R, Hicks C, Fuentes F, Smalling R, Gould K. Positron imaging of myocardial infarction with rubidium-82. J Nucl Med. 1986;27:1824–9.
10. Di Carli MF, Hachamovitch R. Should PET replace SPECT for evaluating CAD? The end of the beginning. J Nucl Cardiol. 2006;13(1):2–7.
11. Tillisch J, Brunken R, Marshall R, et al. Reversibility of cardiac wall-motion abnormalities predicted by positron tomography. N Engl J Med. 1986;314:884–8.
12. Allman KC, Shaw LJ, Hachamovitch R, Udelson JE. Myocardial viability testing and impact of revascularization on prognosis in patients with coronary artery disease and left ventricular dysfunction: a meta-analysis. J Am Coll Cardiol. 2002;39:1151–8.
13. Camici P, Ferrannini E, Opie LH. Myocardial metabolism in ischemic heart disease: basic principles and application to imaging by positron emission tomography. Program Cardiovasc Dis. 1989;32:217–38.
14. Yamagishi H, Shirai N, Takagi M, et al. Identification of cardiac sarcoidosis with $^{13}N-NH_3/^{18}F$-FDG PET. J Nucl Med. 2003;44:1030–6.
15. Shoup TM, Elmaleh DR, Bohab AA, Fischman AJ. Evaluation of trans-9-^{18}F-fluoro-3,4-Methyleneheptadecanoic acid as a PET tracer for myocardial fatty acid imaging. J Nucl Med. 2005;46(2):297–304.
16. Yu M, Bozek J, Kagan M, Guaraldi M, Silva P, Azure M, Onthank D, Robinson SP. Cardiac retention of PET neuronal imaging agent LMI1195 in different species: impact of norepinephrine uptake-1 and -2 transporters. Nucl Med Biol. 2013;40(5):682–8.
17. Cho ZH, Chan JK, Ericksson L, Singh M, Graham S, MacDonald NS, Yano Y. Positron ranges from biomedically important positron-emitting radionuclides. J Nucl Med. 1975;16:1174–6.
18. Katz L, Penfold AS. Range-energy relations for electrons and the determination of beta-ray end-point energies by absorption Rev. Mod Phys. 1952;24:28–44.
19. King MM, Chou WT. NDS. 1994;76:285.
20. Esteves FP, Nye JA, Khan A, Folks RD, Raghuveer KH, Garcia EV, Schuster DM, Lerakis S, Raggi P, Votaw JR. Prompt-gamma compensation in Rb-82 myocardial perfusion 3D PET/CT. J Nucl Cardiol. 2010;17(2):247–53.
21. Hsu B, Helmuth P, McGhie I, Bateman T, Case J. Is 3D-only PET/CT scanner ready to acquire rest/stress Rb-82 myocardial blood flow using the same infusion for clinical images? J Nucl Med. 2009;50(Supplement 2):600.
22. Weber MJ, Monchamp RR. Luminescence of Bi4Ge3O12: spectral and decay properties. J Appl Phys. 1973;44:5495–9.
23. Melcher CL, Schweitzer JS. Cerium-doped lutetium orthosilicate: a fast, efficient new scintillator. IEEE Trans Nucl Sci. 1992;NS-39:502–5.
24. Ter-Pogossian MM, Mullani NA, Ficke DC, et al. Photon time-of-flight-assisted positron emission tomography. J Comput Assist Tomogr. 1981;5:227–39.
25. Cherry SR, Dahlborn M, Hoffman EJ. 3D PET using a conventional multislice tomography without septa. J Comput Assist Tomogr. 1991;15(4):655–68.
26. Case JA, Hsu BA, Cullom SJ. Attenuation and scatter correction in cardiac PET. In: Heller GV, Mann A, Hendel RC, editors. Nuclear cardiology: technical applications. 2009.
27. Loghin C, Sdringola S, Gould KL. Common artifacts in PET myocardial perfusion images due to attenuation-emission misregistration: clinical significance, causes, and solutions. J Nucl Med. 2004;45(6):1029–39.

28. Gould L, Pan T-S, Laghin C, Johnson NP, Guha A, Sdringola S. Frequent diagnostic errors in cardiac PET/CT due to misregistration of CT attenuation and emission PET images: a definite analysis of causes, consequences and corrections. J Nucl Med. 2007;48(7):1112–21.
29. Hsu BL, Case JA, Moser KW, Bateman TM, Cullom SJ. Reconstruction of rapidly acquired Germanium-68 transmission scans for cardiac PET attenuation correction. J Nucl Cardiol. 2007;14:706–14.
30. Kinahan PE, Townsend DW, Beyer T, Sashin D. Attenuation correction for a combined 3D PET/CT scanner. Med Phys. 1998;25(10):2046–53.
31. Kalender WA, Wolf H, Suess C. Dose reduction in CT by anatomically adapted tube current modulation: phantom measurements. Med Phys. 1999;26:2248–53.
32. DiFilippo FP, Brunken RC. Do pacemaker leads and ICDs cause metal-related artifact in cardiac PET/CT. J Nucl Med. 2005;46(3):436–43.
33. Abdoli M, Dierckx RAJO, Zaidi H. Metal artifact reduction strategies for improved attenuation correction in hybrid PET/CT imaging. Med Phys. 2012;39:3343–61.
34. Alessio AM, Kohlmyer S, Branch K, Chen G, Caldwell J, Kinahan P. Cine CT for attenuation correction in cardiac PET/CT. J Nucl Med. 2007;48(5):794–801.
35. de Juan R, Seifert B, Berthold T, von Schulthess GK, Goerres GW. Clinical evaluation of a breathing protocol for PET/CT. Eur Radiol. 2004;14:1118–23.
36. Beyer T, Antoch G, Blodgett T, Freudenberg LF, Akhurst T, Mueller S. Dual-modality PET/CT imaging: the effect of respiratory motion on combined image quality in clinical oncology. Eur J Nucl Med Mol Imaging. 2003;30:588–96.
37. Ollinger JM. Model-based scatter correction for fully 3D PET. Phys Med Biol. 1996;41(1):153–76.
38. Watson C, Newport D, Casey M, DeKemp R, Beanlands R, Schmand M. Evaluation of simulation-based scatter correction for 3-D PET cardiac imaging. IEEE Nucl Sci Symp Conf Rec. 1997;44:90–7.
39. Case J, Patil H, Courter SA, Bateman TM. Comparison of a lower-dosimetry 3D Rb-82 PET myocardial perfusion imaging protocol versus the conventional 2D protocol. Circulatory. 2012;126, A18016.
40. King MM, Chou WT. NDS 76285(1995), 11 Feb 1994.
41. Casey ME, Hoffman EJ. Quantitation in positron emission computed tomography: a technique to reduce noise in accidental coincidence measurements and coincidence efficiency calibration. J Comput Assist Tomogr. 1986;10:845–50.
42. Hudson HM, Larkin RS. Accelerated image reconstruction using ordered subsets of projection data. IEEE Trans Med Imaging. 1994;13(4):601–9.
43. Dilsizian V, et al. ASNC imaging guidelines for nuclear cardiology procedures: PET myocardial perfusion and metabolism clinical imaging. J Nucl Cardiol. 2009;16(4):651. http://www.asnc.org/imageuploads/ImagingGuidelinesPETJuly2009.pdf.
44. Henzlova MJ, Cerqueria MD, Mahmarian JJ, Yao S-S. Stress protocols and tracers. J Nucl Cardiol. 2006;13(6):e80–90.
45. Hutchins GD, Schwaiger M, Rosenspire KC, Krivokapich J, Shelbert H, Kuhl DE. Noninvasive quantification of regional blood flow in the human heart using N-13 ammonia and dynamic positron emission tomographic imaging. J Am Coll Cardiol. 1990;5:1032–42.
46. Yoshida K, Mullani N, Gould KL. Coronary flow and flow reserve by PET simplified for clinical applications using rubidium-82 or nitrogen-13-ammonia. J Nucl Med. 1996;37(10):1701–12.
47. Lortie M, Beanlands RS, Yoshinaga K, Klein R, DaSalvia JN, deKemp RA. Quantification of myocardial blood flow with 82Rb dynamic PET imaging. Eur J Nucl Med Mol Imag. 2007;34(11):1765–74.
48. Heller GV, Case JA, Reibsane J, Irvine T, Karnish J, Nakao C, Frey B, Bateman TM, Borgatta L. Feasibility of a low dosage 3D dedicated Rb-82 PET imaging protocol: an image quality comparison against high-dose traditional 2D imaging in obese patients. J Nucl Cardiol.

49. Case JA, Van Vickle S, Courter SA, Burgett EV, Bateman TM. A rapid acquisition protocol for measuring perfusion, gating and absolute blood flow using dedicated frame-mode 3D PET scanners. J Nucl Cardiol. 2014.
50. Bateman TM, Heller GV, McGhie AI, et al. Diagnostic accuracy of rest/stress ECG-gated Rb-82 myocardial perfusion PET: comparison with ECG-gated Tc-99m sestamibi. J Nucl Cardiol. 2006;13:24–33.
51. Goudarzi B, Fukushima K, Bravo P, Merrill J, Bengel FM. Comparison of the myocardial blood flow response to regadenoson and dipyridamole: a quantitative analysis in patients referred for clinical 82Rb myocardial perfusion PET. Eur J Nucl Med Mol Imaging. 2011;38(10):1908–16.
52. Cullom S, Hsu B, Courter S, Luangamath M, Case J, Bateman T. Comparison of quantitative perfusion and function between dipyridamole and regadenoson for pharmacologic rubidium-82 PET. J Nucl Cardiol. 2013;20:76–83.
53. Case JA, Heller GV, Cullom SJ, Hsu BL, Noble GL, Masse M, Bateman TM. Sensitivity of myocardial perfusion PET/CT imaging scan appearance on accurate transmission/emission registration. J Nucl Cardiol. 2005;12:S117.
54. Martinez-Moller A, Souvatzoglou M, Navab N, Schwaiger M, Nekolla SG. Artifacts from misaligned CT in cardiac perfusion PET/CT studies: frequency, effects, and potential solutions. J Nucl Med. 2007;48:188–93.
55. Martinez-Möller A, Souvatzoglou M, Navab N, Schwaiger M, Nekolla SG. Artifacts from misaligned CT in cardiac perfusion PET/CT studies: frequency, effects, and potential solutions. J Nucl Med. 2007;48:188–93.
56. Goerres GW, Kamel E, Heidelberg TN, Schwitter MR, Burger C, von Schulthess GK. PET-CT image co-registration in the thorax: influence of respiration. Eur J Nucl Med Mol Imag. 2002;29:351–60.
57. Woo J, Cheng V, Dey D, Lazewatzky J, Ramesh A, Hayes S, Berman D, Germano G, Slomka P. Automatic 3D registration of dynamic stress and rest (82)Rb and flurpiridaz F 18 myocardial perfusion PET data for patient motion detection and correction). Med Phys. 2011;38(11): 6313–26.
58. Hsu BLBL, Saha K, Bateman TM, Case JA. Frequency and appearance of image artifacts in cardiac PET/CT imaging utilizing fast CT scans for attenuation correction. J Nucl Cardiol. 2007;14:S32.
59. Di Carli M, Czernin J, Hoh CK, Gerbaudo VH, Brunken RC, Huang SC, et al. Relation among stenosis severity, myocardial blood flow, and flow reserve in patients with coronary artery disease. Circulation. 1995;91:1944–51.
60. Ziadi MC, deKemp RA, Williams K, Guo A, Renaud JM, Chow BJW, et al. Does quantification of myocardial flow reserve using rubidium-82 positron emission tomography facilitate detection of multivessel coronary artery disease? J Nucl Cardiol. 2012;19(4):670–80.
61. Hutchins GD, Caraher JM, Raylman RR. A region of interest strategy for minimizing resolution distortions in quantitative myocardial PET studies. J Nucl Med. 1992;33:1243–50.
62. Senthamizhchelvan S, Bravo PE, Lodge MA, Merrill J, Bengel FM, Sgouros G. Radiation dosimetry of 82Rb in humans under pharmacologic stress. J Nucl Med. 2011;52:485–911.
63. Stabin MG. Radiopharmaceuticals for nuclear cardiology: radiation dosimetry, uncertainties, and risk. J Nucl Med. 2008;49:1555–63.
64. Einstein AJ, Moser KW, Thompson RC, Cerqueira MD, Henzlova MJ. Radiation dose to patients from cardiac diagnostic imaging. Circulation. 2007;116:1290–305.
65. Cerqueira MD, Allman KA, Ficaro EP, Hansen CL, Nichols KJ, Thompson RC, Van Decker WA, Yakovlevitch M. Recommendations for reducing radiation exposure in myocardial perfusion imaging 2010. J Nucl Cardiol. 2010;15:1071–8.
66. Tilkemeier PL, Cooke CD, Ficaro EP, Glover DK, Hansen CL, McCallister BD. American Society of Nuclear Cardiology information statement: standardized reporting matrix for radionuclide myocardial perfusion imaging. J Nucl Cardiol. 2006;13(6):e157–71.

67. Dorbala S, Vangala D, Sampson U, Limaye A, Kwong R, Di Carli MF. Value of vasodilator left ventricular ejection fraction reserve in evaluating the magnitude of myocardium at risk and the extent of angiographic coronary artery disease: a 82Rb PET/CT study. J Nucl Med. 2007;48(3):349–5.
68. Dorbala S, Hachamovitch R, Curillova Z, Thomas D, Vangala D, Kwong RY, Di Carli MF. Incremental prognostic value of gated Rb-82 positron emission tomography myocardial perfusion imaging over clinical variables and rest LVEF. J Am Coll Cardiol Img. 2009;2: 846–54.
69. Johnson NP, Kirkeeide RL, Gould KL. Is discordance of coronary flow reserve and fractional flow reserve due to methodology or clinically relevant coronary pathophysiology. J Am Coll Cardiol Img. 2012;5:193–202.
70. Murthy VL, Di Carli MF. Non-invasive quantification of coronary vascular dysfunction for diagnosis and management of coronary artery disease. J Nucl Cardiol. 2012;19:1060–72.

Chapter 18
Cardiac PET Quality Improvement

James A. Case and Gary V. Heller

Abstract Maintaining a high quality laboratory in Cardiac PET requires continual evaluation and improvement. This chapter will examine methods of establishing a Quality Improvement Program in Cardiac PET including key components to the program such as instrumentation, reports, and patient care matters.

Keywords Cardiac PET • Quality improvement • Physician measures • Data evaluation

Introduction

Laboratory quality should not be considered a static goal; rather it is a process that continually identifies problems with quality and opportunities for improvement. Processes must go beyond policy and training to include review feedback and methods for improvement. There is not one solution that will work for all laboratories. Each laboratory is responsible for establishing their own system for quality improvement to insure that all aspects of patient care is continually being addressed.

Quality improvement extends beyond the appearance of the clinical images. The Intersocietal Commission for the Accreditation of Nuclear Laboratories identifies three major areas for quality maintenance and improvement [1]:

1. Administrative quality: Examples of this would be patient scheduling, document completeness and patient satisfaction (See Table 18.1).
2. Technical Quality: Examples of this are imaging quality and protocol adherence, as well as attention to new advancements and recommendations that may apply to a given laboratory (see Table 18.2).

J.A. Case, PhD
Technical Director, Cardiovascular Imaging Technologies, Kansas City, MO, USA
e-mail: jcase@cvit.com

G.V. Heller, MD, PhD (✉)
Gagnon Cardiovascular Institute, Morristown Medical Center, Atlantic Healthcare System, Morristown, NJ, USA

Research Section, Intersocietal Accreditation Commission, Ellicott City, MD, USA
e-mail: garyvheller@gmail.com

P.L. Tilkemeier et al. (eds.), *Quality Evaluation in Non-Invasive Cardiovascular Imaging*, DOI 10.1007/978-3-319-28011-0_18

Table 18.1 Quality improvement measures: administrative [2]

Item	Sample variables	Evaluation method
Patient satisfaction	Hours of operation, convenience of the facility location, cleanliness, waiting time, comfort, explanation of the procedure, questions answered, friendliness of the staff, knowledge and professionalism of the staff, respect for modesty, confidentiality, overall impression of visit, willingness to return, likelihood of referring others	Patient surveys
Referral physician satisfaction	Transcription of reports, availability/timeliness of reports, procedure scheduling process, phone hospitality, billing/insurance/pre-authorization instructions, quality of the images, timeliness of scheduling, quality/accuracy of the reports, availability for consultation, interactions with the patient, convenience for patient, staff courtesy, frequency of patient complaints, response to complaints	Physician questionnaires and method for collecting issues in real time. Review of reporting times
Documentation	Patient information; physician information; procedure information report accuracy: clinical indication; description of the procedure; pharmaceutical data, and route of administration; physician signature, report approved with 4 working days, pertinent positive and negative findings; other findings, if applicable; succinct impression	Review of reports

Table 18.2 Quality improvement measures: technical quality measures [2]

Item	Sample variables	Evaluation method
Image quality	Patient motion; breast attenuation; diaphragmatic attenuation; superimposed bowel artifact, hot liver, low count study, gating error, overall quality, imaging technologist	Review of raw and processed data for at least 30 random patients
Patient preparation	NPO, caffeine withheld >18 h, no theophylline containing products, beta blockers withheld, calcium channel blockers withheld, patient appropriately dressed	Review of patient histories and checklists
Adequacy of stress tests	85 of maximum stress on exercise tests, protocol adherence on pharmacological tests	Review of stress test reports

3. Physician Performance: Examples would be interobserver agreement, adherence to Appropriate Use Criteria and correlation with cardiac catheterization (See Table 18.3).

These broad categories all work to further the patient experience, from the moment they are told they need an imaging study until they are discussing the recommendations with their physician. For continued IAC accreditation, nuclear laboratories

Table 18.3 Quality improvement measures: physician performance [2]

Item	Sample variables	Evaluation method
Interobserver variability	Overall result; defect size, severity and type; defect location using a 17 segment model; ejection fraction, regional wall motion abnormality; and artifact	Comparison of reports from all reading physicians
Intraobserver variability	Overall result; defect size, severity and type; defect location using a 17 segment model; ejection fraction, regional wall motion abnormality; and artifact	Review of reports from the same physician
Correlation with other studies	Accuracy with angiography (50 % and 70 % thresholds), LVEF with ECHO, MRI, Cath, etc. Negative predictive value	Review of nuclear report with reports from other modalities
Appropriateness of care	Percentage of appropriate, inappropriate and uncertain indications; referring physician name and practice according to AUC [11]	Review of indications in at least 30 patients

must conduct regular assessments of their quality improvement program to insure that problems are addressed and improvements are made. It is stated in the IAC Nuclear Standards that quarterly meetings need to be held, and at least 2/year specific to QI measures. Attendance of each technologist and physician as well as other personnel (PA, APRN) must be 50 % of the meetings [1].

Quality improvement relies upon establishing a system that can recognize problems and correct them. In order to recognize quality improvement opportunities, it is essential to identify measurements that can be used for determining quality and how it can be improved. The US Department of Health and Human Services lists three characteristics of a good quality measures [2]:

1. Importance of the measure.
2. Soundness of the scientific measurement.
3. Feasibility of the measurement.

Quality measurements need to be objective and reproducible for them to be meaningful. Each facility should employ measurements that fit their particular situation and provides actionable information to help in decision making.

The Quality Improvement process (PDSA) can be summarized in four process steps [3]:

1. Plan: An opportunity for improvement is identified and a plan is developed.
2. Do: Collection of data to establish the metrics to be measured.
3. Study: Analyze the data to develop the intervention strategy
4. Act: Execute the intervention and measure the metrics to establish if quality goal has been met.

This process should be seen as continual: actions restart the process as a site continually looks for opportunities for improvement. Once a problem has been identified and addressed, another QI project should begin.

It is also essential that staff understand that a quality improvement program needs their buy-in and is designed to improve their work environment as well as the patient experience.

Establishing Measurable Metrics for Cardiac PET

Patient-Centered Imaging

In 2012, the American Society of Nuclear Cardiology published a practice statement entitled, "Patient Centered Imaging" [4]. In this article, the importance of tailoring imaging procedures to patient needs was highlighted. This includes choices such as radiation dosage, stress testing options, appropriateness of the test, accuracy of interpretation etc.

In establishing an image quality metric, it is important to track that the right protocol is being applied to the right patient. Specifically, for SPECT in the information statement of ASNC in 2010 high radiation dosage protocols, such as dual isotope protocols, should be strongly discouraged in favor of lower dosage protocols [5]. Very low dosage protocols, such as stress only imaging with attenuation correction, should be favored for younger, lower risk patients [5].

Similarly in PET, higher dosage protocols should be avoided. When using PET/CT, the lowest mAs and kVp should be used for acquiring a patient's attenuation map and diagnostic quality CT studies should only be used when medically necessary. New technologies, such as 3D imaging should also be considered as a vehicle for reducing patient dosage.

In the end, radiation dosage should be adapted to the needs of the patient to insure and the right study is done to answer the appropriate question. A one-size-fits-all approach to nuclear imaging is not in the interests of patients or laboratories striving to achieve real quality improvements.

The metrics for measuring personalized approaches should track patient dosage as a function of age and pre-test risk. It also should track when abbreviated protocols, such as stress only, are used. Patients have become more aware of their lifetime radiation exposure and laboratories should consider methods for tracking this information.

Image Quality as a Quality Metric

Image quality is an essential part of any diagnostic imaging center; however the identification of reasonable measures of image quality is more challenging. An approach to measuring and tracking image quality issues can be broken down into several broad categories: (1) Camera performance, (2) protocol adherence, (3) image processing and (4) reader performance.

Camera performance can be tracked in terms of daily, weekly or monthly quality measurements, such as floods; however the quality program can only be effective if values are recorded and tracked. Nuclear laboratories should record daily QC values from instrumentation and have clear procedures in place for when instrumentation does not meet specifications, including cancelling patients until the instrumentation can be brought into compliance. These procedures should be included with the written procedures for the laboratory. For new systems, it may be important to involve equipment manufacturers in the development of camera QC procedure to insure approaches are relevant to the site's instrumentation.

Patient image quality can be more difficult to measure, however there are certain metrics that should be considered. Practitioners should consider recording and tracking instances of preventable image artifacts such as significant patient motion, non-cardiac uptake and poor ECG signals. Technologists should record when post acquisition corrections, such as motion correction, are applied and efforts should be made to minimize reliance on post acquisition correction software. When preventable imaging problems arise, constructive feedback needs to be provided to the personnel in the imaging suite.

Administrative Quality

Administrative quality is used to describe those activities that relate to the satisfaction of entities that use the services of the laboratory: for example, patients and referral physicians. Some examples that impact patients are scheduling, patient wait times and timeliness of reporting. A sample survey for patient satisfaction is shown in Fig. 18.1. Referral physician satisfaction also relates to administrative quality. The completeness of reports, timeliness of reports, and usefulness of the information provided all should be tracked to insure the satisfaction of referring physicians. Table 18.1 list examples of measurements that can be made to track administrative quality.

Administrative quality metrics are typically straightforward to measure. One of the most frequent complaints of patients is wait time; wait times for setting an appointment, wait times when they arrive and time until they receive their results. Scheduling procedures should include processes for capturing wait time information at time points important for referral physician and patient satisfaction. Real time interrogation of the data is also important for identifying when a patient or referral physician has fallen through the cracks.

During nuclear testing, there is unavoidable waiting involved with the nuclear stress testing: delays for a tracer to clear non-cardiac structures, redistribution of tracer or the surprise when a stress only study necessitates a return on a different day for rest imaging. However, unnecessary waiting should be avoided. Patient imaging time slots must be realistic and any quality improvement programs should include a review of patient wait times between arrival and scanning. Stress only imaging and

Cardiovascular Care Center (Sample) Patient Satisfaction Survey Data Collection							
Question	Great 5	Good 4	OK 3	Fair 2	Poor 1	No response	Total
Facility and Convenience							
Hours of Operation							
Location							
Cleanliness							
Waiting time in Reception							
Comfort of Waiting Room							
Staff							
Explanation of Procedure							
Questions Answered							
Friendly and Helpful							
Knowledgeable and Professional							
Modesty Respected							
Confidentiality Respected							
Overall							
Overall Impression of Visit							
Willingness to Return							
Likelihood of Referring Others							
What did you like about our facility?							
What did you like least about out facility?							
Suggestions for improvement?							
About You:	Gender?	Age?	Number of visits to our facility?				

Fig. 18.1 Suggested patient satisfaction survey (Source of data: Intersocietal Accreditation Commission: http://www.intersocietal.org/)

positron emission tomography (PET) can also be used to reduce a patient's time in the nuclear laboratory, due to faster protocols.

A mentioned earlier, referral physician satisfaction is another key metric for assessing the quality of an imaging program. A sample of a physician satisfaction survey is shown in Fig. 18.2. Nuclear laboratories must consider monitoring report quality, timeliness of scheduling, procedures for pre-authorization, timeliness of report, follow-through on high risk studies, and responsiveness to complaints. All of these metrics are crucial for referral physician satisfaction and quality patient care.

Cardiovascular Care Center (Sample) Referral Physician Satisfaction Survey Data Collection							
Question	Great 5	Good 4	OK 3	Fair 2	Poor 1	No response	Total
Clerical Services							
Transcription of reports							
Availability and timeliness of reports							
Scheduling process							
Phone "hospitality"							
Billing/Insurance explanations							
Professional Staff							
Quality of images							
Timeliness of scheduling							
Timeliness of completion of exam							
Quality/accuracy of reports							
Availability for consultation							
Interactions with patients							
Overall							
Convenience for patients							
Staff courtesy							
Frequency of patient complaints							
Response to your complaints							
What did you like about our facility?							
What did you like least about out facility?							
Suggestions for improvement?							

Fig. 18.2 Sample physician satisfaction survey (Source of data: Intersocietal Accreditation Commission: http://www.intersocietal.org/)

Technical Quality

Quality Control and Maintenance of the PET Imaging System

The technical quality of images produced by PET and PET/CT is directly related to the instrumentation that is used, proper maintenance, training of staff on the imaging protocols and patient cooperation. ACR-NEMA provides guidance for the maintenance of PET and PET/CT systems using in clinical practice [6]. In addition, the International Atomic Energy Agency also has provided guidance on the maintenance of these systems [7].

The daily routine for maintaining the equipment in the PET and PET/CT quality begins with the review of daily blank scans and CT data. Quality control of this image data should be visually and quantitatively inspected to confirm the proper functioning of the system. Careful attention should paid to QC image variations that could be missed by the automated programs, such as subtle changes in detector efficiency across the field of view or artifacts that could masked in quantitative data. It is essential that the quality values be recorded and regularly inspected to confirm the system is in working order. In addition to measuring the day to day working consistency, systems must be regularly upgraded to meet the evolving quality standards. This includes replacing outdated instrumentation.

Most manufacturers define the quality maintenance program for their PET system. These programs include daily uniformity measurements, and quantitative integrity. Though the measurements are important, they should not be considered the only measurements necessary to maintain the equipment. Rod sources used for attenuation correction decay, x-ray tubes fail and supporting equipment such as ECG monitoring and acquisition computers can fail. Faulty supportive equipment can corrupt images as easily as a bad blank scan. In designing a quality improvement program, all equipment should be regularly inspected for proper performance and replaced as necessary.

Appropriate software is essential to maintaining a high quality nuclear PET program. At each step (acquisition, processing, and interpretation) computer systems much be maintained. The quality improvement program for these systems should review:

1. Appropriateness of software for tasks, for example: 3D imaging, ECG gating, misregistration correction, iterative reconstruction options, adjustable filtering.
2. Security of systems: Login control, security updates
3. Backup and disaster recovery plans.
4. Current support contract for all equipment and whether proper maintenance is occurring.

All of the equipment used should be regularly assessed to assure it can execute protocols that are consistent with the current standard of care including dosage, data corrections and interpretation.

Monitoring Program

The monitoring of the performance of imaging instrumentation is only valuable if the staff is aware of the actionable alerts situations, and what actions should be taken when a quality problem is discovered. This requires written protocols that explicitly define acceptable performance standards of equipment and what user actions are necessary when a deviation occurs. For PET and PET/CT at a minimum, the quality monitoring program for the instrumentation should include:

1. Daily blank scan evaluation: In particular visual and quantitative variations in the daily blank scan.
2. Daily CT or line source evaluation.
   (a) For PET/CT: CT number, low contrast, uniformity and resolution.
   (b) For line source: Daily blank scan and line source strength.
3. Post service quality assurance program: review of service report, norm file evaluation and phantom study that tests clinical acquisition protocol.
4. Image review of pre and post service visit QC and clinical images

Data Storage

A quality program must also include the storage of a patient's medical data. In assessing the archiving computer backup needs of a cardiac PET program, it is important to separate the goals of archiving into two distinct tasks: archiving and disaster recovery. Disaster recovery backup solutions should provide real time protection of the workstation environment to insure that in the event of computer failure, no patient data would be lost. The second task is the long term archiving and retrieval of patient data sets.

Disaster Recovery

In assessing the disaster recovery need of a department, it is important to match the information technology capabilities to the disaster recovery technology employed. Though there are many approaches to disaster recovery, they all revolve around the same principle of creating a duplicate copy of the hard drive of a computer so that in the event the drive fails, the backup can be used to restore the system.

The simplest of these approaches is to use a separate, external hard drive, like a USB drive to create a real time mirror of the systems hard drive. These USB drives have the advantage of being very low cost, easy to install and maintain. In most cases the USB drive has backup software pre-loaded to support real time mirroring of a system's hard drive. There are several limitations of that approach. First, USB drives can be unreliable over a long period of time. Another serious concern about external USB drive is the ease in which they can be removed from systems. According to the US Department of Health and Human Services [8], USB drives are one of the major sources of major HIPAA violations. As a result, practices should consider the encryption on all data detachable data drives [9].

A more reliable technique is to use a disk array to provide data security. A disk array uses multiple disk drives to create a single, virtual disk drive. In addition to the obvious advantage of increased the disk space available users, this technique also allows for a high level of real time data protection. When these drives are arranged into a "redundant array of independent disks" (referred to as a "RAID"), an entire hard drive can fail and the system can continue to function normally. In addition, most RAID system can be configured with a fail-over drive that can automatically be brought online when a hard drive fails.

The configuration of the RAID (the RAID level), describes how the RAID is arranged to protect the user data. The simplest RAID configuration (RAID Level 0), uses two, identical drives in which identical data is written to both drives. This configuration provides the user with only half of the total disk space for use. More sophisticated RAID configurations can leverage the symmetries of digital data to provide much larger usable space, while using less disk space. For a description of higher RAID levels.

Whenever a site accepts the responsibility for managing their own data, storage of physical backups to off-site facilities must be used. Regular audits and random retrievals from the storage service should be performed to insure data can be retrieved and is being stored in a manner consistent with laws and regulations.

More recently, cloud-based services have become more widely available and inexpensive enough to allow users and institutions to leverage large internet based storage providers. These services provide for high levels of redundancy, security and on-demand expansion of storage space. When investigating the feasibility a cloud based service it is essential to investigate the data security policies of the provider, their up-time records and ability to comply with the requirements of all applicable laws and regulates for handling medical information (including HIPAA).

Physician Performance

Quality improvement of a Cardiac PET program is the direct responsibility of the Medical Director. However, a successful laboratory seeks input from its entire staff including the chief technologists, all technologists, all interpreting physicians and other ancillary personnel. There are several means of improving quality, as listed below:

1. *Awareness of new procedures, technologies*. The field of cardiac PET is rapidly evolving with new tracers, applications and methods to reduce radiation exposure. For example, software solutions for enabling cameras to perform high sensitivity 3D imaging are now available to reduce radiation exposure and maximize image quality in large patients. Applications for FDG imaging, such the imaging myocardial viability and sarcoidosis, are emerging which should be considered for an individual practice. The Medical Director should regularly attend professional education meetings, webinars, etc. to remain current as to these changes and how they may be applied in his/her laboratory.
2. *Monitoring of image quality of the laboratory*. It is the responsibility of the Medical Director to monitor acquisition practices, processing, and patient preparation to maintain a high quality laboratory. There should be continual communication with technologists and testing personnel. Formal surveys from

	MPI Findings						Cath Results					Agreement			
Study	Chart ID	Nuclear Scan Date	Overall	LAD	LCx	RCA	Cath Date	Overall	LAD	LCx	RCA	Overall	LAD	LCx	RCA
1	14321	15-Mar-15	Abn	N	Rev	Part-Rev	20-Mar-15	Abn	N	N	80%	TP	TN	FP	TP

Fig. 18.3 Sample myocardial perfusion imaging and coronary catheterization correlation

patients, referring physicians are particularly important in identifying opportunities for improving quality.

3. *Quality Improvement Projects relating to Physician Performance*. It is reasonable to measure physician performance based on the accuracy of image interpretation to a gold standard, such as cardiac catheterization. It is now a mandate of IAC Nuclear that a quality improvement project is in place for re-accreditation, using such projects as listed in Table 18.3. Quarterly meetings to evaluate the laboratory performance on QI projects are also mandated with at least 50 % attendance by all involved in the cardiac PET program. Several QI projects are suggested by IAC but do not need to be confined to those alone. A sample of data collection and analysis for correlation between perfusion imaging results and cardiac catherization findings are illustrated in Figs. 18.3 and 18.4. A brief discussion of potential projects is listed below.

(a) Cardiac catheterization and blood flow. A comparison of PET imaging results with those patients going onto cardiac catherization is an important QI project and should be done on a continuing basis. Such a catherization project should evaluate individual physician performance. The program should provide the opportunity to evaluate images in where differences between anatomy and physiology occur with the entire group in a quarterly meeting setting. In addition, additive information such as TID, reversible wall motion findings and myocardial blood flow should be considered in evaluating the effectiveness of the cardiac PET program. If myocardial blood flow is being reported, it is important to correlate blood flow results with cardiac catheterization, particularly in those reported as normal. Normal blood flow rates and blood flow reserve values from the medical literature can differ from a practice's experience if software, imaging protocol and patient population are difference. Laboratories that implement absolute blood flow measurements should establish meaningful limits of normal based on their own patients and instrumentation, and software used.

(b) Appropriate Use Criteria Study. The Appropriate Use Criteria (AUC) are now being used extensively in Cardiology, including non-invasive testing/imaging, catheterization procedures and electrophysiology. Standards are being developed by payers that will evaluate how many patients meet criteria. They will also closely evaluate when patients are deemed "rarely appropriate" and if the percentage is too high, practices may be penalized in the future. These standards are also being incorporated into re-accreditation standards. Thus, an AUC project is of great importance. There are many "application" aps that can easily

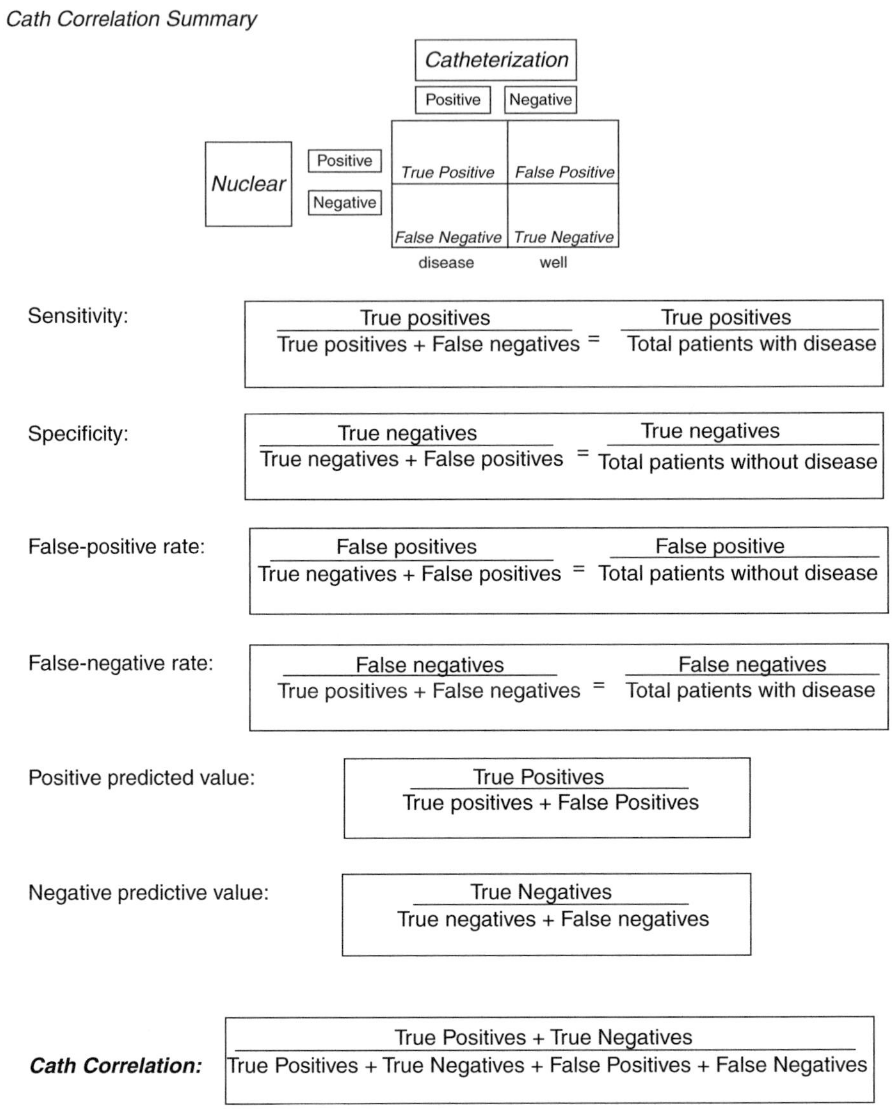

Fig. 18.4 Sample MPI and coronary catherization correlation: data analysis

calculate the AUC category. Such a project should determine the percentage of "appropriate, rarely and usually appropriate categories. For those in the "rarely" category, the referring physician should be identified if the percentage is particularly high and disturbing, and contacted for discussion. This may be a delicate matter if the physician/allied personnel are not in the group performing the test, but data suggest patients in the "rarely" category are far more likely to have a normal study, indicating the study to be of little value.

(c) Observer agreement: A high quality laboratory should maintain consistency of interpretation between all readers and within all readers. The former, consistency between readers is aided if the Medical Director establishes a report system in which all agree upon terminology as well as the size and severity of the defects when noted. The ASNC 17 segment system [10] is generally considered optimal for all to use. Similarly, there should be consistency of reporting within the individual reader. Both intra and inter observer variability can be a QI project.

Summary

For a quality improvement program to be successful, it must be comprehensive and involve all stakeholders: medical director, technologists, nurses, referring physicians. It must be a continual process of identification of opportunities for improvement and executing plans to achieve those goals. It ultimate goal is providing the best possible outcome for the patient, both in terms of accuracy while minimizing testing risk and incontinence. It is upon each laboratory to evaluate its procedures, instrumentation, personnel and protocol to develop a quality improvement program that can fit their needs.

References

1. The Intersocietal Accreditation Commission (IAC). Standards and guidelines for nuclear/PET accreditation [internet]. 2012. Intersocietal Accreditation Commission, Published online. Available from: http://intersocietal.org/nuclear/standards/IACNuclearPETStandards2012.pdf.
2. National Quality Measures Clearinghouse. Template of measure attributes [internet]. 2015. Available from: http://www.qualitymeasures.ahrq.gov/tutorial/attributes.aspx.
3. Cochran C. The continual improvement process: from strategy to the bottom line. Chico: Patton Professional; 2003. p. 71–91.
4. DePuey EG, Mahmarian JJ, Miller TD, Einstein AJ, Hansen CL, Holly TA, Miller EJ, Polk DM, Wann LS. Patient centered imaging. J Nucl Cardiol. 2012;19:185–215. http://www.asnc.org/media/PDFs/PatientCenteredImagingFINAL.pdf.
5. Cerqueira MD, et al. Recommendations for reducing radiation exposure in myocardial perfusion imaging. J Nucl Cardiol. 2010;17:709–18. www.asnc.org/section_73.cfm.
6. National Electronics Manufacturers Association. Performance measurements of Gamma Cameras. NEMA NU 1–2007. 2007.
7. International Atomic Energy Agency. Quality assurance for SPECT systems [internet]. 2009. Veinna. Available from: http://wwwpub.iaea.org/MTCD/publications/PDF/Pub1394_web.pdf.
8. Department of Health and Human Services. HIPAA security guidance. [Internet] 2006. Available from: http://www.hhs.gov/ocr/privacy/hipaa/administrative/securityrule/remoteuse.pdf.
9. Scarfone K, Souppaya M Sexton M. Guide to storage encryption technologies for end user devices: recommendation of the National Institute of Standards and Technology. Special Publication 800–111, [Internet] 2007. Available from: http://www.hhs.gov/ocr/privacy/hipaa/administrative/securityrule/nist800111.pdf.

10. Cerqueira MD, Weissman NJ, Dilsizian V, et al. Standardized myocardial segmentation and nomenclature for tomographic imaging of the heart. A statement for healthcare professionals from the Cardiac Imaging Committee of the Council on Clinical Cardiology of the American Heart Association. Circulation. 2002;105(4):539–42.
11. Hendel RC, Berman DS, Di Carli MF, Heidenreich PA, Henkin RE, Pellikka PA, Pohost GM, Williams KA. ACCF/ASNC/ACR/AHA/ASE/SCCT/SCMR/SNM 2009 appropriate use criteria for cardiac radionuclide imaging. J Am Coll Cardiol. 2009;53(23):2201–29.

Part V
SPECT

Chapter 19
SPECT: Clinical Applications

Cesia Gallegos and Robert C. Hendel

Abstract The knowledge about quality control and the development of quality initiatives provide techniques for the optimal performance of SPECT imaging and therefore maximize the clinical value of this important non-invasive technique. Given the increasing volume in cardiac imaging and its related expense, it is critical to provide clinically relevant data and do so in a cost-effective manner. This section will focus on the clinical implications of SPECT myocardial perfusion imaging. We will review the evaluation of multiple patient populations including those with suspected coronary artery disease, risk stratification, preoperative risk assessment, evaluation of therapy in patients with known coronary disease, risk stratification of the diabetic patient, assessment of women and additional unique patient cohorts. The body of evidence supporting each of these indications is very strong and will be reviewed.

Keywords SPECT • Patient populations • Coronary artery disease • Risk stratification • Diagnostic value

Background

Coronary artery disease (CAD) remains the leading cause of death worldwide. In America, it is estimated that every 34 s one individual will have a coronary event, and every 83 s one will die from one [1]. The detection of ischemia is of paramount importance for early diagnosis and risk stratification of patients with known or suspected CAD, so as to intervene in order to reduce subsequent cardiac events. Radionuclide myocardial perfusion imaging (MPI) has been established as means

C. Gallegos, MD
Department of Medicine, University of Miami Miller School of Medicine, Miami, FL, USA
e-mail: cesia.gallegos@jhsmiami.org

R.C. Hendel, MD, FACC, FAHA, FASNC (✉)
Cardiovascular Division Chief (Interim), University of Miami Miller School of Medicine, 1120 NW 14th Street, Suite 1123, CRB, Miami, FL 33136, USA
e-mail: RHendel@med.miami.edu

P.L. Tilkemeier et al. (eds.), *Quality Evaluation in Non-Invasive Cardiovascular Imaging*, DOI 10.1007/978-3-319-28011-0_19

of evaluating patient with diagnosed or suspected CAD and remains one of the most widely used and readily available method [2–5].

SPECT myocardial perfusion imaging is a powerful and useful tool for the clinical diagnosis, risk stratification, and management of cardiac disease, with widespread utilization [5]. Its clinical impact in decision-making has been well established, and the evidence for its clinical applications continues to grow. SPECT MPI has robust literature supporting its use for patients with suspected or known CAD, in the determination of prognosis, for preoperative risk assessment, and in the evaluation of therapy. In addition to examining these clinical states, this chapter we will also review the use of SPECT MPI in various patient subgroups.

Evaluation of Patient with Suspected CAD

The initial step for evaluation of patients with known/suspected CAD is usually a pretest assessment of the likelihood of CAD and subsequent risk of cardiac events. This involves the evaluation of traditional risk factors, both modifiable and non-modifiable and the use of clinical prediction models to stratify patients into low, intermediate, and high-risk categories for CAD and cardiac death. The Adult Treatment Panel III in particular, defines absolute risk for CAD as any hard cardiac event (MI or death) over the next 10 years. These risks can be categorized as low (10-year absolute CAD risk less than 10 %), moderate (10-year absolute CAD risk between 10 and 20 %), and high (10-year absolute CAD risk of greater than 20 %) [6]. Other indices, such as the Framingham risk score (FRS) and the Reynolds score have been developed and shown predictive value with regards to outcomes [7–9].

When symptoms that may represent obstructive CAD and the associated risk factors are evaluated, the pretest probability of CAD should be assessed. For example, Diamond and Forrester provided a clinical relevant assessment of the probability of significant CAD based on gender, age and type of chest pain, as noted in Table 19.1. The determination of a patient's likelihood of CAD using this approach provides four categories:

Table 19.1 Pretest probability of coronary artery disease by age, gender, and symptoms

Age (years)	Gender	Typical/definite angina pectoris	Atypical/probable angina pectoris	Nonanginal chest pain	Asymptomatic
30–39	Men	Intermediate	Intermediate	Low	Very low
	Women	Intermediate	Very low	Very low	Very low
40–49	Men	High	Intermediate	Intermediate	Low
	Women	Intermediate	Low	Very low	Very low
50–59	Men	High	Intermediate	Intermediate	Low
	Women	Intermediate	Intermediate	Low	Very low
60–69	Men	High	Intermediate	Intermediate	Low
	Women	High	Intermediate	Intermediate	Low

Adapted from Hendel et al. [17] with permission from Elsevier
High >90 %, *Intermediate* 10–90 %, *low* <10 %, *very low* <5

- Very low likelihood: <5 %
- Low likelihood: <10 %
- Intermediate likelihood: 10–90 %
- High likelihood: >90 %

All risk models have deficiencies, included this often utilized method for the determination of pre-test likelihood for CAD, as several clinical risk factors, including diabetes are not included and even models of coronary heart disease risk such as the FRS, do not include family history or presence of end-stage renal disease (ESRD) Therefore, non-invasive cardiac testing is often necessary and improves the classification of risk beyond clinical factors.

ECG exercise tolerance testing (ETT) remains an important method for the detection of CAD, but possesses limited diagnostic accuracy. SPECT MPI has a higher diagnostic accuracy and allows for the elucidation of the size, severity, and extent of disease. Additionally, SPECT MPI permits the assessment of known or suspected CAD even when factors are present which confound the analysis of the ECG, such as conduction abnormalities, left ventricular hypertrophy, or the use of digoxin are present.

In patients who are incapable of maximum exercise, SPECT MPI may be performed with pharmacologic stress, either with vasodilators (adenosine, dypiridamole or regadenoson) or a catecholamine, such as dobutamine. Vasodilators increase coronary blood flow, which is less pronounced in arteries that are flow-restricted causing heterogeneous myocardial perfusion. This can be observed using a tracer that follows coronary blood flow. Dobutamine, which may be used in patients with contraindications to vasodilators (primarily reversible airway disease), increases myocardial oxygen demand thereby increasing coronary blood flow, again demonstrating heterogeneous blood flow in stenotic areas.

The diagnostic accuracy of pharmacologic stress is similar to that obtained with exercise SPECT, although it is preferable to perform exercise whenever possible so as to assess functional capacity, evaluate symptoms, blood pressure response, and arrhythmias.

Risk Stratification

Risk stratification is vital for clinical decision-making. High-risk patients for subsequent events should be considered for aggressive treatment, including coronary revascularization; patients identified as low-risk should be the targeted for medical therapy, including risk factor modification.

Risk stratification is usually defined by three categories [10]:

- High Risk (>3 % annual cardiac death or MI)
- Intermediate Risk (1–3 % of annual cardiac death or MI)
- Low risk (<1 % of annual cardiac death or MI)

Clinical parameters, such as cardiac risk factors and symptoms, as well as the resting ECG may be used to define risk, although these may provide only limited stratification. The evaluation of functional capacity also provides substantial prognostic value. Nonetheless, using clinical parameters and treadmill data will often place more than 55 % of the patients into the intermediate risk, requiring further evaluation [4]. Moreover, coronary angiography considered the "gold standard" for diagnosing CAD, often does not provide physiologic information and may not optimize risk assessment, especially in the setting of borderline lesions (50–70 %).

SPECT MPI provides physiologic significance of a known or suspected coronary stenosis and determines the extent, severity and location of ischemia and infarction, as well as predicts functional recovery after revascularization. For example, a normal SPECT heralds an excellent prognosis, even in the setting of chronic ischemic heart disease [11, 12]. An abnormal SPECT study, in the other hand, suggests an increased risk for cardiac events [4]. The value of MPI comes from its capacity to identify and quantify the degree of affected myocardium during stress, which provides powerful prognostic information. Other key SPECT indicators of prognosis include the following [4]:

- Perfusion defect
- Extensive and/or severe defect
- Multivessel distribution
- Reversibility
- Postinfart ischemia
- Transient ischemia dilation
- Left ventricular dilation
- Left ventricular dysfunction

Overall, SPECT MPI has shown great value in clinical decision-making and serves as a "gatekeeper" to the cath lab and coronary revascularization. Furthermore, it has been shown to be cost-effective, a critical consideration in the current era [13–15].

Preoperative Risk Assessment for Non-cardiac Surgery

Preoperative risk assessment is a vital tool for the evaluation of patients prior to any surgery, which will guide management both before and after the procedure including further lifestyle modifications. It should begin with emphasis on clinical risk and exercise capacity, along with the nature of the surgical procedure. In selected patients, further data may be beneficial to stratify them into low or high-risk group and for prediction of long-term cardiac events related to the procedure. Most importantly, the starting point in deciding if a patient requires a SPECT study or further work-up at all, is to first categorize the type of surgery he or she will undergo as described below.

As noted in Fig. 19.1 [16] non-invasive testing for preoperative assessment is recommended in the following situations [16, 17]:

1. Patient has poor functional capacity (<4 METS) **AND**
2. One or more clinical risk factors (ischemic heart disease, compensated or prior heart failure, diabetes mellitus, renal insufficiency or cerebrovascular disease), **AND**
3. Is undergoing intermediate or high-risk surgery.

Taking this into consideration, SPECT MPI can stratify patients into low- or high-risk groups, which is helpful for both short and long-term prediction of cardiac events. Since ischemia on SPECT identifies patients at higher risk, larger perfusion defects have been associated with higher event rates and worse prognosis.

Evaluation of Therapies in Patients with Known CAD

SPECT MPI is an important tool in following patients with known CAD, in particular when there is a change in the frequency or pattern of symptoms.

Groups that benefit incrementally with the use of SPECT MPI include:

- Patients with known CAD with symptoms, to assess risk for future events
- Patients with previous myocardial infarction or revascularization procedures such as PCI or CABG, in which medication optimization is sought
- Patients with prior angiography demonstrating significant disease that may require CABG
- High-risk individuals for future events, such as diabetic patients
- Patients with previous positive radionuclide scan

In post-CABG patients, the indication for stress MPI depends [17] on the presence or absence of symptoms and the timing after the procedures. A threshold of 5 years has been applied to the asymptomatic post-CABG patient [18, 19]. In patients who have undergone CABG more than 5 years beforehand, SPECT is effective for risk stratification regardless of symptoms [19]. Zellweger et al. demonstrated that asymptomatic patients ≤5 years post-CABG have a low cardiac death rate of 1.3 %, and would not usually benefit from routine nuclear testing.

The timing of SPECT MPI after PCI remains controversial. Early studies performed in the times of balloon angioplasty demonstrated high rate of false-positives tests after performing imaging in the first few weeks after PCI [20]. Hence patients with typical symptoms early after PCI are better evaluated by repeat angiography. Although there are no randomized trial to support this, when MPI is done >6 months after PCI it can identify patients at highest risk of poor outcomes [20]. Currently, MPI is considered to be appropriate in any patient either with atypical symptoms or in those who require further ischemia work-up, as well as those who are symptomatic or are thought to be incompletely revascularized [17]. However, there appears to be little indication for SPECT MPI within 2 years of PCI unless new or recurrent symptomatology is present.

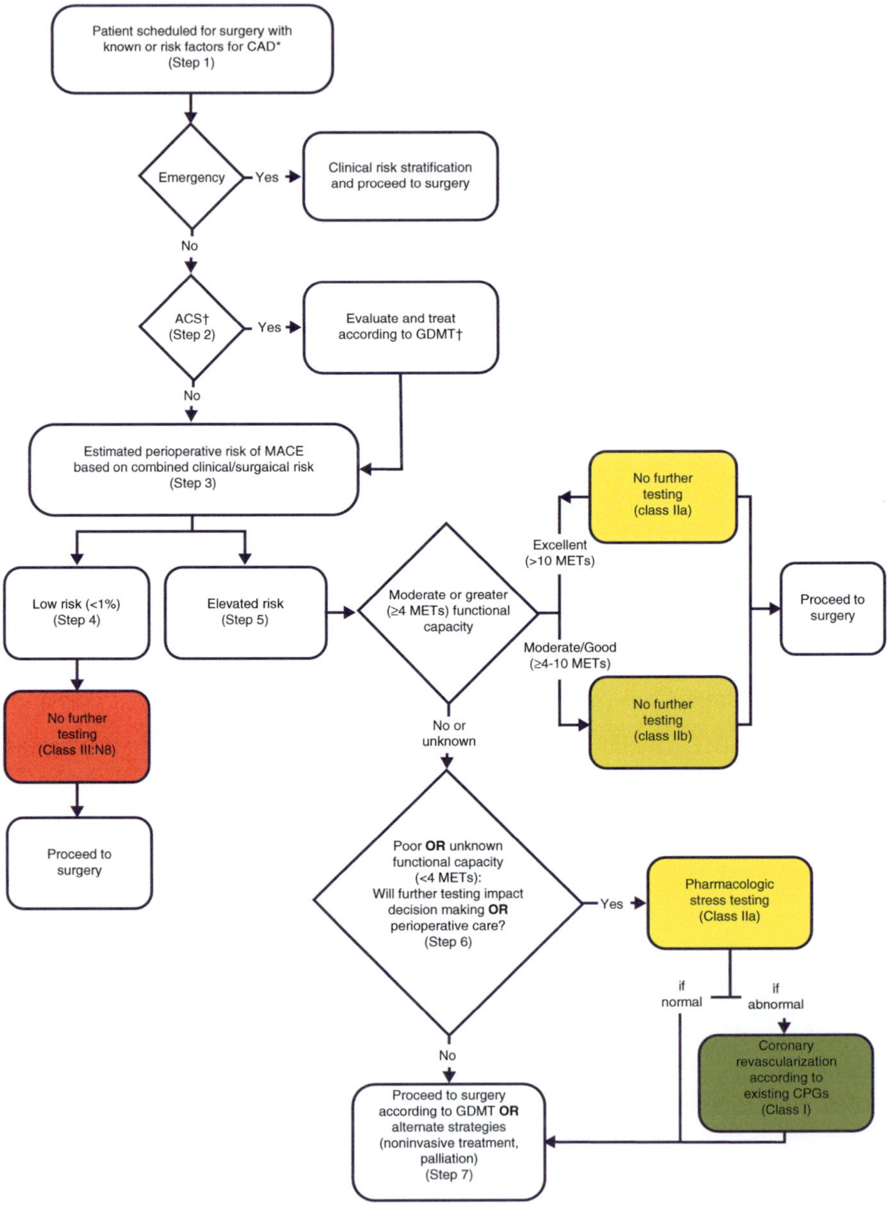

SPECT MPI is also useful in patients who survive an acute MI, many of whom have an increased incidence of re-infarction or cardiac-related death. Studies have demonstrated that it can be done as early as 2–4 days after an uncomplicated myocardial infarction [21–23]. This approach can shorten hospital stay and has excellent prognostic value. Furthermore, for risk stratification, a large area of ischemia (>10 % of the LV) on MPI using adenosine performed after an uncomplicated MI is superior to coronary angiography in stratifying patient to increased risk for cardiac events versus low risk [23] The INSPIRE trial showed that SPECT MPI can be used to monitor changes in ischemia after revascularization or intensive medical therapy following an acute coronary syndrome without intervention and help to guide additional therapeutic intervention [23].

Risk Stratification in the Diabetic Patient

It is well known that patients with type 2 diabetes mellitus have a high risk for a first coronary event and also have a poor prognosis for recurrent events and cardiac death, validating the classification of diabetes as a CAD equivalent [6, 24, 25]. In addition to more frequent occurrence, myocardial ischemia is often asymptomatic in these patients [26, 27] with more diffuse and accelerated disease. In the case of diabetic women, in particular those who are insulin dependent, their risk for cardiovascular death is up to 7.5 times that of a woman without diabetes [28].

The goal of evaluating asymptomatic diabetic patients is to identify those at increased risk for cardiovascular events, which may benefit from early intervention. SPECT MPI has been demonstrated to be of value to evaluate symptoms or other conditions to be worthy of testing for CAD. In a study, Bell and al demonstrated that

Fig. 19.1 Stepwise approach to perioperative cardiac assessment for CAD. Step 1: in patients scheduled for surgery with risk factors for or known CAD, determine the urgency of surgery. Step 2: if the surgery is urgent or elective, determine if the patient has an ACS. If yes, then refer patient for cardiology evaluation and management. Step 3: if the patient has risk factors for stable CAD, then estimate the perioperative risk of major cardiovascular events (MACE) on the basis of the combined clinical/surgical risk. Step 4: if the patient has a low risk of MACE (<1 %), then no further testing is needed, and the patient may proceed to surgery. Step 5: If the patient is at elevated risk of MACE, then determine functional capacity. If the patient has moderate, good, or excellent functional capacity (≥4 METs), then proceed to surgery without further evaluation. Step 6: if the patient has poor (<4 METs) or unknown functional capacity, then the clinician should consult with the patient and perioperative team to determine whether further testing will impact patient decision making (e.g., decision to perform original surgery or willingness to undergo CABG or PCI, depending on the results of the test) or perioperative care. If yes, then pharmacological stress testing is appropriate. In those patients with unknown functional capacity, exercise stress testing may be reasonable to perform. If the stress test is abnormal, consider coronary angiography and revascularization depending on the extent of the abnormal test. If the test is normal, proceed to surgery according to GDMT. Step 7: if testing will not impact decision making or care, then proceed to surgery according to GDMT or consider alternative strategies, such as noninvasive treatment of the indication for surgery (e.g., radiation therapy for cancer) or palliation (Reprinted from Fleisher et al. [16] with permission from Elsevier)

SPECT MPI had a sensitivity of 97 % with a predictive value of 88 % [29]. However, the DIAD trial raised questions about the use of SPECT imaging in asymptomatic diabetic patients with normal rest ECG's, and demonstrated that routine testing with MPI is not recommended as subsequent cardiac events were not predicted by imaging in this low risk cohort [5, 30].

Assessment of Women

The primary cause of death among American women remains ischemic heart disease [1]. Therefore, the assessment of heart disease in women poses an important challenge to a clinician, particularly given the differences in presentation of heart disease between men and women.

Exercise ECG testing (ETT) remains the most common test to detect CAD, although false positive studies are common, likely due to lower burden of disease, baseline physiologic gender differences in response to exercise, altered exercise capacity, ECG changes related to estrogen or lower pretest probability of heart disease. Moreover, as demonstrated by the WOMEN trial, an ETT in low-risk women who are able to exercise provides similar prognostic data regarding 2-year outcomes as compared to SPECT MPI, while doing so with significant cost savings [31]. However, in women with limited exercise capacity, pharmacologic stress is an important alternative. Stress MPI had been shown to have good predictive value to improve the diagnostic accuracy of ETT alone, but is affected by several factors, in particular, breast attenuation and small heart size. Risk stratification also is an essential tool for evaluating CAD in women and SPECT MPI has demonstrated substantial prognostic value in women [4].

Additional Unique Patient Groups

Several additional medical conditions are associated with an elevated risk for cardiovascular events and cardiac death. Therefore, the detection of coronary artery disease in this population may improve outcomes by identifying patients who might benefit from aggressive medical therapy or revascularization, even when no symptoms are present. This group includes those patients with diabetes, chronic kidney disease, Human Immunodeficiency Virus (HIV), autoimmune diseases and use of antiarrhythmic medications [32].

Cardiovascular disease is also the leading cause of death in patients with chronic kidney disease (CKD). In addition to a high prevalence of conventional CAD risks, the pathogenesis of CKD impacts in coronary atherosclerosis and plaque rupture. Even in asymptomatic subjects with CKD, SPECT MPI has independent prognostic value for the prediction of cardiac events and all-cause mortality. In completely asymptomatic patients, the value of radionuclide imaging has demonstrated an incidence of perfusion defects between 10 and 22 % [32]. Hence, these patients have an intermediate likelihood of having occult CAD, and SPECT MPI provides superior diagnostic accuracy and prognosis.

HIV patients are known to have accelerated coronary atherosclerosis and in 77 % of the patients, myocardial infarction is the initial presentation. Although some HIV medications may increase the risk for cardiac events, there is no evidence available to support the use of SPECT MPI for detection of occult CAD in asymptomatic patients.

Regarding patients with autoimmune disease, there is insufficient evidence to recommend SPECT MPI to detect asymptomatic CAD. Hence, these patients have to be taken in the clinical context, with evaluation of potential ischemic symptoms.

SPECT MPI in the Emergency Department

In patients with acute chest pain arriving to the ED, the goal is to promptly evaluate them to further categorize the possible etiology into cardiac or non-cardiac. This generally starts with assessment of symptoms as well as a 12-lead ECG. Once that cardiac chest pain is assumed, the decision to appropriately discharge or admit a patient must be made. However, in the absence of diagnostic ECG changes with or without symptoms, the decision becomes challenging. Acute rest MPI has emerged as an excellent tool for diagnosis and prognosis of patient with acute coronary syndrome and uninterpretable ECG. It has a good sensitivity and a very high negative predictive value for the diagnosis of both acute myocardial infarction and unstable angina and had demonstrated cost-effectiveness [33]. Current American Heart Association Guidelines recommend acute rest SPECT myocardial perfusion imaging as Class I indication for evaluation of chest pain presenting to the ED [10].

Myocardial Viability

Coronary heart disease (CHD) remains the most common cause of left ventricular dysfunction, although this is not always an irreversible process [34]. Individuals with CHD and HF may have dysfunctional viable myocardium, which may benefit from revascularization or other forms of therapy [35, 36]. Hence, the definition and differentiation of viable vs. non-viable myocardium is of high clinical importance, as revascularization may lead to improvement in quality of life, regional and global LV function, and survival [37]. Although this topic has become controversial in the past few years, it was initially demonstrated in a meta-analysis performed by Allman et al. that the use of noninvasive imaging techniques could identify patients with CAD and LV dysfunction who are at high risk of death and would benefit from revascularization, guiding the difficult decision making of further interventions in these category of patients [4, 35, 38]. However, questions have arisen about the utility of viability testing after the results of the STITCH trial were published in 2011, suggesting that patients with viable myocardium undergoing CABG did not have survival benefits, disputing the results of the aforementioned meta-analysis.

Nevertheless, STICH was originally designed to test the influence of viability assessment on all-cause mortality. As viability testing hampered the recruitment of patients for the study, it ultimately became optional, thereby introducing bias into patients undergoing SPECT imaging Furthermore, SPECT methodology was not standardized. Therefore STICH contained many concerns regarding statistical adequacy and applicability of the results to the general population [37]. The results of STITCH once again serve as a matter of reflection and recognition that appropriate selection is critical, especially in patients with severely depressed LV dysfunction, in which the perioperative mortality may be as high as the potential benefit.

Neuronal Imaging

In addition to the use of SPECT MPI in the setting of ischemic heart disease, tomographic radionuclide imaging may also be used to assess cardiac neuronal function, which may have important implications in the management of heart failure and sudden cardiac death [39]. The major uses of neurohormonal imaging are the assessment of heart failure, arrhythmias, and ischemic heart disease, as impairment of cardiac autonomic function can reflect the severity of cardiac disease and in many cases may contribute to the worsening of any of the aforementioned conditions.

Imaging of cardiac sympathetic innervation focuses on the synaptic junction. Since norepinephrine (NE) is ultimately stored at high concentration in presynaptic vesicles, most tracers being studied have used analogs of NE, including I-123 metaiodobenzylguanine (I-mIBG). There is evidence that among heart failure patients, mIBG will help identify patients with lower mortality risks, as indicated by a heart to mediastinal ratio (HMR) of $\geq$1.6 [40, 41].

The current approach for HF focuses on neurohormonal changes that may contribute or worsen the condition, in which the sympathetic adrenergic system and the renin-angiotensin system are activated, with the release of modulators that worsen the cardiac function and activate this cycle even further, subsequently worsening cardiac function. Multiple recent studies have evaluated the association between MIBG HMR and LVEF and mortality, as a decreased HMR has been consistently associated with a poor prognosis [41].

Another promising application of ^{123}I-mIBG imaging is to monitor response to medical therapy for heart failure. For example, studies have demonstrated how ^{123}I-mIBG improves after therapy with β-Blockers [42]. Other medications that have shown improvement in cardiac uptake are spironolactone, angiotensin-converting enzyme inhibitors (ACE-I) and angiotensin receptor blockers (ARBs) [43–45].

Currently, LVEF is used to assess which patients will benefit from an ICD, however its ability to predict sudden cardiac death (SCD) is limited. The cardiac autonomic system also plays a crucial factor in sudden cardiac death and ^{123}I-mIBG imaging appears to assist in defining which patients are at risk for SCD [40, 46].

References

1. Hendel RC, Heller GV. Nuclear cardiology: practical applications. 2nd ed. McGraw-Hill Professional. 2011. p. 416.
2. Go AS, Mozaffarian D, Roger VL, Benjamin EJ, Berry JD, Blaha MJ, et al. Heart disease and stroke statistics – 2014 update: a report from the American Heart Association. Circulation. 2014;129(3):e28–292. PubMed.
3. Metz LD, Beattie M, Hom R, Redberg RF, Grady D, Fleischmann KE. The prognostic value of normal exercise myocardial perfusion imaging and exercise echocardiography: a meta-analysis. J Am Coll Cardiol. 2007;49(2):227–37. PubMed.
4. Jaarsma C, Leiner T, Bekkers SC, Crijns HJ, Wildberger JE, Nagel E, et al. Diagnostic performance of noninvasive myocardial perfusion imaging using single-photon emission computed tomography, cardiac magnetic resonance, and positron emission tomography imaging for the detection of obstructive coronary artery disease: a meta-analysis. J Am Coll Cardiol. 2012;59(19):1719–28. PubMed.
5. Shaw LJ, Hage FG, Berman DS, Hachamovitch R, Iskandrian A. Prognosis in the era of comparative effectiveness research: where is nuclear cardiology now and where should it be? J Nucl Cardiol Off Publ Am Soc Nucl Cardiol. 2012;19(5):1026–43. PubMed.
6. National Institutes of Health: National Heart L, and Blood Institute. Third Report of the National Cholesterol Education Program (NCEP) expert panel on detection, evaluation, and treatment of high blood cholesterol in adults (adult treatment panel III). NIH Publication No. 02–5215; Sept 2002.
7. Cook NR, Paynter NP, Eaton CB, Manson JE, Martin LW, Robinson JG, et al. Comparison of the Framingham and Reynolds risk scores for global cardiovascular risk prediction in the Multiethnic Women's Health Initiative. Circulation. 2012;125(14):1748–56.
8. DeFilippis AP, Blaha MJ, Ndumele CE, Budoff MJ, Lloyd-Jones DM, McClelland RL, et al. The association of Framingham and Reynolds risk scores with incidence and progression of coronary artery calcification in MESA (Multi-Ethnic Study of Atherosclerosis). J Am Coll Cardiol. 2011;58(20):2076–83. PubMed Pubmed Central PMCID: 4079464.
9. Diamond GA, Forrester JS. Analysis of probability as an aid in the clinical diagnosis of coronary-artery disease. N Engl J Med. 1979;300(24):1350–8. PubMed.
10. Fihn SD, Gardin JM, Abrams J, Berra K, Blankenship JC, Dallas AP, et al. 2012 ACCF/AHA/ACP/AATS/PCNA/SCAI/STS guideline for the diagnosis and management of patients with stable ischemic heart disease: a report of the American College of Cardiology Foundation/American Heart Association Task Force on Practice Guidelines, and the American College of Physicians, American Association for Thoracic Surgery, Preventive Cardiovascular Nurses Association, Society for Cardiovascular Angiography and Interventions, and Society of Thoracic Surgeons. J Am Coll Cardiol. 2012;60(24):e44–164. PubMed.
11. Shaw LJ, Hendel R, Borges-Neto S, Lauer MS, Alazraki N, Burnette J, et al. Prognostic value of normal exercise and adenosine (99 m)Tc-tetrofosmin SPECT imaging: results from the multicenter registry of 4,728 patients. J Nucl Med Off Publ Soc Nucl Med. 2003;44(2):134–9. PubMed Epub 2003/02/07. eng.
12. Hachamovitch R, Hayes S, Friedman JD, Cohen I, Shaw LJ, Germano G, et al. Determinants of risk and its temporal variation in patients with normal stress myocardial perfusion scans: what is the warranty period of a normal scan? J Am Coll Cardiol. 2003;41(8):1329–40. Apr 16, PubMed Epub 2003/04/23. eng.
13. Shaw LJ, Hachamovitch R, Berman DS, Marwick TH, Lauer MS, Heller GV, et al. The economic consequences of available diagnostic and prognostic strategies for the evaluation of stable angina patients: an observational assessment of the value of precatheterization ischemia. Economics of Noninvasive Diagnosis (END) Multicenter Study Group. J Am Coll Cardiol. 1999;33(3):661–9. PubMed Epub 1999/03/18. eng.

14. Shaw L, Heller G, Travin M, Lauer M, Marwick T, Hachamovitch R, et al. Cost analysis of diagnostic testing for coronary artery disease in women with stable chest pain. J Nucl Cardiol. 1999;6(6):559–69. 1999/11/01, English.
15. Shaw LJ, Hachamovitch R, Heller GV, Marwick TH, Travin MI, Iskandrian AE, et al. Noninvasive strategies for the estimation of cardiac risk in stable chest pain patients. Am J Cardiol. 2000;86(1):1–7.
16. Fleisher LA, Fleischmann KE, Auerbach AD, Barnason SA, Beckman JA, Bozkurt B, et al. 2014. ACC/AHA guideline on perioperative cardiovascular evaluation and management of patients undergoing noncardiac surgery: a report of the American College of Cardiology/American Heart Association Task Force on Practice Guidelines. J Am Coll Cardiol. 2014. PubMed.
17. Hendel RC, Berman DS, Di Carli MF, Heidenreich PA, Henkin RE, Pellikka PA, et al. ACCF/ASNC/ACR/AHA/ASE/SCCT/SCMR/SNM 2009 appropriate use criteria for cardiac radionuclide imaging: a report of the American College of Cardiology Foundation Appropriate Use Criteria Task Force, the American Society of Nuclear Cardiology, the American College of Radiology, the American Heart Association, the American Society of Echocardiography, the Society of Cardiovascular Computed Tomography, the Society for Cardiovascular Magnetic Resonance, and the Society of Nuclear Medicine. J Am Coll Cardiol. 2009;53(23):2201–29. PubMed.
18. Palmas W, Bingham S, Diamond GA, Denton TA, Kiat H, Friedman JD, et al. Incremental prognostic value of exercise thallium-201 myocardial single-photon emission computed tomography late after coronary artery bypass surgery. J Am Coll Cardiol. 1995;25(2):403–9.
19. Zellweger MJ, Lewin HC, Lai S, Dubois EA, Friedman JD, Germano G, et al. When to stress patients after coronary artery bypass surgery? Risk stratification in patients early and late post-CABG using stress myocardial perfusion SPECT: implications of appropriate clinical strategies. J Am Coll Cardiol. 2001;37(1):144–52.
20. Manyari DE, Knudtson M, Kloiber R, Roth D. Sequential thallium-201 myocardial perfusion studies after successful percutaneous transluminal coronary artery angioplasty: delayed resolution of exercise-induced scintigraphic abnormalities. Circulation. 1988;77(1):86–95. January 1, 1988.
21. Brown KA, Heller GV, Landin RS, Shaw LJ, Beller GA, Pasquale MJ, et al. Early dipyridamole 99mTc-sestamibi single photon emission computed tomographic imaging 2 to 4 days after acute myocardial infarction predicts in-hospital and post discharge cardiac events: comparison with submaximal exercise imaging. Circulation. 1999;100(20):2060–6.
22. Mahmarian JJ, Mahmarian AC, Marks GF, Pratt CM, Verani MS. Role of adenosine thallium-201 tomography for defining long-term risk in patients after acute myocardial infarction. J Am Coll Cardiol. 1995;25(6):1333–40. PubMed Epub 1995/05/01. eng.
23. Mahmarian JJ, Shaw LJ, Olszewski GH, Pounds BK, Frias ME, Pratt CM, et al. Adenosine sestamibi SPECT post-infarction evaluation (INSPIRE) trial: a randomized, prospective multicenter trial evaluating the role of adenosine Tc-99 m sestamibi SPECT for assessing risk and therapeutic outcomes in survivors of acute myocardial infarction. J Nucl Cardiol Off Publ Am Soc Nucl Cardiol. 2004;11(4):458–69. PubMed.
24. Hammoud T, Tanguay J-F, Bourassa MG. Management of coronary artery disease: therapeutic options in patients with diabetes. J Am Coll Cardiol. 2000;36(2):355–65.
25. Haffner SM, Lehto S, Rönnemaa T, Pyörälä K, Laakso M. Mortality from Coronary Heart Disease in subjects with type 2 diabetes and in nondiabetic subjects with and without prior myocardial infarction. N Engl J Med. 1998;339(4):229–34. PubMed.
26. Dweck M, Campbell IW, Miller D, Francis CM. Clinical aspects of silent myocardial ischaemia: with particular reference to diabetes mellitus. Br J Diabetes Vasc Dis. 2009;9(3): 110–6.
27. Xanthos T, Ekmektzoglou KA, Papadimitriou L. Reviewing myocardial silent ischemia: specific patient subgroups. Int J Cardiol. 2008;124(2):139–48.
28. Zuanetti G, Latini R, Maggioni AP, Santoro L, Maria Grazia F. Influence of diabetes on mortality in acute myocardial infarction: data from the GISSI-2 study. J Am Coll Cardiol. 1993;22(7):1788–94.

29. Bell DS, Yumuk VD. Low incidence of false-positive exercise thallium 201 scintigraphy in a diabetic population. Diabetes Care. 1996;19(2):185–6. PubMed Epub 1996/02/01. eng.
30. Young LH, Wackers F, Chyun DA, et al. Cardiac outcomes after screening for asymptomatic coronary artery disease in patients with type 2 diabetes: the diad study: a randomized controlled trial. JAMA. 2009;301(15):1547–55.
31. Shaw LJ, Mieres JH, Hendel RH, Boden WE, Gulati M, Veledar E, et al. Comparative effectiveness of exercise electrocardiography with or without myocardial perfusion single photon emission computed tomography in women with suspected coronary artery disease: results from the What Is the Optimal Method for Ischemia Evaluation in Women (WOMEN) trial. Circulation. 2011;124(11):1239–49. PubMed.
32. Hendel RC, Abbott BG, Bateman TM, Blankstein R, Calnon DA, Leppo JA, et al. The role of radionuclide myocardial perfusion imaging for asymptomatic individuals. J Nucl Cardiol Off Publ Am Soc Nucl Cardiol. 2011;18(1):3–15. PubMed.
33. Udelson JE, Beshansky JR, Ballin DS, Feldman JA, Griffith JL, Handler J, et al. Myocardial perfusion imaging for evaluation and triage of patients with suspected acute cardiac ischemia: a randomized controlled trial. JAMA. 2002;288(21):2693–700. PubMed Epub 2002/12/04. eng.
34. Shabana A, El-Menyar A. Myocardial viability: what we knew and what is new. Cardiol Res Pract. 2012;2012:607486. PubMed Pubmed Central PMCID: 3440854.
35. Chareonthaitawee P, Gersh BJ, Araoz PA, Gibbons RJ. Revascularization in severe left ventricular dysfunction: the role of viability testing. J Am Coll Cardiol. 2005;46(4):567–74. PubMed.
36. Allman KC. Noninvasive assessment myocardial viability: current status and future directions. J Nucl Cardiol. 2013;20(4):616–7.
37. Bonow RO, Mauer G, Lee KL, Holly TA, Binkley PF, Desvigne-Nickens P, et al. Myocardial viability and survival in ischemic left ventricular dysfuction. N Engl J Med. 2011;364: 1617–25.
38. Allman KC, Shaw LJ, Hachamovitch R, Udelson JE. Myocardial viability testing and impact of revascularization on prognosis in patients with coronary artery disease and left ventricular dysfunction: a meta-analysis. J Am Coll Cardiol. 2002;39(7):1151–8.
39. Carrió I. Cardiac neurotransmission imaging*. J Nucl Med. 2001;42(7):1062–76.
40. Jacobson AF, Senior R, Cerqueira MD, Wong ND, Thomas GS, Lopez VA, et al. Myocardial iodine-123 meta-iodobenzylguanidine imaging and cardiac events in heart failure. Results of the prospective ADMIRE-HF (AdreView Myocardial Imaging for Risk Evaluation in Heart Failure) study. J Am Coll Cardiol. 2010;55(20):2212–21. PubMed.
41. Al Badarin F. The utility of ADMIRE-HF risk score in predicting serious arrhythmic events in heart failure patients: incremental prognostic benefit of cardiac 123I-mIBG scintigraphy. J Nucl Cardiol. 2014;21(4):753–5. PubMed.
42. Agostini D, Belin A, Amar MH, Darlas Y, Hamon M, Grollier G, et al. Improvement of cardiac neuronal function after carvedilol treatment in dilated cardiomyopathy: a 123I-MIBG scintigraphic study. J Nucl Med. 2000;41(5):845–51.
43. Carrio I, Cowie MR, Yamazaki J, Udelson J, Camici PG. Cardiac sympathetic imaging with mIBG in heart failure. J Am Coll Cardiol Img. 2010;3(1):92–100. PubMed.
44. Kasama S, Toyama T, Kumakura H, Takayama Y, Ichikawa S, Suzuki T, et al. Effect of spironolactone on cardiac sympathetic nerve activity and left ventricular remodeling in patients with dilated cardiomyopathy. J Am Coll Cardiol. 2003;41(4):574–81.
45. Takeishi Y, Atsumi H, Fujiwara S, Takahashi K, Tomoike H. ACE inhibition reduces cardiac iodine-123-MIBG release in heart failure. J Nucl Med Off Publ Soc Nucl Med. 1997;38(7): 1085–9. PubMed eng.
46. Kelesidis I, Travin MI. Use of cardiac radionuclide imaging to identify patients at risk for arrhythmic sudden cardiac death. J Nucl Cardiol Off Publ Am Soc Nucl Cardiol. 2012;19(1): 142–52; quiz 53–7. PubMed Epub 2011/12/02. eng.

Chapter 20
SPECT: Patient Selection

Robert C. Hendel and Cesia Gallegos

Abstract Patient selection plays an important role in the appropriate utilization of SPECT myocardial perfusion imaging in order to maximize clinical impact. The indications and contraindications for specific patient populations with regard to myocardial perfusion imaging as well as appropriate stress modalities will be examined. Applications of the appropriate use criteria will also be presented and provide a basis for optimization of SPECT MPI use.

Keywords SPECT • Appropriate use criteria • Indications/contraindications • Cost efficiency

Patient Selection

Quality in cardiovascular imaging begins with the selection of an appropriate and useful test for a specific clinical scenario. Despite advances in the technology, and extension of the clinical applications, minimal value for SPECT MPI will be realized unless this powerful tool is applied to the correct patient cohort and is designed to answer a relevant clinical question. In the absence of such a selection process, overuse and misuse are possible, resulting in potential patient harm and increased societal costs. This chapter will discuss the importance of test and patient selection for the clinical applications, as well as contraindications for stress SPECT MPI. An overview of the appropriate use criteria will be provided, so as to guide the selection of the right test, for the right patient, at the right time.

R.C. Hendel, MD, FACC, FAHA, FASNC (✉)
Cardiovascular Division, University of Miami Miller
School of Medicine, 1400 NW 12th Avenue, Suite 2022, Miami, FL 33136, USA
e-mail: rhendel@med.miami.edu

C. Gallegos, MD
Department of Medicine, University of Miami Miller School of Medicine, Miami, FL, USA
e-mail: cesia.gallegos@jhsmiami.org

P.L. Tilkemeier et al. (eds.), *Quality Evaluation in Non-Invasive Cardiovascular Imaging*, DOI 10.1007/978-3-319-28011-0_20

Test Selection and Contraindications for Stress Testing

The choice of testing modality, including SPECT MPI should depend on several issues:

- The ability of the patient to exercise
- The base line ECG characteristics
- The patient's body habitus
- History of prior revascularization.

Patients who are unable to exercise, are deconditioned, have musculoskeletal problems, or are unable to achieve adequate heart rate response to exercise, pharmacological stress SPECT may be implemented. It is most advantageous in older patients who are at highest risk of CAD, who are unable to perform maximal exercise.

In general, specific contraindications for stress testing will depend on the type of physiologic stress, with general exclusions for all form of stress [1] The absolute and relative contraindications for stress testing SPECT MPI are shown in Table 20.1. Additionally, exercise should not be performed in the setting of uncontrolled hypertension (>200/110 mmHg) or known aortic aneurysm >5 cm in diameter.

Exercise testing should be terminated when the circumstances depicted in Table 20.2 are present. Additionally, for exercise testing, a decrease in systolic blood pressure >10 mmHg from baseline, despite an increase in workload, in addition to other evidence of ischemia should be considered a contraindication.

In the case of pharmacologic stress testing, the contraindication will depend whether dobutamine or a vasodilator is used. There are currently three vasodilator agents available: dipyridamole, adenosine, and regadenoson. Contraindications specific for vasodilator stress testing include the following [2]:

Table 20.1 Contraindications for stress testing

Absolute contraindications to stress testing
• Acute myocardial infarction within the last 4 days
• High-risk unstable angina, active chest pain
• Decompensated heart failure
• Cardiac arrhythmias
• Severe symptomatic aortic stenosis
• Acute myocarditis, pericarditis or myopericarditis
• Acute aortic dissection
• Acute pulmonary embolism
• Severe pulmonary hypertension
• Recent neurologic event, i.e. CVA, TIA
Relative contraindications for stress testing
• Moderate aortic stenosis
• Hypertrophic cardiomyopathy or other form of outflow tract obstruction
• Known left main stenosis
• High-degree atrioventricular (AV) block

Table 20.2 Indications for the termination of stress testing

Moderate-to-severe angina pectoris
Dyspnea or fatigue
Patient's request to terminate the test
Signs of poor perfusion
Marked ST-segment depression (>2 mm)
ST-segment elevation (>1 mm) in leads without diagnostic Q waves (except for leads V1 or aVR)
Development of new LBBB or intraventricular conduction delay
Excessive hypertensive response (systolic blood pressure >250 mmHg and/or diastolic pressure >115 mmHg)
Ataxia, dizziness, or near-syncope
Technical difficulties in monitoring hemodynamic parameters like systolic blood pressure or electrocardiogram

- Asthmatic patient with active wheezing
- Systolic blood pressure <90 mmHg
- 2nd or 3rd degree AC block or sick sinus syndrome, without a pacemaker, or sick sinus syndrome
- Known hypersensitivity to the agent
- Use of methylxanthine, including caffeine within 24 h of the test
- For regadenoson or adenosine, the recent use of dipyridamole, or dipyridamole-containing medications

The development of symptomatic hypotension, persistent AV block, severe chest pain with associated ST elevation, signs of poor perfusion, should result in the early termination of pharmacologic stress and/or aminophylline administration. Other indications for early termination include patient's request and technical difficulties in monitoring [1].

Dobutamine is usually recommended for SPECT MPI in patients who cannot exercise and those who have contraindications to vasodilator agents, in particular with reactive airway disease. Contraindications specific to the use of dobutamine include:

- Atrial tachyarrhythmias with uncontrolled ventricular response
- Prior history of ventricular tachycardia
- Uncontrolled hypertension
- Patients with aortic dissection or large aortic aneurysm
- Patients on β-blockers (*relative as may affect diagnostic accuracy with failure to achieve 85 % MPHR*)

Appropriate Use Criteria (AUC) for Patient Selection

Clinical practice guidelines attempt to provide clinicians with information regarding applications of a technology such as SPECT myocardial perfusion imaging. However, guidelines are often not readily translating into guiding clinical practice.

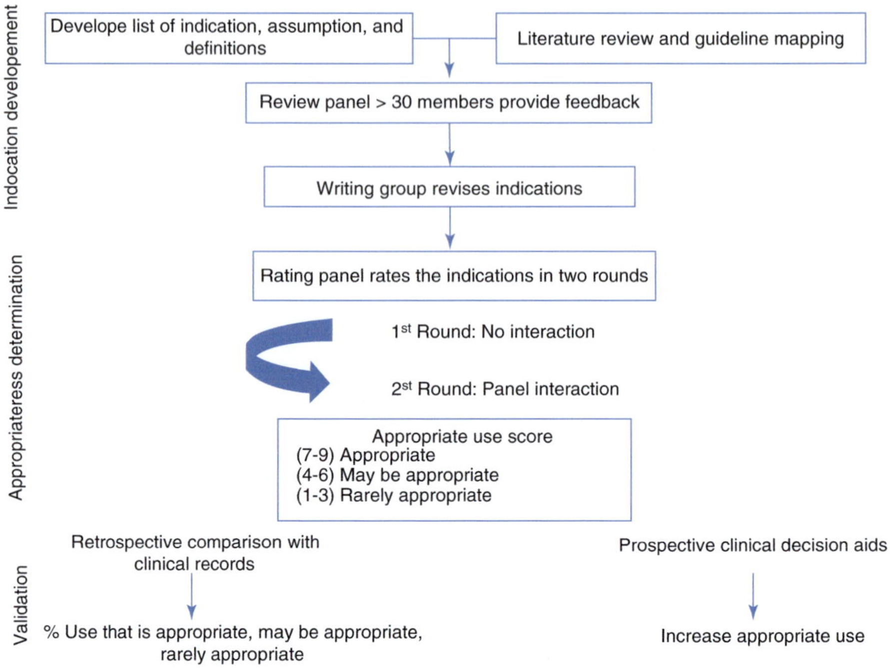

Fig. 20.1 Methodology for the development of the ACC appropriate use criteria (Reprinted from Ref. [6] with permission from Elsevier)

With increasing concern about care optimization and cost-effectiveness, the AUC were developed with the goal of encouraging the use of a test/procedure to be performed on the right patient and at the right time.

Appropriate use criteria American Society of Nuclear Cardiology (ASNC) developed for SPECT MPI by the American College of Cardiology Foundation and ASNC were the first in a series of documents aimed at guiding clinicians, patients, and payers, in the rationale of use of cardiac imaging procedures [3]. The purpose of AUC is to help clinicians with decision-making, supporting the practice of high-quality patterns of procedure use and to serve as a reimbursement policy. Initially published in 2005 [3], the SPECT AUC were subsequently revised in 2009 [4] to provide an expanded list of applications and reflect changes in the medical literature. AUC were updated in 2013 to include other testing modalities [5], as well as to reflect changes in the methodology for the development of AUC. Notably, these 2013 multimodality AUC are focused exclusively on ischemic heart disease and replace the preceding documents, except when the indication is not present in these 2013 Criteria.

The development of these AUC is complex and well routed in a scientific method [6]. Using the UCLA Rand methodology and a modified Delphi approach, the specific clinician indications are carefully constructed and rated as Appropriate, May Be Appropriate, or Rarely Appropriate, for a specific indication. The methodology

Table 20.3 Most common inappropriate indications for SPECT MPI

Indication	Inappropriate indications (%)	Total studies (%)
Detection of CAD	44.5	6.0
Asymptomatic, low CHD risk		
Asymptomatic, post-revascularization	23.8	3.2
<2 years after PCI, symptoms before PCI		
Evaluation of chest pain, low probability point	16.1	2.2
Interpretable ECG and able to exercise		
Asymptomatic or stable symptoms, known CAD	3.9	0.5
<1 year after catheterization or abnormal prior SPECT		
Preoperative assessment	3.8	0.5
Low risk surgery		
Total	92.1	12.4

is outlined in Fig. 20.1. These predominately evidenced-based criteria are a practical and essential tool for making patient-centered imaging decisions, which also encourages competent patient care by permitting the selective use of more invasive procedures. The primary goal of AUC is to optimize patient care with a clear emphasis on reduction of inappropriate imaging tests, thereby reducing cost and radiation exposure.

Several general trends are noted with regards to the appropriate use of SPECT MPI. In general, it is rarely appropriate for asymptomatic patients who have low CHD risk or those with intermediate risk and interpretable ECG to undergo SPECT MPI. However, when equivocal or discordant findings are noted on other studies, SPECT imaging becomes appropriate. In those patients with a calcium score >400, or when 100–400 in a high-risk patient, SPECT MPI is appropriate. Serial imaging was also addressed by the AUC. It is rarely appropriate when performed within 2 years of prior testing if symptoms are stable. Nevertheless, if new symptoms are present, then SPECT would be appropriate if the prior study was normal or may be appropriate if the preceding evaluation was normal. Table 20.3 lists some of the most common inappropriate indications for SPECT MPI [7].

AUC for the Evaluation of Suspected Coronary Artery Disease and Risk Stratification

As previously discussed, the use of SPECT for evaluation of patients with suspected CAD should begin with the delineation of symptoms. Subsequently, one must determine the pretest risk for coronary artery disease and for the assessment of coronary heart disease (CHD) risk. In the case of an asymptomatic patient, absolute risk is defined as the probability of developing, CHD including myocardial

Indication test		Excercise ECG	Stress RNI	Stress echo	Stress CMR	Calcium scoring	CCTA	Invasive coronary angiography
1.	. Low pre-test probability of CAD . ECG interpretable AND able to excercise	A	R	M	R	R	R	R
2.	. Low pre-test probability of CAD . ECG uninterpretable or unable to excercise		A	A	M	R	M	R
3.	. Intermediate pre-test probability of CAD . ECG interpretable AND able to excercise	A	A	A	M	R	M	R
4.	. Intermediate pre-test probability of CAD . ECG uninterpretable or unable to excercise		A	A	A	R	A	M
5.	. High pre-test probability of CAD . ECG interpretable AND able to excercise	M	A	A	A	R	M	A
6.	. High pre-test probability of CAD . ECG uninterpretable or unable to excercise		A	A	A	R	M	A

Fig. 20.2 Multimodality AUC. This figure reflects options for testing, ranging from exercise ECG, stress radionuclide imaging (RNI), and invasive coronary angiography for symptomatic patients with suspected coronary artery disease. *A* appropriate, *M* may be appropriate, *R* rarely appropriate (Reprinted from Ref. [5] with permission from Elsevier)

infarction or cardiac death over a given period. As mentioned previously, the ATP III report specifies absolute risk over the next 10 years as low, moderate or high risk. In the setting of patients with symptoms which may represent obstructive CAD, the pretest probability of CAD for each patient should be assessed, and should be determined as very low, low, intermediate, or high pretest probability, as this will guide the choice of study to be performed [4, 5, 8]. An example of AUC for symptomatic patients with suspected CAD is shown in Fig. 20.2.

Cost-Efficiency of Radionuclide Imaging

Guidelines and even AUC, however, do not formally gauge the financial impact of the imaging study or whether there is true value in terms of cost-effectiveness. Cost efficiency is also contingent upon the study's ability to stratify those with or without the disease, along with its cost and health benefits related to the testing procedure [9]. As SPECT MPI may identify those patients at high risk for subsequent cardiac event, this technique may be used to guide further testing and revascularization procedures, functioning as a gatekeeper for more resource-intense techniques [10, 11]. SPECT imaging may help guide which patients undergo coronary angiography and thereby reduce "unnecessary" cardiac catheterizations, which obviously has important cost-effective implication [10, 12]. A recent cohort study, in which the impact of AUC on the cost-effectiveness SPECT was evaluated with the subsequent post-SPECT testing or interventions, the cost associated with inappropriate MPI, was about 1.5 times that of appropriate/uncertain use; inappropriate testing seems to impair cost-effective risk stratification [13].

Conclusion

In conclusion, the available evidence supports the use MPI for cost-effective risk stratification of patients at intermediate risk suspected CAD or for subsequent CV complications. For low-risk patients, no testing or the use of exercise ECG is likely the most cost-effective strategy, while for high-risk patients; cardiac catheterization may be the most effective diagnostic approach.

References

1. Henzlova MJ, Cerqueira MD, Hansen CL, Taillefer R, Yao S-S. ASNC imaging guidelines for nuclear cardiology procedures. J Nucl Cardiol. 2009;16(2):331–43.
2. Jaarsma C, Leiner T, Bekkers SC, Crijns HJ, Wildberger JE, Nagel E, et al. Diagnostic performance of noninvasive myocardial perfusion imaging using single-photon emission computed tomography, cardiac magnetic resonance, and positron emission tomography imaging for the detection of obstructive coronary artery disease: a meta-analysis. J Am Coll Cardiol. 2012;59(19):1719–28. PubMed.
3. Brindis RG, Douglas PS, Hendel RC, Peterson ED, Wolk MJ, Allen JM, et al. ACCF/ASNC appropriateness criteria for single-photon emission computed tomography myocardial perfusion imaging (SPECT MPI): a report of the American College of Cardiology Foundation Quality Strategic Directions Committee Appropriateness Criteria Working Group and the American Society of Nuclear Cardiology endorsed by the American Heart Association. J Am Coll Cardiol. 2005;46(8):1587–605. PubMed.
4. Hendel RC, Berman DS, Di Carli MF, Heidenreich PA, Henkin RE, Pellikka PA, et al. ACCF/ASNC/ACR/AHA/ASE/SCCT/SCMR/SNM 2009 appropriate use criteria for cardiac radionuclide imaging: a report of the American College of Cardiology Foundation Appropriate Use Criteria Task Force, the American Society of Nuclear Cardiology, the American College of Radiology, the American Heart Association, the American Society of Echocardiography, the Society of Cardiovascular Computed Tomography, the Society for Cardiovascular Magnetic Resonance, and the Society of Nuclear Medicine. J Am Coll Cardiol. 2009;53(23):2201–29. PubMed.
5. Wolk MJ, Bailey SR, Doherty JU, Douglas PS, Hendel RC, Kramer CM, et al. ACCF/AHA/ASE/ASNC/HFSA/HRS/SCAI/SCCT/SCMR/STS 2013 multimodality appropriate use criteria for the detection and risk assessment of stable ischemic heart disease: a report of the American College of Cardiology Foundation Appropriate Use Criteria Task Force, American Heart Association, American Society of Echocardiography, American Society of Nuclear Cardiology, Heart Failure Society of America, Heart Rhythm Society, Society for Cardiovascular Angiography and Interventions, Society of Cardiovascular Computed Tomography, Society for Cardiovascular Magnetic Resonance, and Society of Thoracic Surgeons. J Am Coll Cardiol. 2014;63(4):380–406. PubMed.
6. Hendel RC, Patel MR, Allen JM, Min JK, Shaw LJ, Wolk MJ, et al. Appropriate use of cardiovascular technology: 2013 ACCF appropriate use criteria methodology update: a report

of the American College of Cardiology Foundation appropriate use criteria task force. J Am Coll Cardiol. 2013;61(12):1305–17. PubMed.
7. Hendel RC, Cerqueira M, Douglas PS, Caruth KC, Allen JM, Jensen NC, et al. A multicenter assessment of the use of single-photon emission computed tomography myocardial perfusion imaging with appropriateness criteria. J Am Coll Cardiol. 2010;55(2):156–62. PubMed.
8. Diamond GA, Forrester JS. Analysis of probability as an aid in the clinical diagnosis of coronary-artery disease. N Engl J Med. 1979;300(24):1350–8. PubMed.
9. Goldman L, Garber AM, Grover SA, Hlatky MA. Task force 6. Cost effectiveness of assessment and management of risk factors. J Am Coll Cardiol. 1996;27(5):1020–30.
10. Shaw LJ, Hachamovitch R, Berman DS, Marwick TH, Lauer MS, Heller GV, et al. The economic consequences of available diagnostic and prognostic strategies for the evaluation of stable angina patients: an observational assessment of the value of precatheterization ischemia. Economics of Noninvasive Diagnosis (END) Multicenter Study Group. J Am Coll Cardiol. 1999;33(3):661–9. PubMed Epub 1999/03/18. eng.
11. Des Prez RD, Shaw LJ, Gillespie RL, Jaber WA, Noble GL, Soman P, et al. Cost-effectiveness of myocardial perfusion imaging: a summary of the currently available literature. J Nucl Cardiol Off Publ Am Soc Nucl Cardiol. 2005;12(6):750–9. PubMed.
12. Shaw LJ, Hachamovitch R, Heller GV, Marwick TH, Travin MI, Iskandrian AE, et al. Noninvasive strategies for the estimation of cardiac risk in stable chest pain patients. Am J Cardiol. 2000;86(1):1–7.
13. Doukky R, Hayes K, Frogge N, Balakrishnan G, Dontaraju VS, Rangel MO, Golzar Y, Garcia-Sayan E, Hendel RC. Impact of appropriate use on the prognostic value of single-photon emission computed tomography myocardial perfusion imaging. Circulation. 2013;128(15):1634–43.

Chapter 21
SPECT: Quality Control

Patty Reames, Cesia Gallegos, and Robert C. Hendel

Abstract The process of quality control starts with ensuring safe measurement and administration of radiopharmaceuticals to the patient. The mechanisms to ensure this will be reviewed. Optimal functioning nuclear cardiology imaging equipment is also essential. Methods to evaluate and monitor quality performance of the imaging equipment will be described. Finally, variability at the patient level can lead to significant artifacts in the images. Mechanisms to recognize and reduce these artifacts will be discussed.

Keywords SPECT • Quality control • Radiopharmaceutical administration • Nuclear medicine camera quality control • Patient artifacts

Background

Quality Assurance (QA), Quality Control (QC), and Quality Improvement (QI) are terms that all medical personnel, including imaging technologists, need to understand. These terms are often used interchangeably, likely due to incomplete understanding of quality control matters in general and the importance of these types of activities.

Quality assurance and quality improvement are programs for an internal assessment with pre-defined indicators and thresholds ensuring that standards of quality

P. Reames, ARRT, CNMT, NCT, FASNC
Practice Manager, Ohio State University Heart and Vascular Center,
2220 Timber Trail, Bellefontaine, OH 4331, USA
e-mail: patty.reames@osumc.edu

C. Gallegos, MD
Department of Medicine, University of Miami Miller School of Medicine, Miami, FL, USA
e-mail: cesia.gallegos@jhsmiami.org

R.C. Hendel, MD, FACC, FAHA, FASNC (✉)
Cardiovascular Division Chief (Interim), University of Miami Miller
School of Medicine, 1120 NW 14th Street, Suite 1123, CRB, Miami, FL 33136, USA
e-mail: RHendel@med.miami.edu

P.L. Tilkemeier et al. (eds.), *Quality Evaluation in Non-Invasive Cardiovascular Imaging*, DOI 10.1007/978-3-319-28011-0_21

Table 21.1 Quality control procedures for SPECT systems

Test	Priority	Frequency
Acceptance testing per NEMA	Recommended	Upon delivery, after major hardware upgrades
Energy peaking	Mandatory	Daily
Uniformity test	Mandatory	Daily
Resolution and linearity	Mandatory	Weekly
Sensitivity	Mandatory	Weekly/monthly
Center-of-rotation multi-detector registration	Mandatory	Weekly/monthly
Uniformity calibration	Mandatory	Weekly/monthly
Phantom	Recommended	Quarterly

Adapted from Nichols [10] with permission from Springer. © 2007 American Society of Nuclear Cardiology

are met. If falling outside the standard, there should be an action plan for improvement. Quality control is the most important element that we have at our disposal enabling us to produce quality imaging that allow the practitioner to determine a diagnosis and plan the next step in the patients plan of care.

The term quality control as described by Wikipedia states "Quality Control (QC) is a process by which entities review the quality of all factors involved in production." In the nuclear laboratory setting, specific controls are utilized including visual inspections, predefined normal values, and action plans for values that fall outside of the normal threshold. Quality control checks ensure equipment is performing properly to meet the predetermined value and to uncover deficiencies. These values are set by the individual manufacturers following standards published by the Association of Electrical Equipment and Medical Imaging Manufacturers (NEMA) [1].

Best practices have a complete quality control program in place that clearly defines what tests are to be completed, the frequency with which these tests are to be carried out, predefined thresholds for each test, a documentation method for the test results, and an action plan when the results fall outside of the determined threshold.

Before initiating procedures such as SPECT MPI, a quality control program needs to be established in the hot lab, all monitoring equipment and the camera(s). Guidelines have been published by multiple organizations including the American Society of Nuclear Cardiology [2] and the Society of Nuclear Medicine and Molecular Imaging that outline the standard QC procedures that need to be performed (Table 21.1). While these guidelines exist, users must also be familiar with their facility's radioactive license which may direct the frequency and methods of the QC tests to be completed. The ultimate goal of the QC program is to produce the highest quality images possible.

Hot Lab

Hot lab quality control establishes that the equipment is functioning properly allowing the user to determine contamination and measure radioactivity. Completing quality control on the dose calibrator is a vital process that enables the user to determine the exact amount of radioactivity that is delivered to the patient as well as ensuring an acceptable dose for imaging. The GM meter, well counter, and dose calibrator are required to pass their daily tests before measuring and dispensing any radioactive material to a patient. When the QC results fall outside of the expected range, further testing and calibrations are necessary. If these fail to bring the equipment back to normal operating standards, service will need to be completed on the unit.

Camera-Acceptance Testing

Acceptance testing is a process that evaluates the performance of your camera system prior to its first clinical use. It is verification that your system is performing to the specifications as indicated by the manufacturer. These tests are then compared to the standards as defined by the NEMA [4]. This process will test the limitations of the system and provide valuable data for the service engineer, physicist, and technologist to utilize throughout the life of the equipment. The documented data will become the gold standard for comparison for all future tests. Additionally, service engineers will be better equipped to determine the remedy for deterioration of image quality since there is a documented baseline.

Camera-Daily Quality Evaluation

Energy peaking (photo peak analysis) must be performed daily, verifying that the detectors and related electronics are accurately registering the energy of the photons emitting from the radioactive source (Fig. 21.1). A visual inspection of the energy spectrum's shape and the corresponding energy window before use of the system is very important. The procedure for obtaining and adjusting the energy window differs from manufacturer to manufacturer. This simple test can be accomplished either extrinsically with a sheet source on the collimator or intrinsically by placing a syringe with a small radioactive source at least five fields of view (FOV) away from the uncollimated detector. In either case, the source must be strong enough to flood the entire FOV. The computer will then display a diagram, which allows the user to adjust the location and width of the energy window for maximal imaging

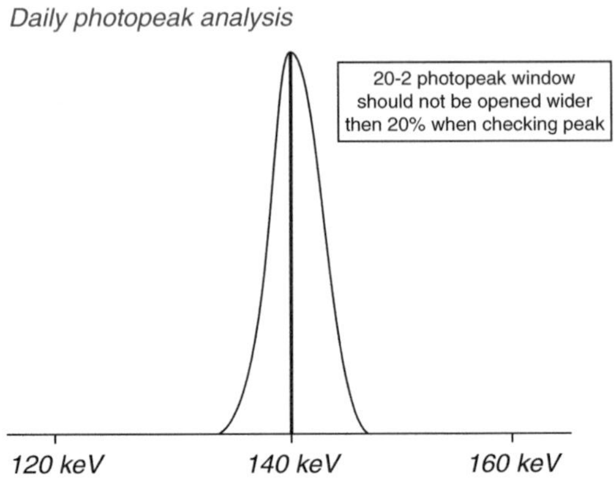

Fig. 21.1 An example of a photopeak analysis, which should be performed daily for optimal camera function

effectiveness. Drifting of the energy window away from the peak of the isotope will lead to significant degradation of image quality secondary to poor count statistics [1–3, 5].

A daily uniformity test is performed to verify the camera's performance and to guarantee that the sensitivity response of the system is uniform across the entire detector(s) face. This test is easily performed by placing a small dose of radiation at least five FOVs away from the uncollimated detector. This method allows testing the source identically to energies used clinically. The "flooding" of the detector is typically performed after peaking the detector for the radioactive energy being utilized.

The point source activity is determined by each manufacturer but is usually in the range of 100–500 μCi in a volume of 0.5 ml. The acquisition parameters for camera set up include a total acquisition of two to five million counts, using a 20 % energy window, when using Tc-99m, with a count rate between 10 and 25 kcps using a 128 × 128 matrix. With a few of the older systems a lead ring is placed on the detector to prevent edge packing on the periphery of the outermost tubes. In some cases it is difficult to achieve the five FOV's distance from the detector. In these situations, some manufacturers provide software to correct for non-uniformities. It may be more practical to perform extrinsic floods in these situations. It is useful to occasionally perform the test with the heads oriented in a different orientation then typical as this may demonstrate some image degradation when the electronics have loosened and may not be making total contact during rotation with an acquisition [1–3, 5].

A daily uniformity can also be performed extrinsically. This test is easily performed by placing a radioactive sheet source of Co-57 or a fillable flood source with Tc-99m on the collimated detector. When multi-detectors are used, all detectors must be tested. The "flooding" of the detector is typically performed after peaking the detector for the radioactive energy being utilized. The Co-57 flood source activity is determined by each manufacturer but is usually in the range of 10 μCi and Tc99m in the range of 100–500 μCi. The acquisition parameters for camera set up include a total acquisition of two to five million counts using a 20 % around the

Table 21.2 Performance parameters for scintillation (or anger) cameras

Parameter	Standard
Integral uniformity	<5 %
Differential uniformity	<5 %
Intrinsic resolution (FWHM)	<6 mm
Note: These values are specific to Anger camera systems using 3/8″ NaI crystal	

Adapted from Nichols [10] with permission from Springer. © 2007 American Society of Nuclear Cardiology

appropriate energy peak for the isotope utilized, with a count rate between 10 and 25 kcps using a 256×256 matrix [1–3, 5].

After the daily flood acquisition is completed (intrinsically or extrinsically), a visual inspection of the flood will determine if any "gross" abnormalities are present. If any change in the visual appearance is noted, a new correction table/uniformity map is acquired and the flood repeated. If the nonuniformity if still present, the camera cannot be used until the service engineer has evaluated the system and corrected the issue. In addition to the visual inspection, a computerized method of analysis will produce recordable results that can be reviewed each day and compared to the previous day's results, enabling the identification of subtle changes before a "gross" abnormality appears. The quantifiable uniformity parameters that are generated include the "integral uniformity" and the "differential uniformity" values. The integral analysis evaluates for global variations in the uniformity over the field of view, while the differential analysis evaluates for local variations in the uniformity over the entire field of view. These values are computed for the UFOV (useful field of view) and the CFOV (central field of view).

- $\text{Integral Uniformity} = (\text{max} - \text{Min}) / (\text{max} + \text{Min}) \times 100\%$
- $\text{Differential Uniformity} = \text{Largest dev}(\text{max} \quad \text{Min}) / (\text{max} + \text{Min}) \times 100\%$

Recordable values should fall within the specifications. If the results fall outside of your standard, the camera should not be utilized and the service engineer should be called to evaluate the system [1–3, 5] (Table 21.2 and Fig. 21.2). Common causes of nonuniformity include outdated correction tables, mistuning (detuning), uncoupling of a PMT, a cracked crystal, or corruption or switching off of one or more of the correction tables of the camera [6].

Camera-Weekly Quality Evaluation

Weekly QC programs include linearity assessments with bar phantoms. Spatial linearity is one of the parameters that affect flood field uniformity. This test is performed to document spatial resolution over time and evaluate the detector's ability to reproduce straight lines. This test should be performed intrinsically so as not to have the collimator's septa interfere with the registration of the photons,

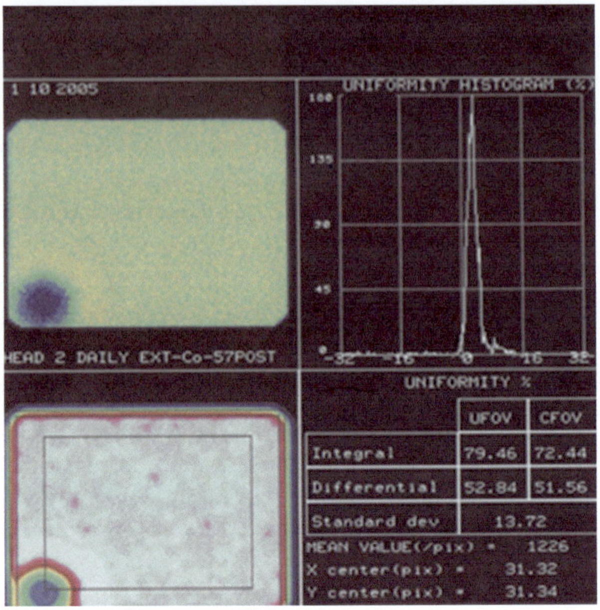

Fig. 21.2 Uniformity flood. An example of nonuniformity, with a *dark blue* area likely indicating an abnormally functioning photomultiplier tube. The graph confirms non-uniformity

allowing for "true" representation of the lines that are produced on the flood. Acquisition parameters for this test are identical to those of the intrinsic daily flood. A point source is placed five FOV's from the uncollimated detector with the bar phantom placed on top of, or as close to the crystal, as possible. There are multiple types of phantoms available, however, the most used is the four-quadrant PLES (parallel line equally spaced) phantom (Fig. 21.3). This phantom contains four distinct areas with varying sizes of lead bars in each quadrant. This type of phantom allows rotation of 90° from the previously placed position with each acquisition so that all four quadrants of the detector can be evaluated the same, enabling the identification of an area that is degrading in quality by comparing the resolution of the bars to the other quadrants. After completion of the acquisition, a visual inspection is required to assess the straightness of the bar images, as well as documenting the smallest bars that are discernible, representing spatial resolution, which is often expressed as the full-width at half maximum (FWHM) of a point spread function. Intrinsic resolution is typically 3.5–4.0 mm. The FWHM may be approximated by multiplying the smallest bar visualized by 1.7. Some manufacturers provide software that calculates this for you. Sources of resolution degradation range from poor alignment of the gains of the photomultiplier tubes (PMTs), defects or deterioration of the crystal, problems with the collimator, and source to detector distance. Should a degradation be noted in the bars that can be seen noting a change in resolution or the lines are no longer straight, the system should not be utilized until the service engineer has an opportunity to evaluate the system.

A Center of Rotation (COR) acquisition is performed for verification that the mechanical and electronic COR's are aligned, i.e. COR offsets are within limits of

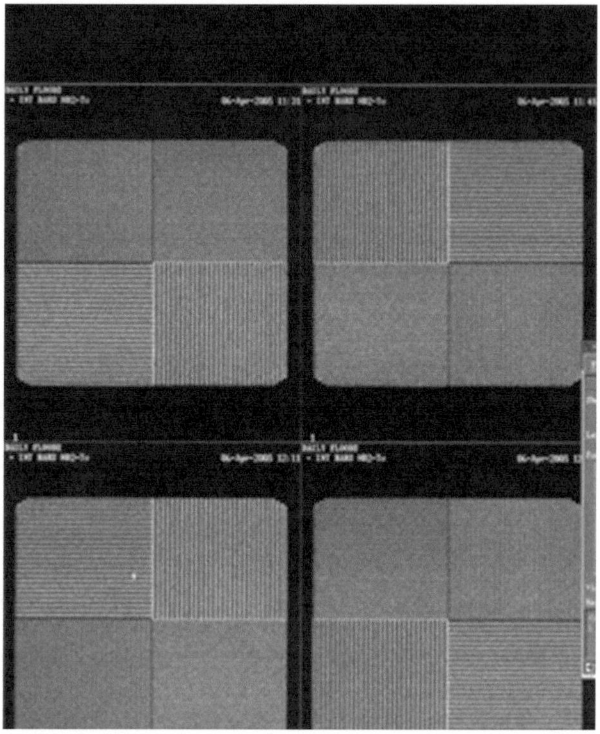

Fig. 21.3 Quadrant bar phantom. An example of a quadrant bar phantom demonstrating rotation of the phantom to test each of the four quadrants at each level of resolution

acceptability, in X and Y directions. An alignment error occurs when the center of the electronic matrix for the camera and the mechanical center-of-rotation (COR) the bed have deviated from the calibrated standard. This misalignment can potentially result in a characteristic "doughnut" (if a 360 orbit and a point source are used) or "tuning fork" artifact (if a 180 orbit is used) in the transverse images, which can appear as patient motion artifact. This is typically seen as a progressive misalignment of the septal and lateral walls. If this artifact is noted with several patients in a row, a COR test should be performed. This type of artifact is most noticeable when greater than two pixels of misalignment exists in a 64×64 matrix. While a smaller misalignment can cause a blurring effect by reduced spatial resolution and image contrast, the artifact is nonetheless important, and is typically seen at the apex.

The performance frequency and recommendations for this test varies from manufacturer to manufacturer depending on the detectors stability. Some recommend that the COR be performed weekly while others suggest monthly. A very specific protocol is followed for determining COR accuracy with recalibration being warranted when the results fall outside of the normal variant. The typically protocol consists of using a 500–750 μCi point source, in a very small volume, which is placed on the patient bed. It is important that the point source has a clean needle placed on the syringe so that the radioactivity appears as a small "dot" during the acquisition. If there is radioactivity in needle or neck of the syringe it may appear as two dots or an elongated dot. This type of result will warrant the test to be repeated, as it is difficult for software applications to calculate accurate results. The detectors are positioned 4–8 in. away from the point source with an acquisition set up similar to that of a standard SPECT protocol. The data is collected for 360°. Most often there is a software application that processes the image and calculates a quantitative result. Once the misalignment is >0.5 pixels on the X-axis, the recalibration procedure should be followed. Anytime service is performed on the system it is important to run a COR test. When test results are outside the expected range and the COR calibration fails to bring the test results back into specification, they camera should not be used and a service engineer will need to be called to evaluate the system.

Camera-Monthly Quality Evaluation

This test is performed to document the sensitivity of the detector and, more importantly, the change in sensitivity over time. A simple test to verify that the camera is counting accurately is the sensitivity test, which consists of calculating detector sensitivity (expressed in terms of counts per minute per megabecquerel) of a known source, calibrated with a dose calibrator. The point source should always be located in the exact same position so that repeat measurements can be compared. A convenient means of measuring sensitivity changes is by recording the time that it takes to acquire the preset counts for an intrinsic (or extrinsic, if more practicable) flood source. Each head will have to be acquired separately. This straightforward test allows the detection of small changes in the system before visual changes are noted on the flood image.

Cameras store flood field correction maps to correct for variations in the sensitivity across the FOV before reconstruction. High-count uniformity correction floods should be performed following the manufacturer's recommendations. The correction is typically performed intrinsically, with 30–100 million count images acquired for each detector using a 128×128 or 256×256 matrix. The frequency varies from once a month to once every 6 months depending on the manufacturer and the stability of the camera. However, when uniformity errors are noted, it is appropriate to acquire a new uniformity correction map and repeat the flood. If the flood still demonstrates nonuniformity the service engineer should be called before the system is used for patient care.

Camera-Quarterly Quality Evaluation

Overall system performance can be evaluated with a fillable multipurpose plexiglass phantom as recommended by The National Electrical Manufacturer's Association (NEMA). There are many commercially available units that will allow for analysis of the acquisition and reconstruction of the phantom images. The phantoms are filled with radioactive water and contain various solid spheres and rod (cold) inserts of different sizes that mimic attenuation and scatter properties of tissue enabling us to evaluate the performance of the systems 3D contrast, resolution, and uniformity similar to imaging a patient in the clinical setting.

This test should be performed quarterly, or whenever the system has undergone significant servicing. Typical acquisition protocol set up includes a 128 × 128 matrix with 128 projections at 40 s per projection, over 360° when using 10 mCi Tc-99m [7]. The detectors are positioned as close to the phantom as is practical acquiring 30 million counts. Once acquired the data is reconstructed and evaluated for resolution of the rods and spheres. When a loss of resolution is noted through solid rod sections, and inappropriate or inadequate flood-field corrections are noted by the appearance of concentric rings, a COR test and uniformity corrections map should be used to correct for the errors and repeat the phantom acquisition.

Camera-Annual Quality Evaluation

As stated previously, extrinsic flood may not need to be performed any more often than once a year, but this is vendor specific. Whether daily extrinsic floods are obtained or not, an annual extrinsic flood that is counted for 100 million counts is needed annually to verify collimator integrity. This is accomplished with a sheet source using the same camera protocol as an extrinsic daily flood. A visual inspection of the FOV will determine if there are any issues with the collimator. Should a visual disturbance be noted, the service engineer will need to be contacted to evaluate the system.

A good quality control program will help to eliminate many potential sources of artifacts and errors that can occur. A well-trained nuclear medicine professional will be able to identify camera artifacts during QC testing as well as identify the potential effects on perfusion images.

Patient Related Artifacts

Although many artifacts may be camera-related as previously discussed, artifacts are also related to acquisition and patient factors as well. Adequate patient preparation is key to obtaining a quality study. In order to reduce patient motion, it is essential that a clear explanation be given to the patient on what to expect during the image acquisition as well as the imagers expectations. It is critical to inform the patient that they must lay still, breath normal and not talk. It is essential that the patient be made as comfortable as possible by supporting their legs, back, arms and head. If a patient has a cough, allowing them to have a cough drop or peppermint often quiets the cough down enabling you to obtain the acquisition. For patients with claustrophobia, allowing a family member or friend into the room and placing a hand on the patient's hand or leg is often times enough to calm the patient down. Additionally utilizing a fan to blow gently on the patients face provides them with a sense of air movement and "freedom". Lastly using any type of distraction such as a radio or small TV helps the patient to settle in and relax. Taking these few precious minutes to maximize the patient's comfort pays of dividends in the end.

Furthermore, all patients should be prepared for the test in a similar fashion. Patients should be called 1–2 days prior to the scheduled exam. This gives plenty of time to do a mini assessment of the patient and adequate time for follow up with the referring physician if needed. Caffeine should be held for everyone for at least 18 h before the stress test. This way if a patient was scheduled for a stress and they need converted to a pharmacological stress, this can easily be done saving a wasted dose, wasted staff time, and down time on the camera. Patients on beta-blockers that are scheduled for a diagnostic exam should have their medication held 24–72 h as determined appropriated by their physician.

The most common causes of patient-related artifacts are caused by soft tissue attenuation, extracardiac activity, patient motion, and an irregular heart rate (R-R interval) on a gated SPECT study. Before any dataset is processed, it must first be evaluated to determine that it contains an acceptable number of acquired counts (count density). As a general rule, peak pixel activity in the left ventricular (LV) myocardium in an anterior planar projection should exceed 100 counts for a Tl-201 study and 200 counts in a Tc-99m study. When acquiring a rest/stress same day study, the stress study should contain three times more counts than the resting study as the radioactivity delivered to the patient is three times more than the resting dose. Failure to acquire this count difference could indicate that a dose was not fully delivered to the patient, the dose was infiltrated, or the acquisition was set up incorrectly. A repeat acquisition should be obtained to acquire the appropriate counts. If the decreased counts remain to be a problem, the study may need to be repeated.

Soft Tissue Attenuation

Soft tissue attenuation is a common source of artifact for both males and females. For females (and occasionally males) the most common type is breast attenuation. The location, size, and severity of the artifact produced are dependent on the size of the patient, the density of the soft tissue, and the photopeak energy. Breast tissue will typically appear as a localized decrease in count density. This decrease in counts may appear over the anterior, anteroseptal, or anterolateral regions depending on the position of the patient's breast tissue during the acquisition. Evaluation of the rotating cines are an excellent way to establish the location of the breast tissue as well as determining if the breast tissue is lying in the same position on both datasets. If, the breast tissue has shifted in location between datasets, it could lead the reader to believe that a reversible defect (ischemia) exist, as review of the gated images will not be able to resolve whether or not this is an artifact. Although controversy is present as to whether the patient should be imaged with bra on or bra off, for whichever method you choose, it is important that the patient is imaged the same way both times. It may useful to record the patient's bra size and whether the patient has implants.

Another source of soft tissue attenuation is from the diaphragm/subdiaphragmatic structures. Imaging a patient to quickly after exercise will induce "upward" creep as the patient's respirations slow. Review of the raw cine data will help the interpreter visualize where the diaphragm is located by tracing the upper line of the liver and following it across the dataset to see where it intersects with the myocardium.

To help with soft tissue artifacts, hardware and software have been commercially developed to help correct for attenuation and scatter. When using this type of correction method, the interpreting physician should review both the corrected and uncorrected datasets before making a final interpretation decision. Another method of "correcting" for breast and diaphragm artifact is to imagine the patient prone [8, 9]. The key to acquiring a quality prone study is to educate the patient on why a prone image is needed and making them as comfortable as possible. The interpreter will review the typical rest and stress datasets, as well as the prone data set at the same time.

Extracardiac Activity

Extra cardiac activity can prove to be a very difficult artifact to overcome. There are many variations discussed among nuclear professionals on the best method to eliminate this artifact from drinking cold water, drink hot water, consuming soda, eating a mini snack, to walking the hallway, but the single most important thing you can do as an imager is to consistently follow your written protocol. It is essential to minimizing this artifact as much as possible. Extracardiac activity may result in a reconstruction artifact seen during filtered back projections and less commonly with iterative reconstruction.

Tracer activity, superimposed bowel loops or liver activity, in very close proximity to the myocardium (heart), may create the appearance of more counts in the adjacent area. This "added" activity may hide a true defect as a result of photon scatter.

When intense tracer is not superimposed, but near the myocardium, it may create a negative reconstruction artifact, which appears as a defect. The production of a "false" defect, such as this, is commonly called a Ramp filter or negative lobe artifact and is minimized by using an interactive reconstruction algorithm. This artifact may appear as a fixed or a reversible defect depending on the activity in the rest and stress datasets.

When performing pharmacological stress studies, there does tend to be greater liver uptake. To help decrease the presence of an artifact due to hepatic activity, it is often useful to perform low-level exercise to help facilitate liver clearance. However, if significant extracardiac activity is present, it is recommended that the acquisition be repeated after waiting for a small period of time, asking the patient to walk for a little bit, or both. Prone imaging may also be useful.

Patient Motion

Patient motion is a common artifact. Patient motion can occur in both the horizontal (side to side) or vertical (head to toe) axis, and occasionally both. A misalignment of the data occurs during filtered back projection that is most commonly noted in the anterior and inferior walls of the myocardium. Review of the raw cine images before allowing the patient to leave is an essential part of a good quality-imaging program. Additionally, the "sinogram" and/or "linogram" may be used to detect patient motion as well. In order to reduce patient motion, it is essential that a clear explanation be given to the patient on what to expect during the image acquisition as well as the imagers expectations. It is critical to inform the patient that they must lay still, breath normal and not talk. It is essential that the patient be made as comfortable as possible from supporting their legs, back, arms and head. Taking these few precious minutes to maximize the patient's comfort pays dividends in the end.

When faced with a dataset that contains motion, it is important to repeat the acquisition if more than a 2-pixel shift due to motion is present. For less severe motion, there are commercially available motion correction programs, which are often quite useful. However, caution should be used when working with these programs, as it is possible to introduce more artifacts into the study. When providing the interpreting physician with a motion corrected study, you must also provide the uncorrected study as well.

Gated SPECT

ECG-gated SPECT requires a stable a stable heart rate and rhythm. Once the three leads are attached correctly it is imperative that the QRS is being "sensed" on the monitor. The sensing must be captured on the QRS segment of the cardiac cycle and not the T wave or P wave. Once sensing is confirmed then the R-to-R "beat length acceptance window" is set up. It can be set with a range of 20–100 % acceptance of the captured beats, keeping in mind that the recommended value is 20 % if an "extra frame" is provided that allows the accumulation of rejected counts. The common set up is to monitor lead II, and set the acquisition to gate the heart for eight frames per cycle. Some facilities are gating for 16 frames and have reported good results with the increased temporal sampling, which enable them to obtain more accurate estimates of LVEF as well as parameters of diastolic function.

It is recommended that "bad" beats are rejected or avoided. Such beats are due to premature or ectopic beats or occur in the setting of atrial fibrillation. Once the reconstruction has been completed, the gated image may appear to be flashy, jumpy, or intermittent secondary to a lack of counts being acquired. You may notice that the end diastolic (ED) and end systolic (ES) values are unexpected and the left ventricular ejection fraction is underestimated. Another source of a gating problem is when the gate is improperly set up and not triggering off of the QRS, but is triggered of the T wave or P wave, resulting in an artifact with an inaccurate time-motion curve.

In conclusion, developing a quality control program for your equipment, and ensuring that it is functioning at its peak performance, will provide the imager and physician with the confidence that the datasets are of the best quality that could be acquired. Developing a quality control program for reviewing the acquired datasets before they are processed provides the imager and physician with the assurance that the processed images are of high quality and the data is dependable. Both of these components, quality control for the equipment and quality control for the dataset, are necessary for producing quality images. This level of quality is needed to for the interpreter to make an interpretation that then leads to the next step in the patient's plan of care.

References

1. NEMA Standarization Policies and Procedures of the National Electrical Manufacturers Association. 2009:54.
2. Henzlova MJ, Cerqueira MD, Hansen CL, Taillefer R, Yao S-S. ASNC imaging guidelines for nuclear cardiology procedures. J Nucl Cardiol. 2009;16(2):331–43.
3. American College of Radiology SoNM, Society for Pediatric Radiology. Practice guidelines for the performance of cardiac scintigraphy. 2009.
4. Hayes-Brown K, Frogge N, Doukky R. The impact of appropriate use on the cost effectiveness of spect myocardial perfusion imaging in the community setting. J Am Coll Cardiol. 2014; 63(12_S).
5. Murphy P. Acceptance testing and quality control of gamma cameras, including SPECT. J Nucl Med. 1987;28:1221.
6. Zanzonico P. Routine quality control of clinical nuclear medicine instrumentation: a brief review. J Nucl Med Off Publ Soc Nucl Med. 2008;49(7):1114–31. PubMed Pubmed Central PMCID: 2703015.
7. Tilkemeier PL, Cooke CD, Grossman GB, McCallister BD, Ward RP. Standardized reporting of radionuclide myocardial perfusion and function. J Nucl Cardiol. 2009;16(4):650.
8. Heden B, Persson E, Carlsson M, Pahlm O, Arheden H. Disappearance of myocardial perfusion defects on prone SPECT imaging: comparison with cardiac magnetic resonance imaging in patients without established coronary artery disease. BMC Med Imaging. 2009;9(1):16. PubMed PMID: doi:10.1186/1471-2342-9-16.
9. Worden N, Lindower PD, Burns T, Chatterjee K, Weiss RM. A second look with prone SPECT myocardial perfusion imaging reduces the need for angiography in patients at low risk for cardiac death or MI. 2014;0(0):1–8.
10. Nichols KJ. Instrumentation quality assurance and performance. J Nucl Cardiol. 2007; 14(6):e61–78.

Chapter 22
SPECT: Reporting

Robert C. Hendel and Cesia Gallegos

Abstract The nuclear cardiology report is the final product of a complex process. The report must contain a number of required elements based on current standards. It is vital to the success of the procedure as it represents the information conveyed to the referring health care person. The standards will be reviewed as they pertain to the key elements of the report. The key elements include patient data, indications, description of the procedure, image findings, and the final impression. The importance of compliance with standards to ensure concise and accurate reporting is emphasized.

Keywords SPECT • Quality • Reporting

The final product of a nuclear cardiology procedure is the report. It reflects the performance of the study and its interpretation. It is also a reflection of the interpreter, the nuclear cardiology laboratory, and nuclear cardiology itself. Most importantly, it is THE critical piece of information that ultimately guides patient management.

Unfortunately, many nuclear cardiology reports lack clarity in their interpretation, and are often variable in content and form. The most important goal of a nuclear cardiology report should be the communication of critical findings to the referring physician and their clinical implications. This should include avoidance of words such as "suggestive of", "possible", or "paradoxical", as well as describing severity of perfusion abnormalities as ">2". Finally, comments such as "clinical correlation is suggested" should also be avoided. The use of standard accepted terminology to describe the imaging findings is also very important [1, 2].

R.C. Hendel, MD, FACC, FAHA, FASNC (✉)
Cardiovascular Division Chief (Interim), University of Miami Miller School of Medicine, 1120 NW 14th Street, Suite 1123, CRB, Miami, FL 33136, USA
e-mail: rhendel@med.miami.edu

C. Gallegos, MD
Department of Medicine, University of Miami Miller School of Medicine, Miami, FL, USA
e-mail: cesia.gallegos@jhsmiami.org

P.L. Tilkemeier et al. (eds.), *Quality Evaluation in Non-Invasive Cardiovascular Imaging*, DOI 10.1007/978-3-319-28011-0_22

The report should serve as a fundamental piece of information, which will not only guide management, but it, should also serve to document information pertinent to reimbursement and accreditation licensure. In the next section, we will discuss the key components in the nuclear cardiology report, as delineated by multiple publications and guidelines [1–6].

Key Elements (Table 22.1)

Patient Data

This includes demographics (age, gender race) and body habitus (height, weight). In this part, relevant clinical information should also be described. It should include current symptoms and patient's clinical status, use of medications, in particular because they may impact on the interpretation of the results, previous cardiac history, (history of CAD, s/p myocardial infarction), previous cardiac procedures and diagnostic tests (echocardiography, PCI, CABG, prior MPI and their findings if available). Cardiac risk factors should also be noted.

Indications

The indication for the procedure should be clearly stated. They major indications include:

- Diagnosis of suspected CAD
- Assessment of extent and severity of known CAD
- Risk assessment
- Determination of myocardial viability
- Evaluation of acute chest pain syndrome

The specific indication may be also referenced to a specific diagnostic code to assist in matters related to reimbursement. If pharmacological testing was performed instead of ETT, it is essential to state the reason for using a medication-induced stress procedure.

Table 22.1 Key components of the SPECT report

Key components of the report
Patient data
Study indication
Procedure
Findings
Impression

Adapted from Hendel et al. [6]. With kind permission from Springer Science+Business Media

Procedures

In this portion of the report, the specifics of the nuclear procedure should be well delineated. This will primarily serve to explain the testing results directly to the referring physician, but will also assist as a reference for subsequent comparisons. The elements that must be included are:

- Type and protocol of stress procedure: If exercise was used, the specific protocol should be noted (Bruce or Naughton); the duration of exercise as well as the stage of protocol achieved, finally the functional status in terms of number of metabolic equivalents (METS) achieved should also be stated.
- Adequacy of the procedure: including heart rate achieved in terms of the maximum predicted heart rate, reasons for test termination such as general fatigue or hypotension. If pharmacological stress testing is performed, the dose and agent should be specified, as well as the use of adjunctive exercise.
- Imaging protocol: The actual imaging protocol should also be stated, whether it was planar or SPECT or if it was performed in supine or prone position. The duration of the protocol should be mentioned either 1 or 2-day protocol
- Symptoms during protocol: Any symptoms recorded during the procedure along with the hemodynamic response, heart rate, and blood pressure changes should be noted.
- ECG: Both resting and stress ECG should be described, including abnormalities such as left bundle branch block (LBBB), left ventricular hypertrophy (LVH), or non-specific ST/T-wave abnormalities, with any subsequent electrocardiographic changes, including those that deviate from baseline.
- Radiopharmaceuticals: The agent and dose utilized for the procedure should be clearly stated. If the stress is continued after the radiopharmaceutical injection, the duration of continuation should be documented.
- Attenuation/scatter correction: If these advanced techniques were performed, they should be also specified.

Image Findings

The results of the procedure should be described comprehensively and should attempt to include all pertinent findings. The first part of this section should be about image quality, which should be termed as excellent, good, fair, or of poor quality, but at least inadequate quality should be noted. Extracardiac activity should also be well described and correlated with clinical information.

The perfusion defect's characteristics should be carefully explained, using the 17-segment model to describe the size, severity and location of the perfusion abnormality including the location in terms of segmentation and vascular territory. Clear delineation between single- and multivessel disease should be performed. Defect size should be described as small (1–2 segments), moderate

(3–4 segments), or large (≥5 segments) [2]. Defect description should also include the type (ischemic, reversible, persistent, or mixed), and severity (mild, moderate, severe), of the finding.

The extent of the disease should be described, such as multivessel distribution or the presence of abnormal tracer distribution. If there is cavity enlargement, either immediately following stress, or on both stress and rest images, it should be carefully noted. If transient ischemic dilation (TID) is present, the ratio should be documented.

Left ventricular function assessment is the important component of contemporary SPECT MPI. Therefore the report should describe both global and regional function, in a qualitative and quantitative manner. The calculated left ventricular ejection fraction (LVEF) should be stated. In particular, if the LVEF is between 50 % and 70 %, the reporter may describe this as normal or may report the quantitative value. Defining function as "hyperdynamic" or >70 % may be superior to nonsensical values. Mild, moderate, or severe LV dysfunction must be also defined as LVEF of 40–49 %, 30–39 % and <30 %, respectively [6]. Regional defects should be carefully described as hypokinetic, akinetic, or dyskinetic, and the location of these findings should be given [6].

Impression

The impression part of the report is the most critical, as this may be the only portion read by the referring physician. The description must be clear and the final conclusions well defined. Most reports should begin with a statement whether the MPI is normal or abnormal, avoiding the terms "equivocal", "possible", or "probable". If there are perfusion abnormalities, but the study is interpreted as normal, this discrepancy should be described by commenting whether this is believed to be due to an artifact, such as soft tissue, LBBB, or patient motion. Functional description should also be documented briefly, whether LV function is reduced and if there are any wall motion abnormalities present. The amount of LV dysfunction should be semiquantitated as mild, moderate or severe. Lastly, the perfusion and function findings must be integrated in the final impression, as wall motion may help to distinguish between an attenuation artifact and a true fixed defect, consistent with a scar [7].

This section in the report serves also for documentation of correlation between perfusion imaging data, clinical information, stress test results, and any angiographical correlation if available. It should also include correlation with previous studies, with a direct statement regarding any important changes. An abnormal ECG response to exercise with normal perfusion images should be considered as a false-positive, since the diagnostic accuracy of perfusion imaging is superior to that of ETT, in particularly in the setting of resting ST-abnormalities. Of note, ECG changes occurring during a vasodilator infusion may indicate a worse prognosis, even in the setting of normal SPECT images [7]. Finally and most importantly, the impression must answer the clinical question that was asked, and should be clear. For example, if the study was requested for preoperative assessment, the report should comment specifically on whether there is an increased risk for perioperative cardiac complications based on the study. For acute imaging procedures, the interpreter should note whether there is any evidence of ongoing ischemia or infarction.

Reporting Pearls

The key elements are essential and are all summarized in the incorporation of the five "C"s: clarity, completeness, consistency, clinical relevancy, and communication (Table 22.2). The final item, communication, is essential for patient care. Once the report is prepared, it is crucial that the information is available as soon as possible to the referring physician. ASNC recommends that all studies be interpreted within one business day of acquisition and that the final report be ready within two business days [8]. These recommendations are also in agreement with the standard of the Intersocietal Commission for the Accreditation of Nuclear Cardiology Laboratories, with the additional requirement that a final signed report should be transmitted to the referring provider within four working days [9]. The report must be transmitted to the referring physician by email, facsimile or intranet. Especially in the setting of high-risk findings, direct telephone notification should occur. Ideally the report should include copies of the images, either embedded within the report or attached to the written document. Also, the report should be included in the electronic health record.

In conclusion, as discussed in this chapter, the report is perhaps the most important aspect of a nuclear cardiology procedure, it should be clear in order to validate the overall value of the procedure. Hence, all laboratories and interpreters should strive for the highest quality report possible to convey the maximum amount of useful clinical information. Examples of recommended reports are shown in Figs. 22.1 and 22.2.

Table 22.2 The five C's of quality reporting [10]

Clarity: Refers to minimizing ambiguity
Completeness: Symptoms, stress test results, perfusion data, and functional data should all be described within the report, relating to the clinical scenario
Consistency: The report should be consistent in term if the individual reader's patterns related to a given laboratory as well
Clinical relevancy: The question that is asked should be directly answered
Communication: All referring physicians should be notified of critical findings, through telephone contact or facsimile. Rapid reporting of findings as recommended by guidelines is essential

STRESS/REST (*OR* REST/STRESS) SINGLE/DUAL ISOTOPE SPECT IMAGING WITH EXERCISE STRESS AND GATED SPECT IMAGING

Indication: (select one)
Diagnosis of coronary disease
Evaluation of extent and severity of coronary artery disease
Evaluation of myocardial viability
Risk stratification-post-MI/preoperative/general
Assessment of acute chest pain

Clinical History:
—— year old man/woman with (no) known coronary artery disease
Cardiac risk factors include: ——
Previous cardiac procedures include: ——
Current symptomatology includes: ——

Procedure:
The patient performed treadmill exercise/bicycle exercise using a modified Bruce/Bruce/Naughton/ —— protocol, completing —— minutes and completing an estimated workload of —— METS. The heart rate was —— beats per minute at baseline and increased to —— beats at peak exercise, which was —— % of the maximum predicted heart rate. The blood pressure response to exercise was normally/hypotensive/hypertensive. The patient did/did not develop any symptoms other than fatigue during the procedure; specific symptoms include ——. The resting electrocardiogram demonstrated —— and did/did not show ST-segment changes consistent with myocardial ischemia.

Myocardial perfusion imaging was performed at rest (—— minutes following the injection of —— mCi of ——). At peak exercise, the patient was injected with —— mCi of and exercise was continued for —— minutes(s). Gating post-stress tomographic imaging was performed —— minutes after stress (and rest).

Findings:
The overall quality of the study is poor/fair/good/excellent.
Left ventricular catity is noted to be normal/enlarged on the rest (and/or stress) studies. There is eviednce of abnormal lung activity. Additionally, the right ventricle is normal/abnormal (specify: ——).

SPECT images demonstrate homogeneous tracer distribution throughout the myocardium *OR* a small/moderate/large perfusion abnormality of mild/moderate/serve

Fig. 22.1 Reporting template for exercise radionuclide myocardial perfusion imaging (Adapted from Hendel et al. [6]. With kind permission from Springer Science+Business Media)

STRESS/REST (*OR* REST/STRESS) SINGLE/DUAL ISOTOPE SPECT IMAGING WITH PHARMACOLOGIC STRESS AND GATED SPECT IMAGING

Indication: (select one)
Diagnosis of coronary disease
Evaluation of extent and severity of coronary artery disease
Evaluation of myocardial viability
Risk stratification-post-MI/preoperative/general
Assessment of acute chest pain

Clinical History:
—— year old man/woman with (no) known coronary artery disease
Cardiac risk factors include: ——
Previous cardiac procedures include: ——
Current symptomatology includes: ——

Procedure:
Pharmacologic stress testing was performed with adenosine/dipyridamole/dobutamine with a dose ——. Additionaly, low level exercise was performed along with the vasodilator infusion (specify: ——). The heart rate was —— at baseline and rose to —— beats per minute during the adenosine/dipyridamole/dobutamine infusion. this corresponds with ——% of the maximum predicted heart rate. Blood pressure response was normally/hypotensive/hypotensive during the stress procedure. The patient developed significant symptoms which included ——. The resting electrocardiogram demonstrated —— and did/did not show ST-segment changes consistent with myocardial ischemia. Myocardial perfusion imaging was performed at rest (—— minutes following the injection of —— mCi of ——). At peak pharmacologic effect, the patient was injected of —— mCi of ——. Gating post-stress tomographic imaging was performed —— minutes after stress (and rest).

Findings:
The overall quality of the study is poor/fair/good/excellent.
Left ventricular catity is noted to be normal/enlarged on the rest (and/or stress) studies. There is eviednce of abnormal lung activity. Additionally, the right ventricle is normal/abnormal (specify: ——).

SPECT images demonstrate homogeneous tracer distribution throughout the myocardium *OR* a small/moderate/large perfusion abnormality of mild/moderate/serve intensity is present in the —— (location) region on the stress images. The rest images reveal ——. Gated SPECT imaging reveals normal myocardial thickening and wall

Fig. 22.2 Reporting template for pharmacologic stress radionuclide myocardial perfusion imaging (Adapted from Hendel et al. [6]. With kind permission from Springer Science+Business Media)

References

1. Tilkemeier PL, Cooke CD, Grossman GB, McCallister BD, Ward RP. Standardized reporting of radionuclide myocardial perfusion and function. J Nucl Cardiol. 2009;16(4):650.
2. Hendel RC, Budoff MJ, Cardella JF, Chambers CE, Dent JM, Fitzgerald DM, et al. ACC/AHA/ACR/ASE/ASNC/HRS/NASCI/RSNA/SAIP/SCAI/ SCCT/SCMR/SIR 2008 key data elements and definitions for cardiac imaging: a report of the American College of Cardiology/American Heart Association Task Force on Clinical Data Standards (Writing Committee to Develop Clinical Data Standards for Cardiac Imaging). Circulation. 2009;119(1):154–86. PubMed.
3. Hendel RC, Wackers FJ, Berman DS, Ficaro E, Depuey EG, Klein L, et al. American Society of Nuclear Cardiology consensus statement: reporting of radionuclide myocardial perfusion imaging studies. J Nucl Cardiol: Off Publ Am Soc Nucl Cardiol. 2003;10(6):705–8. PubMed.
4. Gonzalez P, Canessa J, Massardo T. Formal aspects of the user-friendly nuclear cardiology report. J Nucl Cardiol. 1998;5(3):365–6. English.
5. Cerqueira M. The user-friendly nuclear cardiology report: what needs to be considered and what is included. J Nucl Cardiol. 1996;3(4):350–5. English.
6. Hendel RT, Wackers F, Berman D, Ficaro E, DePuey EG, Klein L, et al. American Society of Nuclear Cardiology consensus statement: reporting of radionuclide myocardial perfusion imaging studies. J Nucl Cardiol. 2006;13(6):e152–6. English.
7. Jaarsma C, Leiner T, Bekkers SC, Crijns HJ, Wildberger JE, Nagel E, et al. Diagnostic performance of noninvasive myocardial perfusion imaging using single-photon emission computed tomography, cardiac magnetic resonance, and positron emission tomography imaging for the detection of obstructive coronary artery disease: a meta-analysis. J Am Coll Cardiol. 2012;59(19):1719–28. PubMed.
8. Hendel R, Ficaro E, Williams K. Timeliness of reporting results of nuclear cardiology procedures. J Nucl Cardiol. 2007;14(2):266.
9. Intersocietal Commission for the Accreditation of Nuclear Cardiology Laboratories (ICANL). Standards and guidelines for nuclear/PET accreditation 2012.
10. Hendel RC, Heller GV. Nuclear cardiology: practical applications. 2nd ed. New York: McGraw-Hill Professional; 2011.

Chapter 23
SPECT: Quality Improvement Program

Cesia Gallegos, Patty Reames, and Robert C. Hendel

Abstract This chapter focuses on quality issues related to SPECT myocardial perfusion imaging, emphasizing the appropriate use of this technology and reinforcing the use of known performance metrics and standards to improve daily practice. The chapter will provide specific examples in the areas of appropriate use criteria, image acquisition, radiation exposure, intra-modality and image interpretation quality improvement initiatives.

Keywords SPECT • Appropriate use criteria • Quality • Reporting • Accreditation

Quality in cardiovascular imaging remains an indispensable goal. The U.S. Department of Health and Human Services defines quality improvement as "systematic and continuous actions that lead to measurable improvement in health care services and the health status of targeted patient groups". The Institute of Medicine broadens this definition in terms of health care services as symbiosis between improved health care services and the anticipated health outcomes of patients. However it is defined, poor quality in imaging has the potential to be harmful for patients, possibly adversely impacting patient outcome. Therefore, there is a critical need to institute ongoing process improvement so as to optimize SPECT myocardial perfusion imaging and its clinical value.

C. Gallegos, MD
Department of Medicine, University of Miami Miller School of Medicine, Miami, FL, USA
e-mail: cesia.gallegos@jhsmiami.org

P. Reames, ARRT, CNMT, NCT, FASNC
Practice Manager, Ohio State University Heart and Vascular Center,
2220 Timber Trail, Bellefontaine, OH 4331, USA
e-mail: patty.reames@osumc.edu

R.C. Hendel, MD, FACC, FAHA, FASNC (✉)
Cardiovascular Division Chief (Interim), University of Miami Miller
School of Medicine, 1120 NW 14th Street, Suite 1123, CRB, Miami, FL 33136, USA
e-mail: RHendel@med.miami.edu

P.L. Tilkemeier et al. (eds.), *Quality Evaluation in Non-Invasive Cardiovascular Imaging*, DOI 10.1007/978-3-319-28011-0_23

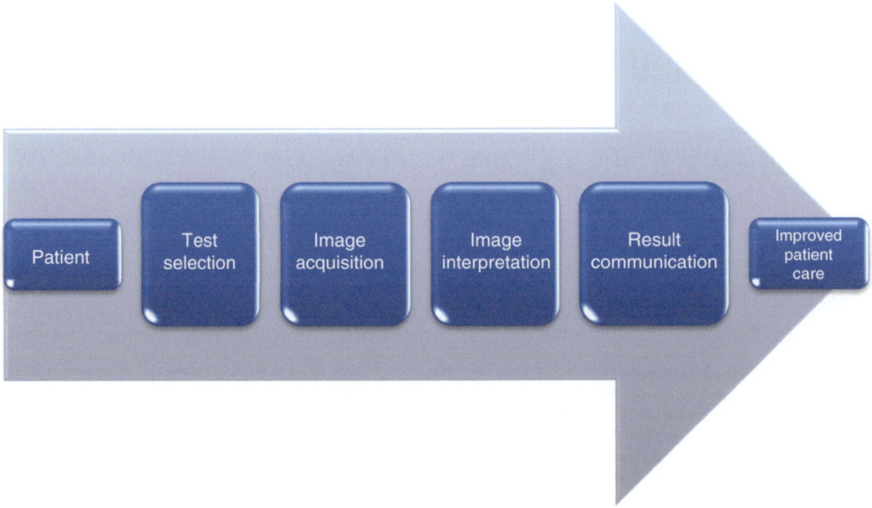

Fig. 23.1 Dimensions of care framework for evaluating quality of cardiovascular imaging (Reprinted from Douglas et al. [2] with permission from Elsevier)

A conference was held to define and focus quality initiatives for cardiovascular imaging [1–3]. The purpose of this conference was to define the key components of quality in cardiovascular imaging and to define measures that may demonstrate quality and improve the practice of imaging which were reassessed 18 months later. The approach consists of the following components:

1. Structural measures: such as equipment and protocols
2. Process measures including patient selection and image acquisition
3. Outcome and impact on decision-making.

This permitted the construction of a plan of quality assessment, with several key steps and a number of quality parameters (Fig. 23.1), which will be outlined in the following sections.

Appropriate Use of SPECT MPI

In recent years, regulators and payers have raised concern about the overuse and misuse of radionuclide imaging, pointing to the high rates of SPECT MPI utilization, as well as the geographic variation in its use. Both of these factors raise suspicion for overuse and misuse of this resource-intensive procedure. The majority of quality statements and guidelines for SPECT imaging focus on either the procedural aspects of imaging or evaluation methods. In order to focus on appropriate utilization of SPECT imaging, Appropriate Use Criteria (AUC) were introduced as discussed earlier this Section. We wish to focus on those AUC developed by the American

Table 23.1 Most common inappropriate indications for SPECT MPI

Indication	Inappropriate indications (%)	Total studies (%)
Detection of CAD Asymptomatic, low CHD risk	44.5	6.0
Asymptomatic, post-revascularization <2 years after PCI, symptoms before PCI	23.8	3.2
Evaluation of chest pain, low probability point Interpretable ECG and able to exercise	16.1	2.2
Asymptomatic or stable symptoms, known CAD <1 year after catheterization or abnormal prior SPECT	3.9	0.5
Preoperative assessment Low risk surgery	3.8	0.5
Total	92.1	12.4

Reprinted from Douglas et al. [2] with permission from Elsevier

College of Cardiology and the American Society of Nuclear Cardiology although other appropriateness criteria were developed by the American College of Radiology. The priority of these documents is to optimize procedural utilization, by highlighting the need to perform the right test, at the right time, for the right patient.

The development and publication of AUC alone is insufficient to impact on utilization. Implementation and evaluation of appropriate use is essential to changing practice patterns. Several publications have focused on the assessment of appropriate use of radionuclide imaging and have demonstrated that current practice contains approximately 10–15 % inappropriate use and the most common reasons for inappropriate use of SPECT are readily identifiable (Table 23.1) [4].

The goal of AUC is to improve patient care, while supporting a cost-effectiveness approach in which the clinician can focus on ordering a specific test based on a specific clinical scenario, to be able to tract appropriateness as a potential metric for quality improvement. The AUC serves to educate caregivers about their practice and feedback provides an opportunity for improvement, as essential quality improvement process.

Accrediting bodies, such as the Intersocietal Accreditation Commission (IAC), require ongoing quality assessment and specifically request applying laboratories to survey the appropriate use of SPECT MPI in their environment [5]. A variety of tools are currently available to help laboratories assess the level of appropriate use, including the FOCUS (Formation of Optimal Cardiovascular Utilization Strategies) instrument, which can be find at www.acc.org/focus and other mobile apps listed http://www.intersocietal.org/nuclear/seeking/sample_qualitycontrol.htm.

Quality initiatives related to AUC should feature the following:

1. Quarterly/Annual review of appropriate use with an audit of at least 30 SPECT examinations categorized as appropriate, may be appropriate, or rarely appropriate
2. Compare individual lab results with national benchmarks
3. Institute an educational program for referring physicians about AUC and provide feedback to these clinicians on their practice habits

Image Acquisition

The next phase of the quality continuum is image acquisition. These metrics deal with the structure and process surrounding the formation of high-quality image. It is a multiple-step process that begins before the patient comes to the laboratory and continues after the patient leaves it. It relies on modality-specific processes, including protocols and sequences that increase the changes of obtaining images that are of diagnostic quality. The American Society of Nuclear Cardiology (ASNC) has developed imaging guidelines that provide detailed information regarding various protocols and its acquisition parameters, as well as what constitutes acceptable practice, to ensure acquisition of high-quality images, consistency, and timeliness as they are critical in image acquisition protocols. The use of these protocols has been shown to provide images of good quality for clinical interpretation and quantitation [6].

Patient-related issues are also included in this domain. Factors related to the patient (soft tissue attenuation, extracardiac activity, motion) should be monitored, as well as specific doses of radiation administered [7]. In addition to defining parameters surrounding image acquisition, quality control procedures should be implemented, such as uniformity flood, and center-of-rotation (COR)-evaluation, which were discussed in Chap. 21 Other aspects of image acquisition include the timely performance of the nuclear procedure and ensuring the comfort and safety of the patient.

Radiation Exposure

SPECT has been shown to be safe, reliable, and widely utilized, serving as a mainstay in the management of known or suspected CAD. However, increasing concern has been raised regarding the use of any test that mandates ionizing radiation, especially when more than one study may be performed [7–10]. There are multiple factors that must be considered regarding SPECT and radiation exposure, the following are three critical factors:

- Appropriateness of the study.
- Lowest radiation dose that will still maintain diagnostic precision (ALARA: As Low As Reasonably Achievable)
- New technologies/protocols/alternate studies that will further reduce radiation dose [9, 11].

Patient selection is the most important constituent for reducing radiation exposure, avoiding unnecessary exams and limiting radiation exposure. The Appropriateness Use Criteria (AUC), have been discussed previously and remain critical to reduce unnecessary radiation exposure [12]. Tracer selection and protocol should be selected based on the specific question for which the study was ordered but dosimetry should always be considered and must be in keeping with ALARA

Table 23.2 Algorithm for weight-adjusted radiopharmaceutical administration

Sestamibi dose chart		
Weight	Two day (mCi)	One day (mCi)
<160 lb	25.0	10/30
160–170 lb	27.5	11/33
170–180 lb	29.2	12/35
180–190 lb	30.0	12/36
190–200 lb	32.5	13/39
200–210 lb	34.0	14/41
210–220 lb	35.7	14/42
220–230 lb	37.3	14/43
240–250 lb	38.9	14/44
>250 lb	40.0	15/45

Courtesy of Gary V. Heller, MD, PhD

principle (as low as reasonably achievable). Patient-centered imaging aims for the lowest dose of radiation that is possible to perform an exam that will yield useful information that will impact in clinical decision-making.

Younger patients tend to have lower likelihood for CAD, but the highest risk of radiation, since the latency between radiation exposure and cancer is believed to be greater than a decade. In these patients, alternate imaging studies should be considered to avoid exposure to ionizing radiation [7, 9]. Likewise, serial testing should be avoided unless there is a significant change in clinical symptoms or status. Clinical judgment is the most important rule in the selection of any test, and must be patient specific. It is also important to remember that the risks of radiation exposure, not only include patients, but also involves medical personnel and public.

Recent advances in nuclear cardiology have further allowed MPI to provide higher quality images with faster scan times, which also contribute to reduction in radiation exposure. New technologies including SPECT cameras and reconstruction software have the potential of reducing radiation through increased photon sensitivity. Multiple studies have been published demonstrating the value of new software algorithms and camera configurations, which permit reduced-dose protocols [11, 13].

An ASNC information statement has recommended a number of measures that should be employed for reducing radiation exposure in SPECT MPI [9]. Firstly, as noted above, the use of AUC will reduce unnecessary exposure by elimination of inappropriate testing. Additionally, laboratories should consider performing stress imaging first and if normal, forgo the rest study. The use of stress-only imaging is likely to have a dramatic impact on dose reduction. Other dose reduction strategies should be employed including the elimination of thallium-201 for use as strictly a perfusion agent and using a weight adjusted dosing regimen for Tc-99m agents (Table 23.2). The ultimate goal should be that 50 % of patients examined with SPECT MPI should have a total exposure of <9 mSv [9].

In conclusion, each laboratory should specify methods for radiation reduction and ALARA, as well as consider all dose-reduction strategies (Table 23.3). Mean, median, and range of doses should be reported on an annual basis, to track

Table 23.3 Radiation reduction strategies for SPECT MPI

AUC to select patients for imaging
Stress-only imaging when possible
Use of short active radiopharmaceuticals; elimination of Tl-201 for perfusion
Weight based dosing of Tc-99m agents
High sensitivity camera
Software modifications including iterative reconstruction

Adapted from Cerqueira et al. [9] with kind permission of Springer.

performance, as well as the percent of patient who receive less than 9 mSv per examination. Additionally, the frequency of the use of thallium-201 and stress-only procedures should be recorded as quality metrics.

Intermodality Comparison and Image Interpretation

Quality improvement requires a systematic approach for the interpretation and reporting of MPI studies in order to provide pertinent information that will guide clinical decision-making as well as management. This component of quality, includes the accuracy of the test, its reproducibility and physician competency. This usually involves correlation with coronary angiography serving as the "gold standard." At least 25 studies should be correlated with angiographic findings each year. Additionally, an assessment of the frequency of normal studies in a group of patients with low likelihood for CAD should be determined (normalcy rate). This may be done by selecting patients who were felt to be at low risk for CAD who had a normal exercise ECG portion of the test and were asymptomatic during the procedure.

Reproducibility of interpretation is also an important quality metric, especially when multiple readers are present in the same laboratory. Therefore, it is recommended that each laboratory select ten cases per quarter to be reviewed by all readers. Further evaluation, could include periodic external review by other nuclear specialists to reduce variability. An evaluation of agreement/concordance should then be performed. It is also recommended that all readers then meet to review the cases as a group, so as to allow for education and improved interpretation. Irrespective of the methodology used, a routine measure of accuracy and reproducibility is critical for maintain quality standards.

Reporting

Another key quality factor is the standardization of data elements. This allows for understandable definitions for concepts such as perfusion defect size and location. It also permits data pooling and registry/database formation encouraging research.

This can be performed by two methods: the standard 17-segment interpretation as recommended by ACC/ASNC and by quantitative programs [14, 15]. Moreover, we want to reinforce that clinical reports should use standard language and be composed clearly, incorporating clinical information that is relevant to the practitioner.

A random sample of reports should be audited each quarter/year for completeness and use of standard terminology. Each report must reflect accurately the content and results of the study, which includes but is not limited to [16]:

1. Identification of the facility
2. Identification of the patient
3. Ordering physician
4. Date of study
5. Clinical indication and pertinent history, prior therapy or administration of radiopharmaceuticals.
6. Name of procedure and mode of exercise/stress
7. Specific Name/Doses/Routes of radiopharmaceuticals
8. Size, severity, and location of any perfusion defects
9. If applicable, the type of attenuation correction
10. A clear, concise conclusion
11. Signed and dated by reader

Communication

Failure to communicate clinically relevant results in a timely fashion detracts from the quality of the imaging procedure, even of all the previously described components are performed well. Hence, as mentioned in the reporting Chap. 22, critical results should be relayed as soon as possible to the referring physician. Current guidelines suggest that the time from study completion to interpretation, and delivery of the report, should be less than two business days [16, 17]. An audit should be performed which provides a determination of the percent of studies with final reports completed within two business days. Results may be transmitted though facsimile, email, intranet transfer, or through the medical record. In the case of high-risk findings, telephone communication should occur, with subsequent documentation of any communication between physicians [16].

Outcomes

If all the components of quality in imaging have been optimized, the final stage of the imaging continuum is improved patient outcomes. This is particularly challenging in terms of cardiac imaging, as many factors and decision occur between the time of the imaging procedure and a specific clinic outcome or events. However, ongoing studies may provide the evidence of the value of quality in nuclear cardiology.

Accreditation/Certification

An important, objective metric, which summarize many aspects of laboratory performance is that of laboratory accreditation, which provides evidence of quality defined as adherence to a standard. In a similar fashion, provider certification demonstrates that an individual has adequate training, experience, and knowledge of nuclear cardiology [18]. Laboratory accreditation and professional certification for nuclear cardiology will be discussion in detail in the next chapter.

References

1. Cook NR, Paynter NP, Eaton CB, Manson JE, Martin LW, Robinson JG, et al. Comparison of the Framingham and Reynolds risk scores for global cardiovascular risk prediction in the multiethnic women's health initiative. Circulation. 2012;125(14):1748–56.
2. Douglas P, Iskandrian AE, Krumholz HM, Gillam L, Hendel R, Jollis J, et al. Achieving quality in cardiovascular imaging: proceedings from the American College of Cardiology-Duke University Medical Center Think Tank on Quality in Cardiovascular Imaging. J Am Coll Cardiol. 2006;48(10):2141–51. PubMed.
3. Douglas PS, Chen J, Gillam L, Hendel R, Hundley WG, Masoudi F, et al. Achieving quality in cardiovascular imaging II: proceedings from the second American College of Cardiology – Duke University Medical Center Think Tank on Quality in Cardiovascular Imaging. J Am Coll Cardiol Img. 2009;2(2):231–40. PubMed.
4. Hendel RC, Cerqueira M, Douglas PS, Caruth KC, Allen JM, Jensen NC, et al. A multicenter assessment of the use of single-photon emission computed tomography myocardial perfusion imaging with appropriateness criteria. J Am Coll Cardiol. 2010;55(2):156–62. PubMed.
5. Intersocietal Commission for the Accreditation of Nuclear Cardiology Laboratories (ICANL). Standards and guidelines for nuclear/pet accreditation 2012.
6. Holly TA, Abbott BG, Al-Mallah M, Calnon DA, Cohen MC, DiFilippo FP, Ficaro EP, Freeman MR, Hendel RC, Jain D, Leonard SM, Nichols KJ, Polk DM, Soman P. ASNC imaging guidelines for nuclear cardiology procedures: single photon-emission computed tomography. [Internet]. 2010 [cited 2014 April 23]. Available from: http://www.asnc.org/imageuploads/ImagingGuidelineSPECTJune2010.pdf.
7. Chen J, Einstein AJ, Fazel R, Krumholz HM, Wang Y, Ross JS, et al. Cumulative exposure to ionizing radiation from diagnostic and therapeutic cardiac imaging procedures: a population-based analysis. J Am Coll Cardiol. 2010;56(9):702–11. PubMed Pubmed Central PMCID: 2952402.
8. Einstein AJ, Moser KW, Thompson RC, Cerqueira MD, Henzlova MJ. Radiation dose to patients from cardiac diagnostic imaging. Circulation. 2007;116(11):1290–305. PubMed.
9. Cerqueira MD, Allman KC, Ficaro EP, Hansen CL, Nichols KJ, Thompson RC, et al. Recommendations for reducing radiation exposure in myocardial perfusion imaging. J Nucl Cardiol: Off Publ Am Soc Nucl Cardiol. 2010;17(4):709–18. PubMed.
10. Einstein AJ, Berman DS, Min JK, Hendel RC, Gerber TC, Carr JJ, et al. Patient-centered imaging shared decision making for cardiac imaging procedures with exposure to ionizing radiation. J Am Coll Cardiol. 2014;63(15):1480–9.
11. Slomka PJ, Dey D, Duvall WL, Henzlova MJ, Berman DS, Germano G. Advances in nuclear cardiac instrumentation with a view towards reduced radiation exposure. Curr Cardiol Rep. 2012;14(2):208–16. PubMed.
12. Hendel RC, Berman DS, Di Carli MF, Heidenreich PA, Henkin RE, Pellikka PA, et al. ACCF/ASNC/ACR/AHA/ASE/SCCT/SCMR/SNM 2009 appropriate use criteria for cardiac

radionuclide imaging: a report of the American College of Cardiology Foundation appropriate use criteria task force, the American Society of Nuclear Cardiology, the American College of Radiology, the American Heart Association, the American Society of Echocardiography, the Society of Cardiovascular Computed Tomography, the Society for Cardiovascular Magnetic Resonance, and the Society of Nuclear Medicine. J Am Coll Cardiol. 2009;53(23):2201–29. PubMed.

13. Miller TD, Askew JW, O'Connor MK. New toys for nuclear cardiologists. Cir: Cardiovasc Imaging. 2011;4(1):5–7.
14. Tilkemeier PL, Cooke CD, Grossman GB, McCallister BD, Ward RP. Standardized reporting of radionuclide myocardial perfusion and function. J Nucl Cardiol. 2009;16(4):650.
15. Hendel RC, Budoff MJ, Cardella JF, Chambers CE, Dent JM, Fitzgerald DM, et al. ACC/AHA/ACR/ASE/ASNC/HRS/NASCI/RSNA/SAIP/SCAI/ SCCT/SCMR/SIR 2008 key data elements and definitions for cardiac imaging: a report of the American College of Cardiology/American Heart Association Task Force on clinical data standards (Writing Committee to Develop Clinical Data Standards for Cardiac Imaging). Circulation. 2009;119(1):154–86. PubMed.
16. Laboratories. ICftAoNM. The intersocietal accreditation commission standards and guidelines for nuclear/PET accreditation 2012. Available from: http://www.intersocietal.org/nuclear/standards/IACNuclearPETStandards2012.pdf.
17. Hendel R, Ficaro E, Williams K. Timeliness of reporting results of nuclear cardiology procedures. J Nucl Cardiol. 2007;14(2):266.
18. National Electrical Manufacturers Association. Standardization policies and procedures of the National Electrical Manufacturers Association. [Internet] Published November 7, 2014. Available from: http://www.nema.org/Standards/About-Standards/Documents/SPP-2014.pdf

Chapter 24
SPECT: Accreditation and Certification

Cesia Gallegos and Robert C. Hendel

Abstract This chapter provides the necessary information and tools for accreditation as part of the quality improvement continuum. The importance of accreditation will be emphasized. Each of the pathways for laboratory accreditation for SPECT imaging will be examined as well as the differences between the pathways. These pathways include the American College of Radiology, the Intersocietal Accreditation Commission, and the Joint Commission. Pathways to physician certification will also be discussed. The importance of both accreditation and certification to laboratory quality will be discussed.

Keywords SPECT • Accreditation • Certification

Accreditation

As the use of cardiac imaging procedures continues to grow, so should the commitment to quality and accepted standards of practice. A nuclear cardiology laboratory's accreditation provides an objective assessment of quality, based on technical quality, safety, and accuracy, performed by an external third party that verifies compliance with regulations and best practice strategies. It is a means to demonstrate that commitment to quality in every aspect: imaging, interpretation, reporting, facility and most importantly, patient care. The optimization of provider and laboratory performance is the key goal for both accreditation and certification.

C. Gallegos, MD
Department of Medicine, University of Miami Miller School of Medicine, Miami, FL, USA
e-mail: cesia.gallegos@jhsmiami.org

R.C. Hendel, MD, FACC, FAHA, MASNC (✉)
Cardiovascular Division Chief (Interim), University of Miami Miller School of Medicine, 1120 NW 14th Street Suite 1123, CRB, Miami, FL 33136, USA
e-mail: RHendel@med.miami.edu

P.L. Tilkemeier et al. (eds.), *Quality Evaluation in Non-Invasive Cardiovascular Imaging*, DOI 10.1007/978-3-319-28011-0_24

Although in the past accreditation was a voluntary process, the ACC, ASNC, United States Center for Medicare Services (CMS) and third-party insurers now mandate accreditation for out-patient and practice-based nuclear cardiology laboratories (MIPPA, 2012). The past decade has further witnessed increasing participation in accreditation by both inpatient and outpatient laboratories, especially in the US, largely due to federal and private payer requirements. Since 2007, nuclear cardiology laboratory accreditation has seen exponential growth due to increasing mandates for accreditation so as to ensure quality and compliance with guidelines and best practices.

Accreditation as a concept in cardiovascular imaging was first introduced in 1990, when the Intersocietal Commission for Accreditation of Vascular Laboratories (ICAVL) was established [1]. Given its success, similar programs were created for other diagnostic procedures including nuclear cardiology. As such, the Intersocietal Commission for the Accreditation of Nuclear Medicine Laboratories (ICANL) established in 1997, is dedicated to quality in nuclear cardiology by providing objective quality metrics and peer review. There are several paths for laboratory accreditation including ICANL, and in January 2010, Medicare announced the three approved accreditation organizations: Intersocietal Accreditation Commission (IAC), American College of Radiology (ACR), and The Joint Commission (previously known as JCAHO) [2].

Joint Commission

The Joint Commission, which was created in 1975, provides accreditation to hospitals and the laboratories within its facility. It was also named by CMS as a designated accreditor of advanced imaging centers. The Joint Commission converges on operational systems that are vital to the safety and quality of health care. An on-site survey by a Joint Commission team is required to obtain and maintain accreditation. This on-site survey serves for evaluation of the facility's performance and it serves as an opportunity to educate and guidance for continuing quality improvement. The team is composed of professionals with advanced medical or clinical degrees with at least 5 years of leadership and training. Once the survey is completed, the facility is given a summary of key points identified during the visit. These are then reviewed by the Joint Commission's Central Office Staff, and subsequently posted to the facility's extranet site. This summary will specify which findings will require an Evidence of Standards Compliance (ESC) submission within a time period of 45 or 60 days. Once the ESC is completed and accepted by The Joint Commission, their decision is posted again to their extranet site and to Quality Check [3]. The Joint Commission provides accreditation information including costs and requirements in its website: www.jointcommission.org/accreditation/ambulatory_healthcare.aspx. Manuals with complete information for accreditation/reaccreditation are available for purchase.

American College of Radiology

Nuclear laboratories may also receive accreditation through the American College of Radiology (ACR), whose program is rigorous and uses a phantom to ensure acceptable camera performance [4]. The ACR also provides accreditation for multiple medical imaging technologies in a similar fashion as IAC. It consists of three modules from which facilities can choose for accreditation: general nuclear medicine (planar imaging), SPECT, and Nuclear Cardiology Imaging. The laboratory must apply for all the modules that are performed in that specific site. For nuclear cardiology, the ACR program is unit based, meaning that every unit used to produce clinical images must pass accreditation testing for the laboratory to be accredited. Moreover, it focuses on imaging systems and the quality of performance, often with the use of phantoms and their corresponding unit, the modules performed at the site and all isotopes. The acquisition of the phantom images encompasses the use of a SPECT phantom designated by the ACR.

The application for accreditation by ACR consists of a two-step process [5]. First, the facility must provide ACR with all the information regarding the practice site characteristics, including modality and specifics about equipment as mentioned above. Information is collected on the quality control and assurance program in place, follow-up, data collection, reporting, and laboratory safety including use of radiopharmaceuticals. Copies of their most recent state of Nuclear Regulatory Commission (NRC) audits must also be submitted. The second step, consists of the submission of clinical images/cases, and may also involve submission of reports, phantom images, scanning protocols, and dose measurements. It is important to note that the phantom and clinical images must not be submitted on the same film, as different teams will be reviewing them. The laboratory must submit two different examination types for each module they are seeking accreditation for. Along with the images, a clinical history must be provided. For nuclear medicine and some other imaging modalities, the ACR now offers the option of electronic submission.

Similar to the IAC, the documentation and application for ACR accreditation undergoes a peer-review process, which not only includes evaluation, but also identifies areas for improvement and other recommendations. Full accreditation for a 3-year period is only granted when all modules or units have passed the complete accreditation process, including notification in writing of any module or unit that has not passed and has been withdrawn from the service. If no module or unit has yet passed the evaluation process but the facility has already applied for accreditation, the facility will be considered "Under Review". Likewise, all interpreting physicians, and technologists must also meet specific requirement for their laboratory to be accredited by ACR. The ACR also provides on-site survey, which includes radiologists and a medical physicist, during the 3-year period of accreditation to ensure continuation of quality. A detailed list of qualifications and requirements for accreditation can be found on www.acr.org.

As will be discussed later in this section, ACR and IAC differ in their focus of review and underlying concept [6]. Unlike IAC, in which the focus is on the quality of the case studies and is camera independent, phantom testing is mandated and normal case studies are preferred for ACR accreditation. It is important to remember that the principal difference between IAC accreditation and ACR: the ACR program was developed for radiology facilities in general with a focus on equipment and imaging, whereas IAC has a primary focus on the clinical aspects of imaging and the final report [6].

Intersocietal Accreditation Commission

The Intersocietal Accreditation Commission (IAC) has a subdivision, the IAC – Nuclear/PET, which provides accreditation for office-based and hospital nuclear cardiology laboratories after a thorough assessment of protocols and procedures, as well as a review of cases and their reports [7]. Accreditation for nuclear cardiology through IAC is focused on myocardial perfusion, equilibrium radionuclide angiography, cardiac PET imaging, and other cardiac imaging. The organization is sponsored by the Academy of Molecular Imaging, the American College of Cardiology, the American College of Nuclear Physicians, along with the American Society of Nuclear Cardiology, and the Society of Nuclear Medicine Technologist Section. Each of the sponsoring societies has stated their commitment for quality, especially through the use of accreditation.

The IAC's main goal is self-assessment through which the laboratories can identify and correct potential issues, thereby validating standards, protocols, and quality assurance programs. In 2000, the IAC accreditation program merged with that of the American College of Nuclear Physicians, adding a mandatory site visit to each applicant laboratory [1]. This was further enhanced through the *IAC Standards and Guidelines for Nuclear/PET Accreditation* and the Online Accreditation application.

The IAC standards have been developed based on guidelines, medical literature and expert consensus documents, which are frequently updated and revised to reflect changing practice and quality measures. The accreditation process aims to provide laboratories with information about their performance in a way to incorporate these findings into constant quality improvement projects. Furthermore, they are able to assess the influence of the quality of imaging services provided to the patient.

The process of accreditation by the IAC consists of multiple phases, all of which must comply with the current Standards: [7] Self-evaluation and case studies' submission, Peer-Review, followed by Board Review evaluation and final decision. The first phase, consists of an in-house, thorough review based on the online application checklist, and a preparation of case studies. The case examples, which are the most important piece of the application, are to be contemporary, that is, performed with current personnel (medical or technical) who interpret or perform any nuclear test on current equipment, they must have been interpreted by as many physicians and technologists as possible, and the Medical Director of the facility must be represented. Furthermore, five cases must be submitted from which one study must be normal, at least one study must be a pharmacological stress and at least one study must be an exercise stress. These cases are then to be submitted along with each application and an IAC Accreditation Agreement to allow reviewers to evaluate the interpretative and technical quality of representative work. Some of the required documentation for submission as part of the Online Accreditation application includes:

- Facility overview
- Procedure Volumes
- Training/Experience Qualification Pathway/Certification documentation
- Physical Medical License
- BLS/ACLS
- CME for all Technologists and Physicians

Further details regarding the application requirements can be found at http://www.intersocietal.org/nuclear/seeking/required_items.htm.

After an application to IAC is submitted, it is assigned to two independent reviewers who simultaneously complete a detailed review of the clinical component. Subsequently, these comments are reviewed by the Director of Accreditation, in preparation for the final discussion with the Board of Directors for the final decision. Accreditation is ultimately based on conformance with published standards and the use of validated and accepted imaging protocols with ongoing commitment to quality [7].

After peer-review, the decision by IAC is made to either (1) Grant, (2) Delay, (3) Perform Site Visit, (4) Deny accreditation. If a site visit is required, it is likely that the information provided was not sufficient to determine compliance. No application is denied on the initial submission. Accreditation is granted for a 3-year period, based on JCAHO recommendations for hospital accreditation. However up to 46 % of laboratories do not receive accreditation based on the initial application [7]. The key reasons for denial of accreditation are listed in Table 24.1.

In an effort to further substantiate continued compliance by accredited facilities and in response to the requirements sanctioned by the Centers for Medicare & Medicaid Services (CMS) for CMS appointed Accreditation Organizations as part of the Medicare Improvements for Patients and Providers Act (MIPPA), the IAC has implemented a policy requiring all accredited facilities to undergo an audit or site

Table 24.1 Common reasons for denial of laboratory accreditation [8]

Common reasons for denial of laboratory accreditation
Lack of documented continuing education
Protocols lacking specific details
Failure to integrate stress and imaging findings
Lack of documented QA activities
Insufficient details regarding image acquisition
Inadequate detail about stress test performance
Absence of detailed description of defect and severity

Courtesy of Mary Beth Farrell IAC

visit at some time during their 3-year accreditation period [7]. It is recommended that information about appropriate use be including as a QA project and include evaluation of a minimum of 30 consecutive patients each year. This should be based on the most recent AUC documents [9, 10].

Another part of their criteria for achieving accreditation by IAC is the fulfillment of certain Continuing Medical Education (CME) by facility staff members as discussed later in this section [11]. It includes 15 h of education every 3 years, AMA Category 1 for physicians and RCEEM-approved for technologists. The content should relate to the performance or interpretation of nuclear cardiology studies, stress testing, or radiation safety. The CME requirement for recent graduations of training programs is waived if the application is within 3 years of graduation. Also, the CME requirement will be waived if board certification by CBNC or ABMS is granted within the prior 3 years.

Reaccreditation

For reaccreditation, the IAC uses the same Online Application required for first-time applicants. It allows facility personnel to access previously submitted information and make updates that have occurred during the 3-year cycle. To maintain uninterrupted accreditation status, the IAC recommends that the reaccreditation application is submitted 3 months prior to expiration date, to allow enough time for the review, which again consists of two independent reviewers, in-site visit if applicable, review by Board of Directors, and a final decision. Furthermore, the IAC requires that the application be submitted by the first of the month, and the case studies no later than the fifth of the month. It is important to note that avoiding expiration is of critical importance, as the use of the Seal of Accreditation on reports or other documents is prohibited. Moreover, expiration impacts on reimbursement policies that require accreditation. However, if the application was submitted prior to expiration, a 60-day grace period is extended to evade a gap in the facility's accreditation due to programming of the Board of Director's decision meeting. The IAC also provides reminders to start preparing the reaccreditation application. The Medical and Technical Directors receive a mailed letter notifying the expiration date 1 year prior to the recommended submission date, along with instructions. Further communications include a reminder postcard, as well as emails for webinars sent at 3 and 6-month intervals from the recommended submission date. The IAC facilitates the reaccreditation process by providing step-by-step guidance for reaccreditation, as well as a list of common pitfalls, frequently asked questions, and informative webinars in their website http://www.intersocietal.org/nuclear/reaccreditation/reaccred_welcome.htm.

In the case of ACR, an Accreditation Renewal Notice is sent about 8 months prior to the expiration date. At that time of renewal, the laboratories are only required to submit updated modality information, which should include personnel certification and qualifications, a new survey agreement, and any other essential laboratory information as detailed in the Accreditation process [5].

Overall, the accreditation process enables the laboratory and its staff to function based on quality standards to provide superior patient care. Furthermore, it has demonstrated that the accreditation process has a positive perceived impact in those involved on it [12], suggesting its impact in quality control and providing new areas for quality improvement projects [13].

Certification

Physician certification requires ensuring that the nuclear cardiologist has had the requisition training and experience, as well as fundamental knowledge as assessed by a focused examination of nuclear cardiology. Although not required for practicing nuclear cardiology or for hospital privileging, the Certification Board of Nuclear Cardiology (CBNC) (www.cbnc.org) provides an objective measure of quality, one that is recognized as an appropriate regulatory pathway by the Nuclear Regulatory Commission (NRC). Additionally, the CBNC certification is being increasingly required for reimbursement of professional services. While a radiologist and nuclear medicine physician often use their Board Certification as evidence of expertise in nuclear cardiology, CBNC provides evidence of an additional lever of competency, and provides objective evidence of expertise in nuclear cardiology for cardiologists.

Certification Board of Nuclear Cardiology

In the CBNC website, there is clear guidance in regards to the documentation required prior to application for certification. For complete information regarding the CBNC Eligibility Requirements for U.S. Applicants may be found in the aforementioned website of CBNC under Certification and Eligibility for US Applicants (http://www.cccvi.org), but are summarized below:

Requirement 1: Training or Experience in the area of Nuclear Cardiology Services. This includes Level 2 nuclear cardiology training, a minimum of 700 h including 80 h of Classroom and Laboratory Training (CLT), which must be completed prior to submission of application

Requirement 2: Licensure. Applicants must hold a current, unconditional, and unrestricted license to practice medicine in the US.

Requirement 3: Board Certification. Applicants must be physicians who are Board Certified in Cardiology, Nuclear Medicine or Radiology.

CBNC's certification is for a period of 10 years and 2 months, before which, the diplomats must recertify. CBNC's recertification process allows candidates to sit for their examination at years, 8, 9, and 10 of their certification period. Applicants have three opportunities to pass their exam within their eligibility without losing their certification status; otherwise, his/her certification will be published as expired. The recertification exam differs from the certification test in that is approximately two-thirds. The Eligibility Requirements for Recertification are detailed in the recertification section of the CBNC's website. These include:

1. Certification in Nuclear Cardiology
2. Licensure: Current, Unconditional and unrestricted license to practice Medicine with a copy of the current license with expiration date.
3. Board Certification: Either in Cardiology, Nuclear Medicine or Radiology
4. Evidence of CME in Nuclear Cardiology
5. Candidate Attestation

In terms of CME, the following applicants must provide documentation of 30 h of CME completed within the 36 months prior to application:

- Certification applications whose Level 2 nuclear cardiology training was completed more than 7 years ago prior to the exam for which they are applying
- Certification applications coming though the Experience Pathway
- Recertification applicants
- Applicants who failed the exam three or more times (These must provide documentation of additional training as well)

As mentioned above, the IAC also has requirements for CME by facility staff members in order to provide accreditation to labs which can be found in their website (http://www.intersocietal.org/nuclear/main/cme_requirements.htm) [7]. For laboratory personnel there are specific requirements, based on laboratory position:

MEDICAL DIRECTOR: at least 15 h if AMA (American Medical Association) Category 1 CME credits, pertinent to nuclear medicine, every 3 years, unless the Medical Director has attained one or more of the following within 3 years prior to the application date, in which the CME requirement will be considered fulfilled:

- Completion of an ACGME approved relevant residency or fellowship
- Initial certification by a relevant ABMS recognized board
- Certification by CBNC (as mentioned above)
- Re-Certification by the American Board of Nuclear Medicine, American Board of Radiology, or CBNC.

TECHNICAL DIRECTOR: at least 15 h of accredited CE relevant to nuclear medicine every 3 years. The IAC requirements will be considered fulfilled if the following have been met within the 3 years prior to application:

- Completion of an accredited nuclear medicine training program
- Attainment if an appropriate technical credential in nuclear medicine; or
- Attainment of advanced technical credential

MEDICAL STAFF: At least 15 h of AMA Category 1 CME credits relevant to nuclear medicine every 3 years, unless the member has successfully attained completion of an ACGME approved relevant residency or fellowship, attaining initial certification by a relevant ABMS recognized board, certification by CBNC, or

4re-certification by the American Board of Nuclear Medicine, American Board of Radiology, or CBNC, to be considered fulfilled.

TECHNICAL STAFF: at least 15 h of accredited CE (must be approved) relevant to nuclear medicine, every 3 years.

American Board of Radiology

The American Board of Radiology (ABR) also provides a pathway for certification of radiologists. For Nuclear Radiology, the initial certification is for those who have not yet been certified in nuclear cardiology, but who are already certified in diagnostic cardiology. The ABR has approved requirement for eligibility of both diagnostic radiology and nuclear cardiology subspecialty certification, in which residents who complete 16 months within a 4-year ACGME accredited radiology program are eligible. As described in their website (http://theabr.org/ic-nuc-landing) the pathway requirements are:

- Sixteen months of nuclear medicine within a 48-month residency, from which 10 must be consecutive
- The supporting diagnostic radiology residency must be in an ACGME-accredited nuclear medicine radiology fellowship or ACGME-accredited nuclear medicine residency program
- Program must fulfill the ABR requirement for NRC training

For accreditation purposes by the ACR, Non-Nuclear Medicine Physician/Radiologist Interpreting Cardiovascular imaging applying for the initial qualification, there are two options: One, they must be either board certified by the American Board of Internal Medicine, American Osteopathic Board of Internal Medicine, Royal College of Physician and of Canada or Le College des Medicins du Quebec AND must have certification un nuclear cardiology by the CBNC OR Completion of at least a Level 2 Core Cardiology Training Symposium (COCATS) in nuclear cardiology, OR if trained prior to 1995, must be certified in Cardiology and have the equivalent of level 2 training. The second option established by ACR is at a minimum completion of an Accreditation Council of Graduate Medical Education (ACGME) approved general nuclear medicine program which must include 200 h n radiation physics and 500 h of preparation n instrumentation, radiochemistry, radiopharmacology, dosimetry, as well as radiation biology, safety and quality control. Moreover, they require 1,000 h of clinical training in general nuclear medicine, which must include technical performance, calculation of dosages, and evaluation of images, intermodality correlation and interpretation [13].

Likewise, certification specific to nuclear cardiology is available for technologists (www.nmtcb.org). The information for certification can be found in this web site. Generally, for continuing education, the NMTCB uses a biennial cycle, in which they require the applicants to document the hours for CE. For Nuclear Cardiology Technologists (NCT), the CNMT requires that the certification is renewed annually and the certificant must always maintain NMTCB certification and/or ARRT (N) and/or CAMRT nuclear medicine credentials either as "Active", "in compliance" or "in good standing". This certification is valid up to 7 years, after which recertification is required through an examination to maintain credentials.

As medicine continues to grow on knowledge and technology, the healthcare system must ensure to provide high quality of care. Overall, provider (physician or technologist) certification provides a structural measure of nuclear cardiology quality and offers the opportunity to excel in the delivery of care in particular, in the area of imaging providing resources and preparing the workforce to better serve patients.

References

1. Heller GV, Katanick SL, Sloper T, Garcia M. Accreditation for cardiovascular imaging: setting quality standards for patient care. J Am Coll Cardiol Img. 2008;1(3):390–7. PubMed.
2. American College of Cardiology. Imaging accreditation FAQ [Internet]. 2011 [cited 2014 Dec 10]. Available from: http://www.cardiosource.org/en/Advocacy/Issues/Imaging/Background-Resources/Imaging-Accreditation-FAQ.aspx.
3. The Joint Commission. Facts about ambulatory care accreditation. [Internet]. 2014 [cited 2014 December 12]. Available from: http://www.jointcommission.org/assets/1/18/Ambulatorycare_1_112.PDF.
4. American College of Radiology. Nuclear medicine accreditation program requirements [Internet]. 2014 [cited 2014 Dec 17]. Available from: http://www.acr.org/~/media/ACR/Documents/Accreditation/Nuclear%20Medicine%20PET/Requirements.pdf.
5. American College of Radiology. Overview for the diagnostic modality accreditation program 2014 [updated 21 Aug 2014]. Available from: http://www.acr.org/~/media/ACR/Documents/Accreditation/Apply/DiagnosticReqs.pdf.
6. Wackers FT. ICANL and ACR nuclear medicine accreditation: a comparison. J Nucl Med Off Publ Soc Nucl Med. 2000;41(5):26N–8. PubMed Epub 2000/06/08. eng.
7. Intersocietal Commission for the Accreditation of Nuclear Cardiology Laboratories (ICANL). Standards and guidelines for nuclear/PET accreditation. 2012.
8. Intersocietal Accreditation Commission. Accreditation Program Policies & Procedures 2012 [updated 07/25/20121]. 30]. Available from: http://www.intersocietal.org/iac/forms/IAC_Operations_P&P_2012.pdf.
9. Palmas W, Bingham S, Diamond GA, Denton TA, Kiat H, Friedman JD, et al. Incremental prognostic value of exercise thallium-201 myocardial single-photon emission computed tomography late after coronary artery bypass surgery. J Am Coll Cardiol. 1995;25(2):403–9.
10. Hendel RC, Patel MR, Allen JM, Min JK, Shaw LJ, Wolk MJ, et al. Appropriate use of cardiovascular technology: 2013 ACCF appropriate use criteria methodology update: a report of the American College of Cardiology Foundation appropriate use criteria task force. J Am Coll Cardiol. 2013;61(12):1305–17. PubMed.
11. Einstein AJ, Moser KW, Thompson RC, Cerqueira MD, Henzlova MJ. Radiation dose to patients from cardiac diagnostic imaging. Circulation. 2007;116(11):1290–305. PubMed.
12. Manning W, Farrell M, Bezold L, Choi J, Cockroft K, Gornik H, et al. How do non-invasive imaging facilities perceive the accreditation process? Results of an Intersocietal Accreditation Commission (IAC) survey. J Am Coll Cardiol. 2014;63(12_S).
13. Jerome S, Farrell M, Godiwala T, Heller G, Bezold L, Choi J, et al. Facility perception of nuclear cardiology accreditation: Results of an Intersocietal Accreditation Commission (IAC) survey. J Nucl Cardiol. 2014;22(3):496–503. English.

Part VI
ECHO

Chapter 25
Elements of the Echocardiographic Exam

Linda D. Gillam and Sofia Shames

Abstract Echocardiography encompasses resting and stress transthoracic cardiac ultrasound as well as transesophageal imaging, applications which collectively are essential for the evaluation and management of virtually every form of heart disease. Quality in echocardiography has many dimensions including patient selection, image acquisition, image interpretation, and results communication/reporting. Quality improvement tools and measures have been developed for each of these elements. This chapter provides an overview of echocardiographic methods and applications including different approaches to the use of cardiac ultrasound, advantages and disadvantages and contraindications to echocardiography.

Keywords Echocardiography • Quality • Clinical approaches • Advantages • Disadvantages • Clinical applications • Contraindications

The term echocardiography, otherwise known as cardiac ultrasound, encompasses a number of applications that use high frequency sound to provide anatomic and functional information about the heart and great vessels. While ultrasound is also used to evaluate the peripheral arterial and venous beds (vascular ultrasound), this section will focus exclusively on echocardiography which is generally broken down into imaging and Doppler components. Although a review of ultrasound physics is beyond the scope of this discussion, it should be noted that M mode, two-dimensional (2-D) and more recently three dimensional (3-D) imaging are all based on reflection of sound when it encounters interfaces between tissues of different acoustic impedances. Echocardiography takes advantage, in particular, of the interfaces between blood and cardiac tissue and, when ultrasound contrast agents are used, on

L.D. Gillam, MD, MPH (✉)
Department of Cardiovascular Medicine, Morristown Medical Center,
100 Madison Avenue, Morristown, NJ 07960, USA
e-mail: linda.gillam@atlantichealth.org

S. Shames, MD
Department of Cardiology, Columbia University Medical Center,
PH 3-342, 622 West 168th street, New York, NY 10032, USA
e-mail: ss3972@cumc.columbia.edu

P.L. Tilkemeier et al. (eds.), *Quality Evaluation in Non-Invasive Cardiovascular Imaging*, DOI 10.1007/978-3-319-28011-0_25

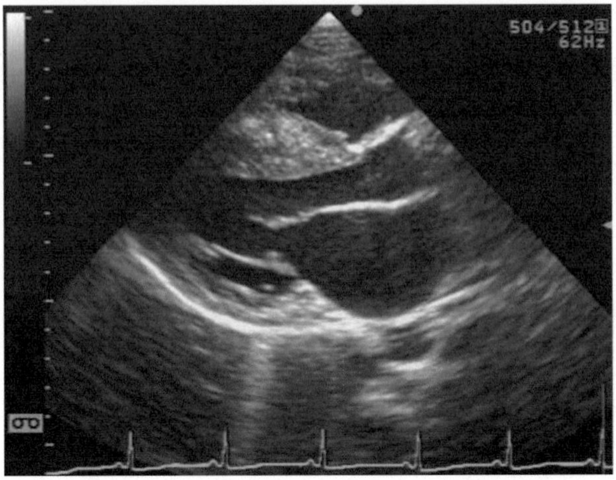

Fig. 25.1 Transthoracic echocardiographic image of a parasternal long axis view. This view shows the aortic and mitral valves as well as the left ventricle and left atrium

the interfaces between blood and the microbubble gaseous contents. An echocardiographic image is generated by plotting the location of specular reflectors relative to the sound source, the ultrasound transducer, based on the assumption that sound is travelling through biologic tissue with a constant speed (Fig. 25.1).

Doppler applications are based on the perceived differences in the frequency of emitted sound when there is a relative change in position of the sound emitter and receiver. In the case of echocardiography, red blood cells or tissue become sound emitters when they reflect sound that has been transmitted toward them from the ultrasound transducer. The transducer simultaneously serves as the sound receiver and, based on the comparison of the frequency it originally emitted and that returned, the echocardiographic system can calculate the velocity of the target of interest (blood cells or tissue). There are different forms of Doppler including continuous wave (CW) and pulsed wave (PW) which are displayed as velocity vs. time maps (Fig. 25.2) and color Doppler, a parametric display of pulsed Doppler information superimposed on M-mode, 3-D or most commonly 2-D imaging displays (Fig. 25.3). Pulsed wave applications are optimized to assess intracardiac/intravascular blood flow or myocardial movement (Doppler tissue imaging) whereas continuous wave is essential for accurate quantitation of high velocity targets and many hemodynamic applications. Recently, speckle tracking echocardiography (STE), has been developed as a method that tracks individual specular reflectors, thereby providing new tools for assessing myocardial function (strain, strain rate, rotation, torsion). Strain and strain rate may also be derived using Doppler tissue imaging (DTI).

Contrast echocardiography takes advantage of the intense ultrasound reflection that occurs at the interface between gas and other materials (blood and tissue). In its simplest application, multiple bubbles of varying sizes (typically up to 30 μm) can be created in intravenously injected solutions, typically saline, by agitating the

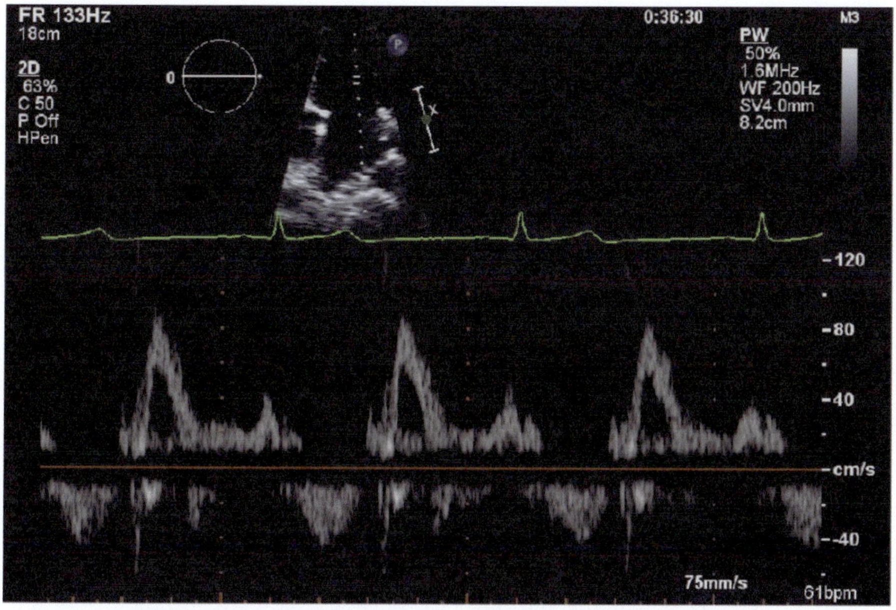

Fig. 25.2 Transthoracic echocardiographic image demonstrating spectral Doppler of mitral valve inflow; sample volume is positioned at the level of mitral valve tips in diastole

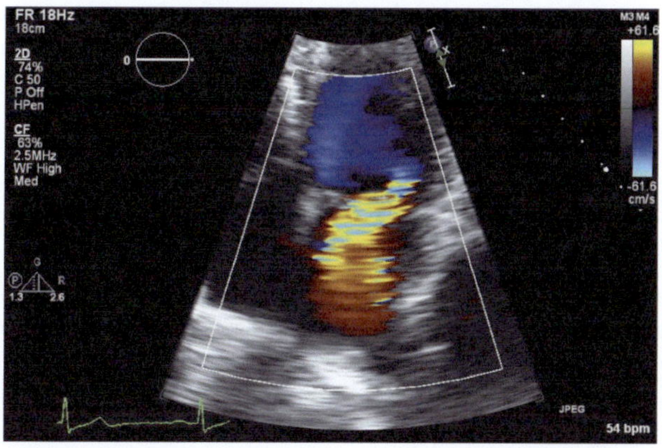

Fig. 25.3 Transthoracic echocardiographic image zoomed on left atrium in apical four chamber view with color flow Doppler demonstrating significant mitral regurgitation in systole

solution prior to injection. Because bubbles thus created vary in size and are usually too large to transit the pulmonary vascular bed and reach the left heart in the absence of an intracardiac or intrapulmonary shunt, their use is limited to the detection of right to left shunts, typically those that occur at the atrial level. Commercial contrast agents consist of uniform small (3–8 μm in diameter) bubbles with either albumin or phospholipid shells that enclose high molecular weight

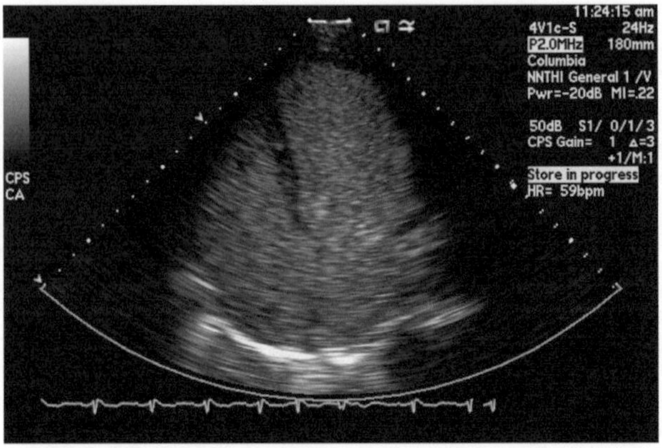

Fig. 25.4 Transthoracic echocardiographic image of the heart in apical four chamber view with injection of left ventricular echo contrast to enhance myocardial definition

gases that promote bubble stability. Because these microbubbles are no larger than red blood cells, they transit the lungs and can be imaged in the left heart blood pool thereby effectively enhancing the interface between the cardiac blood pool and endocardium (Fig. 25.4). These commercial agents are approved for endocardial border definition but also enhance Doppler signals. Additionally these contrast agents will change the echo appearance of perfused myocardium and there are multiple publications attesting to the feasibility of using this property to assess myocardial perfusion. However this ultrasound application, termed myocardial perfusion imaging, remains a research tool.

Echocardiographic Approaches

The most common applications of echocardiography involve positioning the ultrasound transducer, which emits and receives returning ultrasound signals, at various positions on the chest wall, upper abdomen and suprasternal regions. Such imaging, termed transthoracic echocardiography (TTE) (Fig. 25.1) is typically performed by non-physician sonographers. It has the obvious advantage of being non-invasive but is limited by the negative impact on image quality of air and bone and, to a variable degree, soft tissue that intervene between the body surface and the heart. Additionally, a core element of ultrasound physics is that spatial resolution, a key element of image quality, is directly related to ultrasound frequency while penetration, another key element of image quality, is inversely related to frequency. Thus, in an individual patient, the optimum imaging frequency is the highest one that achieves adequate penetration. TTE has no known risks.

Transesophageal echocardiography (TEE) is another common echocardiographic approach in which the imaging transducer/probe is incorporated into an

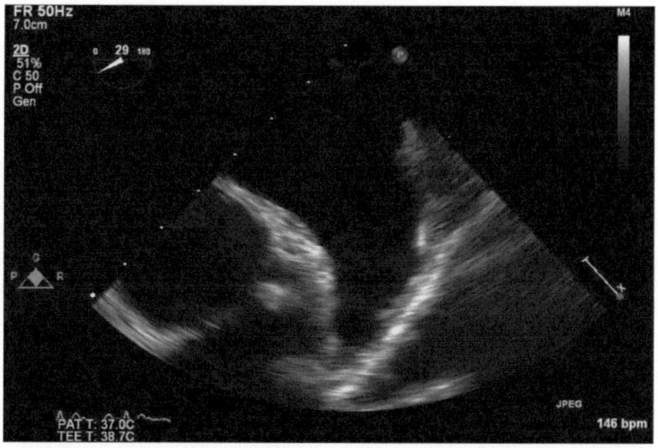

Fig. 25.5 Transesophageal echocardiographic image zoomed on left atrial appendage at 30° angle, midesophageal view

endoscope-like device that can be introduced into the oropharynx and passed along the esophagus into the stomach. This procedure is performed by physicians. From positions along this path, proximity to the heart and the avoidance of interference by intervening tissue permit the use of higher frequencies than can typically be used transthoracically. The result is images of superior quality but with the small risk of infrequent but potentially life threatening complications related to probe insertion and the need for sedation/anesthesia to overcome the gag reflex. TEE is also uniquely able to image the left atrial appendage, an important application in patients undergoing cardioversion for atrial fibrillation (Fig. 25.5).

Intracardiac echocardiography (ICE) relies on miniaturization of ultrasound elements to the point that they can be incorporated into vascular catheters and introduced into the heart by systemic venous access. ICE has 2-D and more recently 3-D capability as well as Doppler applications including color flow mapping. Even smaller catheters are available for use in the coronary arteries (intravascular ultrasound/IVUS) but these are limited to 2-D imaging alone. Because ICE and IVUS are performed by physicians in the cardiac catheterization or electrophysiology labs, these techniques will not be addressed further in this section, which will focus on quality in echocardiography as performed in hospital or office-based echocardiography labs.

A final distinction to be made is that between resting and stress echocardiography. While the vast majority of echocardiograms are performed with the patient at rest, typically in the left lateral decubitus position, stress echocardiography is increasingly commonly used to assess cardiac function during or immediately after stress. Stress may be in the form of exercise, typically treadmill or bicycle, or pharmacologic with the most common agents used being dobutamine which provides inotropic and chronotropic stress or the vasodilators of which the most commonly used is the drug dipyridamole. Vasodilator stress is limited to the identification of ischemia-induced myocardial dysfunction (Fig. 25.6) or, when combined with

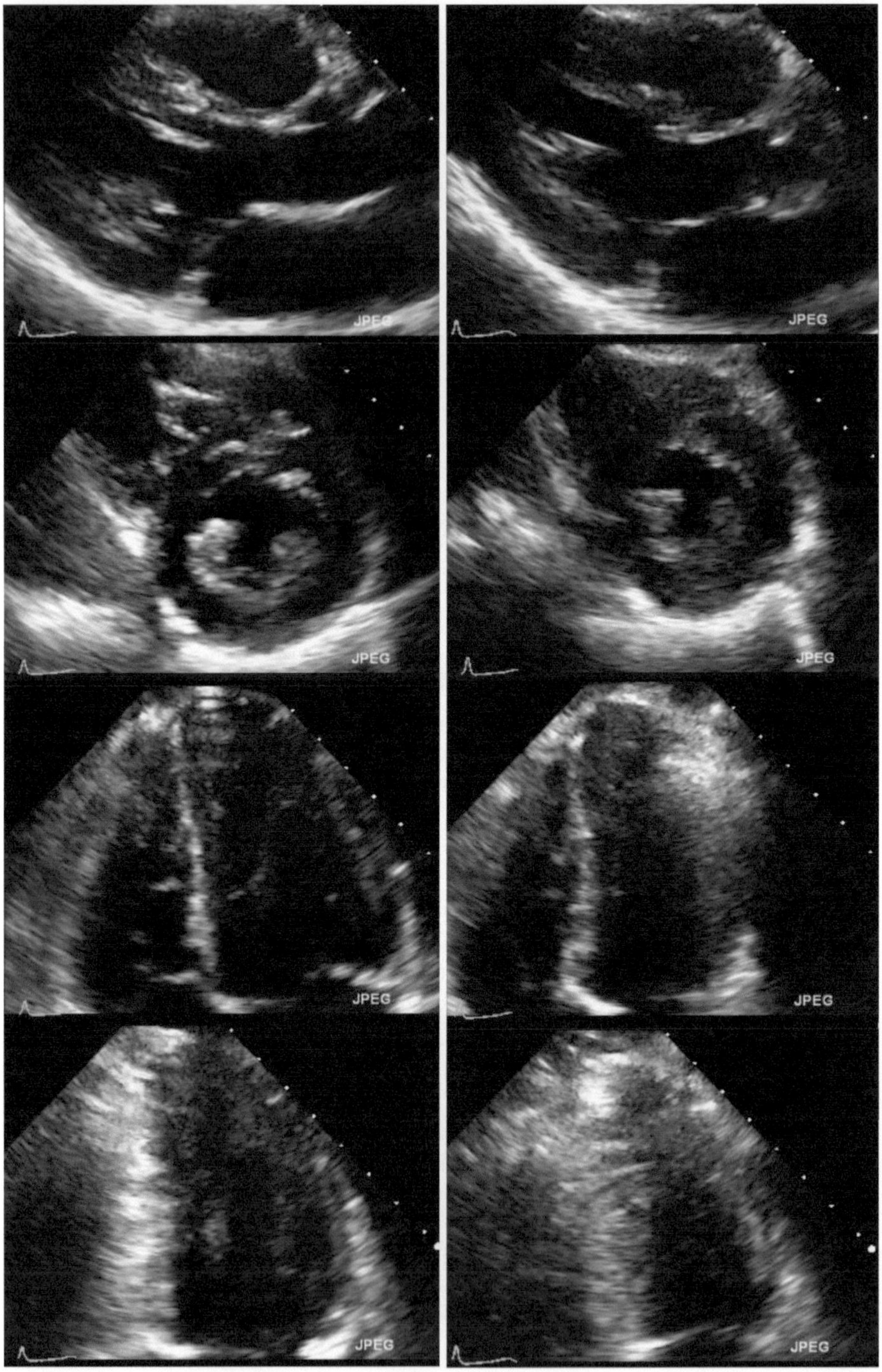

Fig. 25.6 Transthoracic stress echocardiogram displaying baseline images on the left and post exercise images on the right in four standard views

myocardial contrast echocardiography, myocardial perfusions abnormalities, this being considered experimental at present. However exercise and dobutamine stress can also be used to assess for contractile reserve in the context of ischemic or non-ischemic myocardial dysfunction as well as to evaluate the hemodynamic responses to stress in valvular heart disease. The echocardiographic images acquired during stress echocardiography are typically acquired by sonographers with acquisition of the EKG component provided by a stress technologist all under the direct or indirect supervision of a physician.

Advantages of Echocardiography

Echocardiography's widespread use, with applications detailed below, is not surprising given its many strengths:

1. Echocardiography provides images with high spatial and temporal resolution. For TTE and TEE, spatial resolution is approx. 1 mm with optimized temporal resolution >60 frames per second making it ideally suited to assessing the constantly moving heart and capturing rapidly occurring events such as valve motion. While lower, the temporal and spatial resolution of 3-D echo continue to improve.
2. The basic information echocardiography provides is available in real time at the site of image acquisition with more complex measurements (particularly 3D) potentially requiring off-line analysis. It is notable that there is no other imaging modality with the exception of invasive angiography with this real-time capability.
3. Echocardiographic systems are portable with even the most sophisticated systems being movable and routinely taken to the bedside. While newer pocket-sized miniaturized systems with limited functionality may be helpful adjuncts to clinical assessment, studies obtained on such systems are not typically archived or formally reported. Thus they are not included in subsequent sections of this chapter.
4. All echocardiographic techniques employ no ionizing radiation and thus can be repeated without concerns for cumulative radiation exposure.

Disadvantages of Echocardiography

The major disadvantage of echocardiography is that it is operator and patient dependent. The quality of the sonographer, or, in the case of TEE, physician obtaining the studies has enormous impact on image quality, arguably more so than with any other imaging modality. For certain patients, even the best operators may be unable to obtain adequate images with certain patient characteristics such as obesity, hyper-inflated lungs or thoracic skeletal abnormalities challenging even the best operators. For many of these patients, however, commercial contrast agents may be helpful to improve image quality.

Applications of Echocardiography

It would not be an overstatement to say that echocardiography has important applications related to every form of heart disease with its most important limitation being its inability to directly image the coronary arteries. As captured in the ACC/AHA [1] Guidelines for the Clinical Application of Echocardiography, and in subsequent disease focused guidelines published by the American College of Cardiology in partnership with the American Heart Association as well as the European Society of Cardiology, including but not limited to those for Valvular Heart Disease [2, 3], Heart Failure [4], Stable Ischemic Heart Disease [5], and atrial fibrillation [6] echocardiography is an essential tool in the management of acquired diseases of the pericardium, myocardium, valves, coronary arteries, great vessels, and electrical system as well as the full spectrum of congenital heart disease. Its broad application is derived from its ability to provide information about both structure and function including but not limited to ventricular systolic and diastolic function, valvular function (etiology and severity of stenosis and regurgitation) and hemodynamics such as atrial, pulmonary arterial and left ventricular filling pressures.

The following paragraphs provide a snapshot of clinical applications:

- In patients with valvular heart disease, resting TTE, complemented by 2D/3D TEE, is critical for diagnosis and management with stress echocardiography used in some patients to better elucidate symptoms, assess the patient's functional capacity and identify secondary hemodynamic changes such as pulmonary hypertension. It is a critical tool in diagnosing and managing endocarditis and is equally helpful with native and prosthetic valves.
- In patients with known or suspected coronary disease, resting echocardiography can demonstrate left and right ventricular dysfunction that has been caused by ischemia/infarction. This is characteristically regional in a distribution that corresponds to the perfusion bed of the coronary arteries. Echocardiography can also identify mechanical complications of myocardial infarction such as ventricular septal defects, free wall or papillary muscle rupture. Stress echocardiography identifies inducible ischemia by provoking regional wall motion abnormalities and because left ventricular dysfunction is an earlier sign of ischemia than EKG changes or symptoms (chest pain), stress echocardiography has better sensitivity and specificity for epicardial coronary disease than EKG only stress testing particularly if pharmacologic rather than exercise stress has been used. Myocardial contrast perfusion echocardiography offers an approach to assess myocardial perfusion directly with, therefore, reportedly increased sensitivity over conventional stress echocardiography.
- The cardiac myocardium suffers from both primary and secondary abnormalities. Echocardiography is a mainstay in the diagnosis and management of those with primary abnormalities (cardiomyopathies), characterizing the resultant functional and hemodynamic disturbances and frequently pinpointing the diagnosis e.g. the varying phenotypes of hypertrophic cardiomyopathy.

- Pericardial disease is another example of echocardiography's utility. Echocardiography is the principle technique with which pericardial effusion is diagnosed and provides a tool for identifying associated hemodynamic compromise (tamponade physiology). The diagnosis of pericardial constriction is also one in which echocardiography is very helpful.
- In the setting of rhythm disorders, echocardiography may also identify a structural and/or functional root cause and my help screen patients for intervention e.g. excluding intra-atrial thrombus in patients undergoing cardioversion.
- Finally in patients with heart failure, echocardiography distinguishes those with preserved vs. reduced ejection fraction, identifies concomitant secondary valve dysfunction (functional mitral and/or tricuspid regurgitation) and evidence of abnormal filling patterns/pressures that are diagnostically and prognostically important.

A more detailed review of the applications for echocardiography is beyond the scope of this chapter but a rough measure of its role may be the number of indications for echocardiography in ACC/AHA Guidelines. In the 2003 Guidelines for the Clinical Application of Echocardiography [1] there were 192 Class I indications (defined as conditions for which there is evidence and/or general agreement that a given procedure or treatment is useful) and effective and 46 Class IIa indications (defined as conditions for which there is conflicting evidence and/or a divergence of opinion about the usefulness/efficacy but for which the weight of evidence/opinion is in favor of usefulness/efficacy). A review of the substantial literature that supports these recommendations is beyond the scope of this document.

Contraindications

The risk profile for ultrasonic imaging is favorable with their being no identified risk of exposure to ultrasound. Indeed, since echocardiography involves no radiation exposure, transthoracic echocardiography is generally considered to be a risk free procedure.

Stress echocardiography carries the small risks associated with exercise or pharmacologic stress. Transesophageal echocardiography carries a small (<1/2,000) risk of esophageal perforation as well as complications of the associated sedation which can be mitigated with appropriate patient selection (e.g. avoiding its use in patients with known or suspected esophageal pathology) and careful patient monitoring using standard anesthesia protocols. TEE is contra-indicated in those with obstructive esophageal pathology, known esophageal perforation and in those whose have unstable cervical spines.

Contrast echocardiography carries the small risks of adverse reactions to the agents and even smaller risks associated with gaining intravenous access. Given the absence of safety data is pregnant women and the theoretic concern that an intracardiac shunt might allow a "rogue" microbubble larger than the manufactured specified size of approximately 3–8 μm to reach the left heart, contrast agents have always carried these exclusions. However in 2007, based on reports of 11 deaths and 199 adverse events temporally related to echo contrast administration, the FDA issued a class rather than agent specific black box warning that precluded the use of contrast agents in patients with unstable cardiac conditions or pulmonary hypertension and required post-injection monitoring for 30 min. In 2008, these restrictions were relaxed with monitoring required for only high risk patients and removal of most of the 2007 clinical contra-indications with the manufacturers to perform post-market surveillance. Following a series of studies attesting to the safety of contrast agents in even critically ill patients, the warnings were further relaxed in 2011/2012 with the elimination altogether of the requirement for post-injection monitoring, elimination of statements that the safety of contrast agents with exercise or pharmacologic stress has not been established and addition of much less ominous statements to the effect that serious cardiopulmonary reactions, including fatalities, have occurred 'uncommonly' during or following echocardiographic contrast agent administration.

References

1. Cheitlin MD, Armstrong WF, Aurigemma GP, Beller GA, Bierman FZ, Davis JL, et al. ACC/AHA/ASE 2003 guideline update for the clinical application of echocardiography: summary article: a report of the American College of Cardiology/American Heart Association Task Force on Practice Guidelines (ACC/AHA/ASE Committee to Update the 1997 Guidelines for the Clinical Application of Echocardiography). Circulation. 2003;108(9):1146–62.
2. Nishimura RA, Otto CM, Bonow RO, Carabello BA, Erwin JP, Guyton RA, et al. AHA/ACC guideline for the management of patients with valvular heart disease: a report of the American College of Cardiology/American Heart Association Task Force on Practice Guidelines. J Am Coll Cardiol. 2014;63:e57–185. 2014 Mar 7.
3. Vahanian A, Alfieri O, Andreotti F, Antunes MJ, Bar+¦n-Esquivias G, Baumgartner H, et al. Guidelines on the management of valvular heart disease (version 2012): the Joint Task Force on the Management of Valvular Heart Disease of the European Society of Cardiology (ESC) and the European Association for Cardio-Thoracic Surgery (EACTS). Eur Heart J. 2012;33(19):2451–96.
4. Paulus WJ, Tsch+¦pe C, Sanderson JE, Rusconi C, Flachskampf FA, Rademakers FE, et al. How to diagnose diastolic heart failure: a consensus statement on the diagnosis of heart failure with normal left ventricular ejection fraction by the Heart Failure and Echocardiography Associations of the European Society of Cardiology. Eur Heart J. 2007;28(20):2539–50.
5. Fihn SD, Gardin JM, Abrams J, Berra K, Blankenship JC, Dallas AP, et al. 2012 ACCF/AHA/ACP/AATS/PCNA/SCAI/STS guideline for the diagnosis and management of patients with stable ischemic heart disease a report of the American College of Cardiology Foundation/American Heart Association Task Force on Practice Guidelines, and the American College of Physicians, American Association for Thoracic Surgery, Preventive Cardiovascular Nurses Association, Society for Cardiovascular Angiography and Interventions, and Society of Thoracic Surgeons. J Am Coll Cardiol. 2012;60(24):e44–164.
6. January CT, Wann LS, Alpert JS, Calkins H, Cigarroa JE, Cleveland JC, et al. 2014 AHA/ACC/HRS guideline for the-management of patients with atrial fibrillation: executive summary a report of the American College of Cardiology/American Heart Association Task Force on Practice Guidelines and the Heart Rhythm Society. J Am Coll Cardiol. 2014;64(21):2246–80.

Chapter 26
Patient Selection

Linda D. Gillam and Sofia Shames

Abstract Appropriate selection of patients for an echocardiographic study is an important aspect of quality for echocardiography laboratories. Criteria to assist in selecting the right test for the right patients have been developed using the Appropriate Use Criteria methodology employed by the American College of Cardiology. The application of these criteria plays an important role in assuring high quality in patient selection. A number of studies will be reviewed that analyze the application of the appropriate use criteria in different clinical settings.

Keywords Echocardiography • Quality • Intersocietal commission • Appropriate use criteria

Appropriate Use of Echocardiography

Since echocardiography is a test that has broad-ranging indications, carries no or minimal risk and is used in a reimbursement and tort environment that favors testing, it is not surprising that over-utilization has been more of a problem than underutilization. Recognizing the need for prudent use of imaging, the American College of Cardiology, in partnership with subspecialty societies including the American Society of Echocardiography has developed Appropriate Use Criteria (AUC) with an overarching goal of providing the appropriate test for the appropriate patient at the appropriate time. The process addresses commonly occurring scenarios for which echocardiography is categorized as being generally appropriate, may be appropriate or rarely appropriate. Note that this current terminology replaces the original terminology where imaging was categorized as being appropriate, uncertain or inappropriate.

L.D. Gillam, MD, MPH (✉)
Department of Cardiovascular Medicine, Morristown Medical Center, Morristown, NJ, USA
e-mail: linda.gillam@atlantichealth.org

S. Shames, MD
Department of Cardiology, Columbia University Medical Center, New York, NY, USA
e-mail: ss3972@cumc.columbia.edu

P.L. Tilkemeier et al. (eds.), *Quality Evaluation in Non-Invasive Cardiovascular Imaging*, DOI 10.1007/978-3-319-28011-0_26

Tables 26.1, 26.2, and 26.3 include the 2011 AUC criteria for resting transthoracic and transesophageal echocardiography as well as stress echocardiography and the use of contrast echocardiography for left ventricular opacification [1]. This document was published when the original terminology was in place with the tables broken down by indications that are appropriate, uncertain or inappropriate. The use of stress testing for known or suspected cardiac ischemia is also included in a multimodality document that uses the newer terminology and where the use of nuclear cardiology, cardiac magnetic resonance and cardiac CT are addressed along with echocardiography [2]. As such, the appropriate use criteria complement the disease specific guidelines previously referenced.

There have been several studies of the AUC for echocardiography, addressing the degree to which the scenarios addressed by the AUC cover the common indications for echocardiography, the appropriate use of echocardiography in a variety of settings and the degree to which interventions can influence the appropriateness of echocardiographic testing. In a study of the appropriateness of echo ordering in a northeastern regional hospital, Bailey et al. reported that appropriate and inappropriate indications were 97 % and 2 %, respectively using the 2011 guidelines with only 1 % determined to have uncertain indications or a scenario not addressed by the guidelines [3]. Bhatia et al. reported the impact of an intervention consisting of a lecture, pocket reminder card and email feedback on the appropriateness of test ordering by house staff in a major academic medical center. They confirmed that the 2011 AUC address the vast majority of scenarios for test ordering (98 and 99 % in baseline and post-intervention time periods respectively). They also noted that the intervention was associated with a 26 % reduction in the total number of TTEs ordered per day as well as a significantly higher proportion of appropriate TTEs (93 % vs. 84 %) [4]. Addressing a family of indications for which there was a perception of overuse of repeat testing, the serial evaluation of patients with moderate or greater valvular stenosis or regurgitation, Chan et al. reported that only 59 % underwent follow-up echocardiography within the recommended period, rates that were higher when patients were followed by cardiologists or cardiovascular surgeons and, interestingly, when the patients were younger and male [5]. Thus this study identified an area of inappropriate undertesting, rather than anticipated overtesting.

Addressing the appropriateness of pharmacologic stress echocardiography in a single Italian center, Cortigiani et al. noted that only 63 % of the tests performed were considered appropriate by guidelines, 9 % uncertain, and 27 % inappropriate. The tests were much less likely to be abnormal in the inappropriate group providing indirect support for the validity of the appropriateness classification [6]. Similarly high rates of inappropriate use of stress echocardiography were observed in a report from the University of Miami Health System with nearly one-third of stress echocardiograms requested for inappropriate indications. Referrals of inappropriate stress echocardiograms did not decrease over time or with an educational intervention [7].

Table 26.1 Appropriate indications (median score 7–9)

Indication		Appropriate use score (1–9)
TTE for general evaluation of cardiac structure and function suspected cardiac etiology—general		
1.	Symptoms or conditions potentially related to suspected cardiac etiology including but not limited to chest pain, shortness of breath, palpitations, TIA, stroke, or peripheral embolic event	A (9)
2.	Prior testing that is concerning for heart disease or structural abnormality including but not limited to chest X-ray, baseline scout images for stress echocardiogram, ECG, or cardiac biomarkers	A (9)
TTE for general evaluation of cardiac structure and function arrhythmias		
4.	Frequent VPCs or exercise-induced VPCs	A (8)
5.	Sustained or nonsustained atrial fibrillation, SVT, or VT	A (9)
TTE for general evaluation of cardiac structure and function lightheadedness/presyncope/syncope		
7.	Clinical symptoms or signs consistent with a cardiac diagnosis known to cause lightheadedness/presyncope/syncope (including but not limited to aortic stenosis, hypertrophic cardiomyopathy, or HF)	A (9)
9.	Syncope when there are no other symptoms or signs of cardiovascular disease	A (7)
TTE for general evaluation of cardiac structure and function pulmonary hypertension		
15.	Evaluation of suspected pulmonary hypertension including evaluation of right ventricular function and estimated pulmonary artery pressure	A (9)
17.	Routine surveillance (≥1 year) of known pulmonary hypertension without change in clinical status or cardiac exam	A (7)
18.	Re-evaluation of known pulmonary hypertension if change in clinical status or cardiac exam or to guide therapy	A (9)
TTE for cardiovascular evaluation in an acute setting hypotension or hemodynamic instability		
19.	Hypotension or hemodynamic instability of uncertain or suspected cardiac etiology	A (9)
TTE for cardiovascular evaluation in an acute setting myocardial ischemia/infarction		
21.	Acute chest pain with suspected MI and nondiagnostic ECG when a resting echocardiogram can be performed during pain	A (9)
22.	Evaluation of a patient without chest pain but with other features of an ischemic equivalent or laboratory markers indicative of ongoing MI	A (8)
23.	Suspected complication of myocardial ischemia/infarction, including but not limited to acute mitral regurgitation, ventricular septal defect, free-wall rupture/tamponade, shock, right ventricular involvement, HF, or thrombus	A (9)
TTE for cardiovascular evaluation in an acute setting evaluation of ventricular function after ACS		
24.	Initial evaluation of ventricular function following ACS	A (9)
25.	Re-evaluation of ventricular function following ACS during recovery phase when results will guide therapy	A (9)

(continued)

Table 26.1 (continued)

Indication		Appropriate use score (1–9)
TTE for cardiovascular evaluation in an acute setting respiratory failure		
26.	Respiratory failure or hypoxemia of uncertain etiology	A (8)
TTE for cardiovascular evaluation in an acute setting pulmonary embolism		
29.	Known acute pulmonary embolism to guide therapy (e.g., thrombectomy and thrombolytics)	A (8)
31.	Re-evaluation of known pulmonary embolism after thrombolysis or thrombectomy for assessment of change in right ventricular function and/or pulmonary artery pressure	A (7)
TTE for cardiovascular evaluation in an acute setting cardiac trauma		
32.	Severe deceleration injury or chest trauma when valve injury, pericardial effusion, or cardiac injury are possible or suspected	A (9)
TTE for evaluation of valvular function murmur or click		
34.	Initial evaluation when there is a reasonable suspicion of valvular or structural heart disease	A (9)
37.	Re-evaluation of known valvular heart disease with a change in clinical status or cardiac exam or to guide therapy	A (9)
TTE for evaluation of valvular function native valvular stenosis		
39.	Routine surveillance (≥3 year) of mild valvular stenosis without a change in clinical status or cardiac exam	A (7)
41.	Routine surveillance (≥1 year) of moderate or severe valvular stenosis without a change in clinical status or cardiac exam	A (8)
46.	Routine surveillance (≥1 year) of moderate or severe valvular regurgitation without change in clinical status or cardiac exam	A (8)
TTE for evaluation of valvular function prosthetic valves		
47.	Initial postoperative evaluation of prosthetic valve for establishment of baseline	A (9)
49.	Routine surveillance (≥3 year after valve implantation) of prosthetic valve if no known or suspected valve dysfunction	A (7)
50.	Evaluation of prosthetic valve with suspected dysfunction or a change in clinical status or cardiac exam	A (9)
51.	Re-evaluation of known prosthetic valve dysfunction when it would change management or guide therapy	A (9)
TTE for evaluation of valvular function infective endocarditis (native or prosthetic valves)		
52.	Initial evaluation of suspected infective endocarditis with positive blood cultures or a new murmur	A (9)
55.	Re-evaluation of infective endocarditis at high risk for progression or complication or with a change in clinical status or cardiac exam	A (9)
TTE for evaluation of intracardiac and extracardiac structures and chambers		
57.	Suspected cardiac mass	A (9)
58.	Suspected cardiovascular source of embolus	A (9)
59.	Suspected pericardial conditions	A (9)
61.	Re-evaluation of known pericardial effusion to guide management or therapy	A (8)

Table 26.1 (continued)

Indication		Appropriate use score (1–9)
62.	Guidance of percutaneous noncoronary cardiac procedures including but not limited to pericardiocentesis, septal ablation, or right ventricular biopsy	A (9)
TTE for evaluation of aortic disease		
63.	Evaluation of the ascending aorta in the setting of a known or suspected connective tissue disease or genetic condition that predisposes to aortic aneurysm or dissection (e.g., Marfan syndrome)	A (9)
64.	Re-evaluation of known ascending aortic dilation or history of aortic dissection to establish a baseline rate of expansion or when the rate of expansion is excessive	A (9)
65.	Re-evaluation of known ascending aortic dilation or history of aortic dissection with a change in clinical status or cardiac exam or when findings may alter management or therapy	A (9)
TTE for evaluation of hypertension, HF, or cardiomyopathy hypertension		
67.	Initial evaluation of suspected hypertensive heart disease	A (8)
TTE for evaluation of hypertension, HF, or cardiomyopathy HF		
70.	Initial evaluation of known or suspected HF (systolic or diastolic) based on symptoms, signs, or abnormal test results	A (9)
71.	Re-evaluation of known HF (systolic or diastolic) with a change in clinical status or cardiac exam without a clear precipitating change in medication or diet	A (8)
73.	Re-evaluation of known HF (systolic or diastolic) to guide therapy	A (9)
TTE for evaluation of hypertension, HF, or cardiomyopathy device evaluation (including pacemaker, ICD, or CRT)		
76.	Initial evaluation or re-evaluation after revascularization and/or optimal medical therapy to determine candidacy for device therapy and/or to determine optimal choice of device	A (9)
78.	Known implanted pacing device with symptoms possibly due to device complication or suboptimal pacing device settings	A (8)
TTE for evaluation of hypertension, HF, or cardiomyopathy ventricular assist devices and cardiac transplantation		
81.	To determine candidacy for ventricular assist device	A (9)
82.	Optimization of ventricular assist device settings	A (7)
83.	Re-evaluation for signs/symptoms suggestive of ventricular assist device-related complications	A (9)
84.	Monitoring for rejection in a cardiac transplant recipient	A (7)
85.	Cardiac structure and function evaluation in a potential heart donor	A (9)
TTE for evaluation of hypertension, HF, or cardiomyopathy cardiomyopathies		
86.	Initial evaluation of known or suspected cardiomyopathy (e.g., restrictive, infiltrative, dilated, hypertrophic, or genetic cardiomyopathy)	A (9)
87.	Re-evaluation of known cardiomyopathy with a change in clinical status or cardiac exam or to guide therapy	A (9)

(continued)

Table 26.1 (continued)

Indication		Appropriate use score (1–9)
90.	Screening evaluation for structure and function in first-degree relatives of a patient with an inherited cardiomyopathy	A (9)
91.	Baseline and serial re-evaluations in a patient undergoing therapy with cardiotoxic agents	A (9)
TTE for adult congenital heart disease		
92.	Initial evaluation of known or suspected adult congenital heart disease	A (9)
93.	Known adult congenital heart disease with a change in clinical status or cardiac exam	A (9)
94.	Re-evaluation to guide therapy in known adult congenital heart disease	A (9)
98.	Routine surveillance (≥1 year) of adult congenital heart disease following incomplete or palliative repair	A (8)
	With residual structural or hemodynamic abnormality	
	Without a change in clinical status or cardiac exam	
TEE as initial or supplemental test—general uses		
99.	Use of TEE when there is a high likelihood of a nondiagnostic TTE due to patient characteristics or inadequate visualization of relevant structures	A (8)
101.	Re-evaluation of prior TEE finding for interval change (e.g., resolution of thrombus after anticoagulation, resolution of vegetation after antibiotic therapy) when a change in therapy is anticipated	A (8)
103.	Guidance during percutaneous noncoronary cardiac interventions including but not limited to closure device placement, radiofrequency ablation, and percutaneous valve procedures	A (9)
104.	Suspected acute aortic pathology including but not limited to dissection/transsection	A (9)
TEE as initial or supplemental test—valvular disease		
106.	Evaluation of valvular structure and function to assess suitability for, and assist in planning of, an intervention	A (9)
108.	To diagnose infective endocarditis with a moderate or high pretest probability (e.g., staph bacteremia, fungemia, prosthetic heart valve, or intracardiac device)	A (9)
TEE as initial or supplemental test—embolic event		
109.	Evaluation for cardiovascular source of embolus with no identified noncardiac source	A (7)
TEE as initial Test—atrial fibrillation/flutter		
112.	Evaluation to facilitate clinical decision making with regards to anticoagulation, cardioversion, and/or radiofrequency ablation	A (9)
Stress echocardiography for detection of CAD/risk assessment: symptomatic or ischemic equivalent evaluation of ischemic equivalent (nonacute)		
115.	Low pretest probability of CAD	A (7)
	ECG uninterpretable or unable to exercise	

Table 26.1 (continued)

Indication		Appropriate use score (1–9)
116.	Intermediate pretest probability of CAD	A (7)
	ECG Interpretable and able to exercise	
117.	Intermediate pretest probability of CAD	A (9)
	ECG uninterpretable or unable to exercise	
118.	High pretest probability of CAD	A (7)
	Regardless of ECG interpretability and ability to exercise	
Stress echocardiography for detection of CAD/risk assessment: symptomatic or ischemic equivalent acute chest pain		
119.	Possible ACS	A (7)
	ECG: no ischemic changes or with LBBB or electronically paced ventricular rhythm	
	Low-risk TIMI score	
	Negative troponin levels	
120.	Possible ACS	A (7)
	ECG: no ischemic changes or with LBBB or electronically paced ventricular rhythm	
	Low-risk TIMI score	
	Peak troponin: borderline, equivocal, minimally elevated	
121.	Possible ACS	A (7)
	ECG: no ischemic changes or with LBBB or electronically paced ventricular rhythm	
	High-risk TIMI score	
	Negative troponin levels	
122.	Possible ACS	A (7)
	ECG: no ischemic changes or with LBBB or electronically paced ventricular rhythm	
	High-risk TIMI score	
	Peak troponin: borderline, equivocal, minimally elevated	
Stress echocardiography for detection of CAD/risk assessment: asymptomatic (without ischemic equivalent) in patient populations with defined comorbidities new-onset or newly diagnosed HF or LV systolic dysfunction		
128.	No prior CAD evaluation and no planned coronary angiography	(7)
Stress echocardiography for detection of CAD/risk assessment: asymptomatic (without ischemic equivalent) in patient populations with defined comorbidities arrhythmias		
129.	Sustained VT	A (7)
130.	Frequent PVCs, exercise-induced VT, or nonsustained VT	A (7)
Stress echocardiography for detection of CAD/risk assessment: asymptomatic (without ischemic equivalent) in patient populations with defined comorbidities syncope		
134.	Intermediate or high global CAD risk	A (7)
Stress echocardiography for detection of CAD/risk assessment: asymptomatic (without ischemic equivalent) in patient populations with defined comorbidities elevated troponin		
135.	Troponin elevation without symptoms or additional evidence of ACS	A (7)

(continued)

Table 26.1 (continued)

Indication		Appropriate use score (1–9)
Stress echocardiography following prior test results asymptomatic: prior evidence of subclinical disease		
139.	Coronary calcium Agatston score >400	A (7)
Stress echocardiography following prior test results coronary angiography (invasive or noninvasive)		
141.	Coronary artery stenosis of unclear significance	A (8)
Stress echocardiography following prior test results treadmill ECG stress test		
149.	Intermediate-risk treadmill score (e.g., Duke)	A (7)
150.	High-risk treadmill score (e.g., Duke)	A (7)
Stress echocardiography following prior test results new or worsening symptoms		
151.	Abnormal coronary angiography or abnormal prior stress imaging study	A (7)
Stress echocardiography following prior test results prior noninvasive evaluation		
153.	Equivocal, borderline, or discordant stress testing where obstructive CAD remains a concern	A (8)
Stress echocardiography for risk assessment: perioperative evaluation for noncardiac surgery without active cardiac conditions vascular surgery		
161.	≥1 clinical risk factor	A (7)
	Poor or unknown functional capacity (<4 METs)	
Stress echocardiography for risk assessment: within 3 months of an ACS STEMI		
164.	Hemodynamically stable, no recurrent chest pain symptoms, or no signs of HF	A (7)
	To evaluate for inducible ischemia	
	No prior coronary angiography since the index event	
Stress echocardiography for risk assessment: within 3 months of an ACS UA/NSTEMI		
166.	Hemodynamically stable, no recurrent chest pain symptoms, or no signs of HF	A (8)
	To evaluate for inducible ischemia	
	No prior coronary angiography since the index event	
Stress echocardiography for risk assessment: postrevascularization (PCI or CABG) symptomatic		
169.	Ischemic equivalent	A (8)
Stress echocardiography for risk assessment: postrevascularization (PCI or CABG) asymptomatic		
170.	Incomplete revascularization	A (7)
	Additional revascularization feasible	
Stress echocardiography for assessment of viability/ischemia ischemic cardiomyopathy/ assessment of viability		
176.	Known moderate or severe LV dysfunction	A (8)
	Patient eligible for revascularization	
	Use of dobutamine stress only	

Table 26.1 (continued)

Indication		Appropriate use score (1–9)
Stress echocardiography for hemodynamics (includes doppler during stress) chronic valvular disease—asymptomatic		
179.	Severe mitral stenosis	A (7)
185.	Severe mitral regurgitation	A (7)
	LV size and function not meeting surgical criteria	
188.	Severe aortic regurgitation	A (7)
	LV size and function not meeting surgical criteria	
Stress echocardiography for hemodynamics (includes doppler during stress) chronic valvular disease—symptomatic		
190.	Moderate mitral stenosis	A (7)
193.	Evaluation of equivocal aortic stenosis	A (8)
	Evidence of low cardiac output or LV systolic dysfunction ("low gradient aortic stenosis")	
	Use of dobutamine only	
195.	Moderate mitral regurgitation	A (7)
Contrast use in TTE/TEE or stress echocardiography		
202.	Selective use of contrast	A (8)
	≥2 contiguous LV segments are not seen on noncontrast Images	

Reprinted from Reference [1] with permission from Elsevier.
A indicates appropriate

Table 26.2 Uncertain indications (median score 4–6)

Indication		Appropriate use score (1–9)
TTE for general evaluation of cardiac structure and function perioperative evaluation		
14.	Routine perioperative evaluation of cardiac structure and function prior to noncardiac solid organ transplantation	U (6)
TTE for cardiovascular evaluation in an acute setting hypotension or hemodynamic instability		
20.	Assessment of volume status in a critically ill patient	U (5)
TTE for cardiovascular evaluation in an acute setting respiratory failure		
27.	Respiratory failure or hypoxemia when a noncardiac etiology of respiratory failure has been established	U (5)
TTE for evaluation of valvular function native valvular regurgitation		
44.	Routine survelliance (≥3 year) of mild valvular regurgitation without a change in clinical status or cardiac exam	U (4)
45.	Routine survelliance (<1 year) of moderate or severe valvular regurgitation without a change in clinical status or cardiac exam	U (6)
TTE for evaluation of hypertension, HF, or cardiomyopathy hypertension		
69.	Re-evaluation of known hypertensive heart disease without a change in clinical status or cardiac exam	U (4)

Table 26.2 (continued)

Indication		Appropriate use score (1–9)
TTE for evaluation of hypertension, HF, or cardiomyopathy HF		
72.	Re-evaluation of known HF (systolic or diastolic) with a change in clinical status or cardiac exam with a clear precipitating change in medication or diet	U (4)
75.	Routine survelliance (≥1 year) of HF (systolic or diastolic) when there is no change in clinical status or cardiac exam	U (6)
TTE for evaluation of hypertension, HF, or cardiomyopathy device evaluation (including pacemaker, ICD, or CRT)		
77.	Initial evaluation for CRT device optimization after implantation	U (6)
TTE for evaluation of hypertension, HF, or cardiomyopathy cardiomyopathies		
89.	Routine surveillance (≥1 year) of known cardiomyopathy without a change in clinical status or cardiac exam	U (5)
TTE for adult congenital heart disease		
96.	Routine surveillance (≥2 year) of adult congenital heart disease following complete repair	U (6)
	Without residual structural or hemodynamic abnormality	
	Without a change in clinical status or cardiac exam	
97.	Routine surveillance (<1 year) of adult congenital heart disease following incomplete or palliative repair	U (5)
	With residual structural or hemodynamic abnormality	
	Without a change in clinical status or cardiac exam	
TEE as initial or supplemental test—embolic event		
110.	Evaluation for cardiovascular source of embolus with a previously identified noncardiac source	U (5)
Stress echocardiography for detection of CAD/risk assessment: asymptomatic (without ischemic equivalent) general patient populations		
126.	Intermediate global CAD risk	U (5)
	ECG uninterpretable	
127.	High global CAD risk	U (5)
Stress echocardiography for detection of CAD/risk assessment: asymptomatic (without ischemic equivalent) in patient populations with defined comorbidities arrhythmias		
132.	New-onset atrial fibrillation	U (6)
Stress echocardiography following prior test results asymptomatic: prior evidence of subclinical disease		
137.	Low to intermediate global CAD risk	U (5)
	Coronary calcium Agatston score between 100 and 400	
138.	High global CAD risk	U (6)
	Coronary calcium Agatston score between 100 and 400	
140.	Abnormal carotid intimal medial thickness (≥0.9 mm and/or the presence of plaque encroaching into the arterial lumen)	U (5)
Stress echocardiography following prior test results asymptomatic or stable symptoms normal prior stress imaging study		
145.	Intermediate to high global CAD risk	U (4)
	Last stress Imaging study ≥2 year ago	

Table 26.2 (continued)

Indication		Appropriate use score (1–9)
Stress echocardiography following prior test results asymptomatic or stable symptoms abnormal coronary angiography or abnormal prior stress study no prior revascularization		
147.	Known CAD on coronary angiography or prior abnormal stress imaging study	U (5)
	Last stress imaging study ≥2 year ago	
Stress echocardiography following prior rest results new or worsening symptoms		
152.	Normal coronary angiography or normal prior stress imaging study	U (6)
Stress echocardiography for risk assessment: perioperative evaluation for noncardiac surgery without active cardiac conditions intermediate-risk surgery		
157.	≥1 clinical risk factor	U (6)
	Poor or unknown functional capacity (<4 METs)	
Stress echocardiography for risk assessment: postrevascularization (PCI or CABG) asymptomatic		
172.	≥5 year after CABG	U (6)
174.	≥2 year after PCI	U (5)
Stress echocardiography for hemodynamics (includes doppler during stress) chronic valvular disease—asymptomatic		
178.	Moderate mitral stenosis	U (5)
181.	Moderate aortic stenosis	U (6)
182.	Severe aortic stenosis	U (5)
184.	Moderate mitral regurgitation	U (5)
187.	Moderate aortic regurgitation	U (5)
Stress echocardiography for hemodynamics (includes doppler during stress) chronic valvular disease—symptomatic		
189.	Mild mitral stenosis	U (5)
194.	Mild mitral regurgitation	U (4)
Stress echocardiography for hemodynamics (includes doppler during stress) pulmonary hypertension		
198.	Suspected pulmonary hypertension	U (5)
	Normal or borderline elevated estimated right ventricular systolic pressure on resting echocardiographic study	
200.	Re-evaluation of patient with exercise-induced pulmonary hypertension to evaluate response to therapy	U (5)

Reprinted from Reference [1] with permission from Elsevier.

Table 26.3 Inappropriate indications (median score 1–3)

Indication		Appropriate use score (1–9)
TTE for general evaluation of cardiac structure and function arrhythmias		
3.	Infrequent APCs or Infrequent VPCs without other evidence of heart disease	I (2)
6.	Asymptomatic Isolated sinus bradycardia	I (2)
TTE for general evaluation of cardiac structure and function lightheadedness/presyncope/syncope		
8.	Lightheadedness/presyncope when there are no other symptoms or signs of cardiovascular disease	I (3)
TTE for general evaluation of cardiac structure and function evaluation of ventricular function		
10.	Initial evaluation of ventricular function (e.g., screening) with no symptoms or signs of cardiovascular disease	I (2)
11.	Routine surveillance of ventricular function with known CAD and no change in clinical status or cardiac exam	I (3)
12.	Evaluation of LV function with prior ventricular function evaluation showing normal function (e.g., prior echocardiogram, left ventriculogram, CT, SPECT MPI, CMR) In patients in whom there has been no change in clinical status or cardiac exam	I (1)
TTE for general evaluation of cardiac structure and function perioperative evaluation		
13.	Routine perioperative evaluation of ventricular function with no symptoms or signs of cardiovascular disease	I (2)
TTE for general evaluation of cardiac structure and function pulmonary hypertension		
16.	Routine surveillance (<1 year) of known pulmonary hypertension without change in clinical status or cardiac exam	I (3)
TTE for cardiovascular evaluation in an acute setting pulmonary embolism		
28.	Suspected pulmonary embolism in order to establish diagnosis	I (2)
30.	Routine surveillance of prior pulmonary embolism with normal right ventricular function and pulmonary artery systolic pressure	I (1)
TTE for cardiovascular evaluation in an acute setting cardiac trauma		
33.	Routine evaluation in the setting of mild chest trauma with no electrocardiographic changes or biomarker elevation	I (2)
TTE for evaluation of valvular function murmur or click		
35.	Initial evaluation when there are no other symptoms or signs of valvular or structural heart disease	I (2)
36.	Re-evaluation in a patient without valvular disease on prior echocardiogram and no change in clinical status or cardiac exam	I (1)
TTE for evaluation of valvular function native valvular stenosis		
38.	Routine surveillance (<3 year) of mild valvular stenosis without a change in clinical status or cardiac exam	I (3)
40.	Routine surveillance (<1 year) of moderate or severe valvular stenosis without a change in clinical status or cardiac exam	I (3)
TTE for evaluation of valvular function native valvular regurgitation		
42.	Routine surveillance of trace valvular regurgitation	I (1)

Table 26.3 (continued)

Indication		Appropriate use score (1–9)
43.	Routine surveillance (<3 year) of mild valvular regurgitation without a change in clinical status or cardiac exam	I (2)
TTE for evaluation of valvular function prosthetic valves		
48.	Routine surveillance (<3 year after valve Implantation) of prosthetic valve if no known or suspected valve dysfunction	I (3)
TTE for evaluation of valvular function infective endocarditis (native or prosthetic valves)		
53.	Transient fever without evidence of bacteremia or a new murmur	I (2)
54.	Transient bacteremia with a pathogen not typically associated with Infective endocarditis and/or a documented nonendovascular source of Infection	I (3)
56.	Routine surveillance of uncomplicated Infective endocarditis when no change in management is contemplated	I (2)
TTE for evaluation of intracardiac and extracardiac structures and chambers		
60.	Routine surveillance of known small pericardial effusion with no change in clinical status	I (2)
TTE for evaluation of aortic disease		
66.	Routine re-evaluation for surveillance of known ascending aortic dilation or history of aortic dissection without a change in clinical status or cardiac exam when findings would not change management or therapy	I (3)
TTE for evaluation of hypertension, HF, or cardiomyopathy hypertension		
68.	Routine evaluation of systemic hypertension without symptoms or signs of hypertensive heart disease	I (3)
TTE for evaluation of hypertension, HF, or cardiomyopathy HF		
74.	Routine surveillance (<1 year) of HF (systolic or diastolic) when there is no change in clinical status or cardiac exam	I (2)
TTE for evaluation of hypertension, HF, or cardiomyopathy device evaluation (including pacemaker, ICD, or CRT)		
79.	Routine surveillance (<1 year) of Implanted device without a change in clinical status or cardiac exam	I (1)
80.	Routine surveillance (≥1 year) of Implanted device without a change in clinical status or cardiac exam	I (3)
TTE for evaluation of hypertension, HF, or cardiomyopathy cardiomyopathies		
88.	Routine surveillance (<1 year) of known cardiomyopathy without a change in clinical status or cardiac exam	I (2)
TTE for adult congenital heart disease		
95.	Routine surveillance (<2 year) of adult congenital heart disease following complete repair	I (3)
	Without a residual structural or hemodynamic abnormality	
	Without a change in clinical status or cardiac exam	
TEE as initial or supplemental test—general uses		
100.	Routine use of TEE when a diagnostic TTE is reasonably anticipated to resolve all diagnostic and management concerns	I (1)

(continued)

Table 26.3 (continued)

Indication		Appropriate use score (1–9)
102.	Surveillance of prior TEE finding for Interval change (e.g., resolution of thrombus after anticoagulation, resolution of vegetation after antibiotic therapy) when no change in therapy is anticipated	I (2)
105.	Routine assessment of pulmonary veins in an asymptomatic patient status post pulmonary vein Isolation	I (3)
TEE as initial or supplemental test—valvular disease		
107.	To diagnose Infective endocarditis with a low pretest probability (e.g., transient fever, known alternative source of Infection, or negative blood cultures/atypical pathogen for endocarditis)	I (3)
TEE as initial or supplemental test—embolic event		
111.	Evaluation for cardiovascular source of embolus with a known cardiac source in which a TEE would not change management	I (1)
TEE as initial test—atrial fibrillation/flutter		
113.	Evaluation when a decision has been made to anticoagulate and not to perform cardioversion	I (2)
Stress echocardiography for detection of CAD/risk assessment: symptomatic or ischemic equivalent evaluation of ischemic equivalent (nonacute)		
114.	Low pretest probability of CAD	I (3)
	ECG Interpretable and able to exercise	
Stress echocardiography for detection of CAD/risk assessment: symptomatic or ischemic equivalent acute chest pain		
123.	Definite ACS	I (1)
Stress echocardiography for detection of CAD/risk assessment: asymptomatic (without ischemic equivalent) general patient populations		
124.	Low global CAD risk	I (1)
125.	Intermediate global CAD risk	I (2)
	ECG interpretable	
Stress echocardiography for detection of CAD/risk assessment: asymptomatic (without ischemic equivalent) in patient populations with defined comorbidities arrhythmias		
131.	Infrequent PVCs	I (3)
Stress echocardiography for detection of CAD/risk assessment: asymptomatic (without ischemic equivalent) in patient populations with defined comorbidities syncope		
133.	Low global CAD risk	I (3)
Stress echocardiography following prior test results asymptomatic: prior evidence of subclinical disease		
136.	Coronary calcium Agatston score <100	I (2)
Stress echocardiography following prior test results asymptomatic or stable symptoms normal prior stress imaging study		
142.	Low global CAD risk	I (1)
	Last stress imaging study <2 year ago	
143.	Low global CAD risk	I (2)
	Last stress imaging study ≥2 year ago	
144.	Intermediate to high global CAD risk	I (2)
	Last stress imaging study <2 year ago	

Table 26.3 (continued)

Indication		Appropriate use score (1–9)
Stress echocardiography following prior rest results asymptomatic or stable symptoms abnormal coronary angiography or abnormal prior stress study no prior revascularization		
146.	Known CAD on coronary angiography or prior abnormal stress imaging study	I (3)
	Last stress imaging study <2 year ago	
Stress echocardiography following prior test results treadmill ECG stress test		
148.	Low-risk treadmill score (e.g., Duke)	I (1)
Stress echocardiography for risk assessment: perioperative evaluation for noncardiac surgery without active cardiac conditions low-risk surgery		
154.	Perioperative evaluation for risk assessment	I (1)
Stress echocardiography for risk assessment: perioperative evaluation for noncardiac surgery without active cardiac conditions intermediate-risk surgery		
155.	Moderate to good functional capacity (≥4 METs)	I (3)
156.	No clinical risk factors	I (2)
158.	Asymptomatic <1 year post normal catheterization, noninvasive test, or previous revascularization	I (1)
Stress echocardiography for risk assessment: perioperative evaluation for noncardiac surgery without active cardiac conditions vascular surgery		
159.	Moderate to good functional capacity (≥4 METs)	I (3)
160.	No clinical risk factors	I (2)
162.	Asymptomatic <1 year post normal catheterization, noninvasive test, or previous revascularization	I (2)
Stress echocardiography for risk assessment: within 3 months of an ACS STEMI		
163.	Primary PCI with complete revascularization	I (2)
	No recurrent symptoms	
165.	Hemodynamically unstable, signs of cardiogenic shock, or mechanical complications	I (1)
Stress echocardiography for risk assessment: within 3 months of an ACS ACS—asymptomatic postrevascularization (PCI or CABG)		
167.	Prior to hospital discharge in a patient who has been adequately revascularized	I (1)
Stress echocardiography for risk assessment: within 3 months of an ACS cardiac rehabilitation		
168.	Prior to Initiation of cardiac rehabilitation (as a stand-alone indication)	I (3)
Stress echocardiography for risk assessment: postrevascularization (PCI or CABG) asymptomatic		
171.	<5 year after CABG	I (2)
173.	<2 year after PCI	I (2)
Stress echocardiography for risk assessment: postrevascularization (PCI or CABG) cardiac rehabilitation		
175.	Prior to initiation of cardiac rehabilitation (as a stand-alone indication)	I (3)

(continued)

Table 26.3 (continued)

Indication		Appropriate use score (1–9)
Stress echocardiography for hemodynamics (includes doppler during stress) chronic valvular disease—asymptomatic		
177.	Mild mitral stenosis	I (2)
180.	Mild aortic stenosis	I (3)
183.	Mild mitral regurgitation	I (2)
186.	Mild aortic regurgitation	I (2)
Stress echocardiography for hemodynamics (includes doppler during stress) chronic valvular disease—symptomatic		
191.	Severe mitral stenosis	I (3)
192.	Severe aortic stenosis	I (1)
196.	Severe mitral regurgitation	I (3)
	Severe LV enlargement or LV systolic dysfunction	
Stress echocardiography for hemodynamics (includes doppler during stress) acute valvular disease		
197.	Acute moderate or severe mitral or aortic regurgitation	I (3)
Stress echocardiography for hemodynamics (includes doppler during stress) pulmonary hypertension		
199.	Routine evaluation of patients with known resting pulmonary hypertension	I (3)
Contrast use in TTE/TEE or stress echocardiography		
201.	Routine use of contrast	I (1)
	All LV segments visualized on noncontrast images	

Reprinted from Reference [1] with permission from Elsevier.

I Indicates inappropriate

References

1. Douglas PS, Garcia MJ, Haines DE, Lai WW, Manning WJ, Patel AR, et al. ACCF/ASE/AHA/ASNC/HFSA/HRS/SCAI/SCCM/SCCT/SCMR 2011 appropriate use criteria for echocardiography a report of the American College of Cardiology Foundation Appropriate Use Criteria Task Force, American Society of Echocardiography, American Heart Association, American Society of Nuclear Cardiology, Heart Failure Society of America, Heart Rhythm Society, Society for Cardiovascular Angiography and Interventions, Society of Critical Care Medicine, Society of Cardiovascular Computed Tomography, and Society for Cardiovascular Magnetic Resonance Endorsed by the American College of Chest Physicians. J Am Coll Cardiol. 2011;57(9):1126–66.
2. Wolk MJ, Bailey SR, Doherty JU, Douglas PS, Hendel RC, Kramer CM, et al. ACCF/AHA/ASE/ASNC/HFSA/HRS/SCAI/SCCT/SCMR/STS 2013 multimodality appropriate use criteria for the detection and risk assessment of stable ischemic heart disease a report of the American College of Cardiology Foundation Appropriate Use Criteria Task Force, American Heart Association, American Society of Echocardiography, American Society of Nuclear Cardiology, Heart Failure Society of America, Heart Rhythm Society, Society for Cardiovascular Angiography and Interventions, Society of Cardiovascular Computed Tomography, Society for Cardiovascular Magnetic Resonance, and Society of Thoracic Surgeons. J Am Coll Cardiol. 2014;63(4):380–406.

3. Bailey SA, Mosteanu I, Tietjen PA, Petrini JR, Alexander J, Keller AM. The use of transthoracic echocardiography and adherence to appropriate use criteria at a regional hospital. J Am Soc Echocardiogr. 25(9):1015–22.
4. Bhatia RS, Dudzinski DM, Malhotra R, Milford CE, Yoerger Sanborn DM, Picard MH, et al. Educational intervention to reduce outpatient inappropriate echocardiograms: a randomized control trial. JACC Cardiovasc Imaging. 2014;7(9):857–66.
5. Chan RH, Shaw JL, Hauser TH, Markson LJ, Manning WJ. Guideline adherence for echocardiographic follow-up in outpatients with at least moderate valvular disease. J Am Soc Echocardiogr.
6. Cortigiani L, Bigi R, Bovenzi F, Molinaro S, Picano E, Sicari R. Prognostic implication of appropriateness criteria for pharmacologic stress echocardiography performed in an outpatient clinic. Circ Cardiovasc Imaging. 2012;5(3):298–305.
7. Willens HJ, Nelson K, Hendel RC. Appropriate use criteria for stress echocardiography: impact of updated criteria on appropriateness ratings, correlation with pre-authorization guidelines, and effect of temporal trends and an educational initiative on utilization. JACC Cardiovasc Imaging. 2013;6(3):297–309.

Chapter 27
Quality Control: Personnel

Linda D. Gillam and Sofia Shames

Abstract High quality appropriately trained technologists (sonographers) and physicians are key components to the successful performance and interpretation of echocardiograms. This chapter will review the training and certification pathways that are available for cardiac sonographers and interpreting physicians. Insuring high reliability processes to train and evaluate the personnel involved in echocardiographic performance and interpretation is a requirement for a high quality program, as is continuing education to ensure familiarity with developments in the field.

Keywords Echocardiography • Quality • Technologist certification • Physician certification • Intersocietal Accreditation Commission • National Board of Echocardiography • COCATS training documents

Sonographer Credentialing

Sonographer credentialing in the United States is provided by the American Registry of Diagnostic Medical Sonographers (ARDMS) and Cardiovascular Credentialing International (CCI). ARDMS offers credentials exclusively to those involved in ultrasound including the RDCS (registered diagnostic cardiac sonographer) credential for sonographers with options for specialties in adult echocardiography (AE), fetal echocardiography (FE) and pediatric echocardiography (PE) as well as RVT (registered vascular technologist). For each of these credentials, the applicant must pass individual examinations in each discipline in addition to a challenging

L.D. Gillam, MD, MPH (✉)
Department of Cardiovascular Medicine, Morristown Medical Center, 100 Madison Avenue, Morristown, NJ 07962, USA
e-mail: linda.gillam@atlantichealth.org

S. Shames, MD
Department of Cardiology, Columbia University Medical Center, New York, NY 10032, USA

P.L. Tilkemeier et al. (eds.), *Quality Evaluation in Non-Invasive Cardiovascular Imaging*, DOI 10.1007/978-3-319-28011-0_27

common examination which tests knowledge of ultrasound physics and technology – Sonography Principles and Instrumentation (SPI). ARDMS also offers a credential for physicians reading vascular studies – Registered Physician Vascular Interpreter (RPVI).

Prerequisites for sonographer credentialing through ARDMS can be achieved through a number of pathways http://www.ardms.org/Prerequisite%20Charts/generalprerequisites_-_2014-2.pdf that include: successful completion of a 2 year allied health professional program; completion of a sonographer program accredited by the Commission on Accreditation of Allied Health Education Programs (CAAHEP) or the Canadian Medical Association (CMA); 4 year bachelors program in any discipline; or MD/DO or foreign equivalent. Typically clinical experience is also required. A clinical experience pathway that allows those without post-secondary education to become credentialed will sunset 12/31/17.

Cardiovascular Credentialing International (CCI) which also credentials technologists in non-ultrasound disciplines offers the RCS (registered cardiac sonographer) and RCCS (registered congenital cardiac sonographer) as well as the RVS (registered vascular sonographer) credential. CCI offers broader prerequisite options including those for applicants graduating from sonographer programs that are not CAAHEP accredited and likely will continue to provide a clinical experience pathway beyond the ARDMS sunset date. CCI does not independently test physics. http://cci-online.org/content/cci-examination-application-and-overview-booklets. Both CCI and ARDMS require ongoing continuing education for re-credentialing which takes place every 3 (CCI) or 10 (ARDMS) years.

CCI has indicated that it will provide a pilot examination for advanced cardiac sonographers but, for the time being, the basic credentials (ARDMS, RCS) are those that are identified in quality assessment/improvement documents as well as the requirements for lab accreditation through the Intersocietal Commission (see below).

Physician Training and Credentialing in Echocardiography

The typical approach to acquiring and demonstrating expertise in echocardiography for allopathic physicians (MDs) includes level III training in echocardiography as part of or in addition to training in general clinical cardiology followed by Board Certification in Cardiovascular Disease through the American Board in Internal Medicine (ABIM) and Board Certification in Echocardiography through the National Board of Echocardiography (NBE).

Cardiology fellowship training is governed by the Accreditation Council for Graduate Medical Education (ACGME) and includes a minimum of 3 years following preliminary training and Board Certification in internal medicine through the credentialing examination of the ABIM, a member of the American Board of Medical Specialties (ABMS). A credentialing examination in cardiovascular disease is also offered through ABIM.

Fellowship Training Pathway

The elements of training in general cardiology are guided by the Core Cardiology Training Statement (COCATS) of the American College of Cardiology. COCATS Task Force 5 recommendations for training in echocardiography [1], developed in partnership with the American Society of Echocardiography, recognize three levels of training in echocardiography with a minimum of level II required for reading echocardiograms and the expectation that cardiologists should also know how to perform echocardiograms as well. Those interested in becoming experts in echocardiography or directing echocardiography laboratories should complete a minimum of level III training (12 months devoted to echocardiography) with many completing 1–2 years of additional training in echocardiography after the 3 year fellowship. Comparable training may be available through osteopathic training programs currently governed by the American Osteopathic Association (AOA) and American Association of Colleges of Osteopathic Medicine (AACOM). In 2015 both osteopathic organizations announced their intent to become members of ACGME with the goal of standardizing post graduate medical education.

Board Certification in Echocardiography

Board certification in echocardiography is offered by the National Board of Echocardiography (NBE) with the COCATS Echocardiography document stating that, "To confirm competency, trainees should strongly consider preparing for and taking the appropriate National Board of Echocardiography examination." NBE offers examinations in adult echocardiography as well as two exams in peri-operative transesophageal echocardiography targeted to anesthesiologists. To date there is no examination for pediatric or adult congenital echocardiography. The comments in this review will be limited to testing for adult echocardiography for which the examination is administered yearly at computer based testing sites around the world. Any licensed physician is eligible to take the NBE examination and, if successful, is termed a testamur. Additionally testamurs who meet additional requirements for board certification including training and/or practice experience may apply for Board Certification in Echocardiography.

Training requirements for Board Certification in Adult Echocardiography include 2 years of training in adult cardiology, with at least level 2 training in echocardiography and performance of 150 transthoracic echocardiograms, reading of an additional 300 transthoracic echocardiograms, performance and interpretation of 50 transesophageal echocardiograms and supervision and interpretation of 100 stress echocardiograms. The transthoracic requirements are mandatory for all applicants for certification using this training pathway with TEE and stress numbers mandatory for those who seek additional credentials in these modalities. Those who meet all requirements receive comprehensive certification.

Alternate Pathways to Echocardiography Board Certification

Alternate pathways to NBE Board Certification exist for those whose training was completed before June 2009, the so-called practice pathways. Testamur and Board Certification is valid for 10 years from the time of testing. Recertification examinations are shorter but include questions drawn from the same question bank as the initial credentialing exam. In addition to passing the recertification examination, applicants for recertification must provide evidence of ongoing clinical activity (studies read) as well as echocardiography-related continuing medical education.

Details of the certification and recertification processes are available at http://www.echoboards.org/sites/default/files/ASCE%20Cert%20App%20%282%29.pdf. and http://www.echoboards.org/content/reasce-certification respectively. NBE Board Certification is endorsed by the American Society of Echocardiography as a quality measure and is a requirement for Fellowship in the American Society of Echocardiography (FASE) which is, in turn, required for leadership roles within the organization.

In the early days of echocardiography, when many experts were self-taught, some radiologists developed advanced echocardiographic skills. However, current radiology training programs do not typically provide a pathway to expertise in or Board Certification in Echocardiography.

Reference

1. Ryan T, Berlacher K, Lindner JR, Mankad SV, Rose GA, Wang A. COCATS 4 Task Force 5: training in-áEchocardiography. J Am Coll Cardiol. 2015;65(17):1786–99.

Chapter 28
Quality Control: Equipment and Laboratory Structure; Image Acquisition, Review and Analysis; Study Reporting

Linda D. Gillam and Sofia Shames

Abstract The proper performance of high quality echocardiography is dependent on complex sets of equipment and skills being utilized and performed correctly to insure that minimal standards are met for image quality. Quality in image acquisition encompasses standards for laboratory structure and organization, imaging equipment, credentials and skills of sonographers who typically acquire most images and the use of echo contrast agents as needed. Image interpretation is dealt with through physician credentialing and reporting through standards that include obligatory report content, formatting and timeliness. Resources are provided to assist with understanding the standards for each of the processes to insure a high quality echocardiographic study.

Keywords Echocardiography • Quality • Laboratory accreditation • Intersocietal Accreditation Commission • Image interpretation • Reporting standards

Equipment

While echocardiography is a technique that is very dependent on the skills of the sonographer performing the examination, the quality of echocardiographic images is also dependent on the system used to acquire them. While hand held devices with limited but improving functionality have been created to provide a tool for focused ultrasound examinations performed as an adjunct to physical examination, this

---

L.D. Gillam, MD, MPH (✉)
Department of Cardiovascular Medicine, Morristown Medical Center,
100 Madison Avenue, Morristown, NJ 07960, USA
e-mail: linda.gillam@atlantichealth.org

S. Shames, MD
Department of Cardiology, Columbia University Medical Center,
PH 3-342, 622 West 168th street, New York, NY 10032, USA
e-mail: ss3972@cumc.columbia.edu

P.L. Tilkemeier et al. (eds.), *Quality Evaluation in Non-Invasive Cardiovascular Imaging*, DOI 10.1007/978-3-319-28011-0_28

section focuses on the technical capabilities and performance of systems that would typically be used by echocardiography laboratories with the expectation that studies would be recorded and archived and that the results would be formally reported.

The minimum standards for an echocardiographic machine are set out in the ASE Recommendations for Quality Echocardiography Laboratory Operations [1]. These include: transducers with a broad range of frequencies and harmonic capability for both unenhanced and contrast-enhanced imaging; a dedicated non-imaging continuous wave Pedoff probe; multiplane TEE probes (if the lab performs TEE); the ability to record spectral (pulsed and continuous wave) Doppler as well as M-mode and 2-D imaging information using a DICOM (Digital Imaging and Communications in Medicine) standard and, for stress echocardiography, split and quad screen display. Other essentials include the ability to label each image with patient identifiers as well as both the date and time of the study. A clock should make it possible to time the acquisition to the second, particularly important with stress echocardiography where a quality measure is the time of image acquisition relative to the completion of exercise, 60 s for completion of imaging being the goal. Physiologic monitors including single lead EKG and respiratory gating are also imperative. These define the minimum standards of an echocardiographic machine. Additionally, most would agree that a state-of-the-art echocardiography lab should have equipment that is also able to perform Doppler tissue imaging, 3D, and strain/strain rate imaging. Contrast perfusion capability is desirable but not essential.

Echocardiographic equipment should undergo routine maintenance with at least annual testing using phantoms to ensure the accuracy of the calibration on the imaging display. Such service may be performed by the vendor or third party providers of service contracts or through in-house biomedical engineering departments. Probes should be routinely checked to make sure that the casings are intact and transesophageal probes should additionally be tested to ensure that fractures in the probe covering have not resulted in current leaks. Service record logs must be kept.

Transthoracic transducers must be cleaned between each patient contact with transesophageal probes requiring a more extensive disinfection process. Logs that document the required changes in disinfecting solutions should be maintained.

Laboratory Structure

Minimum standards have been recommended for the physical layout of the echocardiography lab with a minimum of 150 ft^2 per scanning room and ready access to, ideally in-room, sinks for hand-washing. Additional requirements include a designated room to disinfect TEE probes as well as access to agents used to clean the TTE transducers between patients [1, 2]. In best conditions, the lab should be equipped with special echo imaging beds that are designed to improve image quality and minimize sonographer work-related injuries. However, such beds are expensive and not routinely available in even the best echocardiography laboratories.

As discussed in more detail below, the current standard for echocardiographic image acquisition and storage is digital using a DICOM standard. Videotape is no longer considered an acceptable alternative due to degeneration of the tape over time and the challenges of comparing images from multiple studies side by side. Optical discs have been replaced by central server storage linked to digital study review and reporting systems. Archival systems must be backed up regularly to eliminate the possibility that images might be lost. Workflow is facilitated by having a single review and reporting system, although the review and reporting functions can be handled on different platforms. The capabilities of the review system are discussed in a later section. However, it should be noted that the review station(s) should be in close proximity to the site of image acquisition to facilitate communication between sonographers and interpreting physicians. The image reading room should be one that can be darkened to facilitate image review and include options for printing and faxing reports.

Image Acquisition

The American Society of Echocardiography provides guidelines and standards for the acquisition/interpretation of images required to assess overall cardiac anatomy and with many of these documents done in collaboration with the European Association of Cardiovascular Imaging, formerly the European Association of Echocardiography. These guidelines can be accessed through the ASE website http://asecho.org/guidelines/guidelines-standards and are also available in poster format as well as through electronic applications for mobile electronic devices. Key documents include: Recommendations for Cardiac Chamber Quantification by Echocardiography in Adults [3], Recommendations for the Evaluation of Left Ventricular Diastolic Function with Echocardiography [4], Guidelines for the Echocardiographic Assessment of the Right Heart in Adults [5], Recommendations for Evaluation of the Severity of Native Valvular Regurgitation with Two-dimensional and Doppler Echocardiography [6], Echocardiographic Assessment of Valve Stenosis [7], and Recommendations for Quantification Methods During the Performance of a Pediatric Echocardiogram [8]. Additionally, a series of consensus statements are also available http://asecho.org/guidelines/guidelines-standards providing guidance for the use of echocardiography in specific clinical scenarios e.g. patients undergoing oncologic treatment with potentially cardiotoxic drugs, hypertrophic cardiomyopathy, etc. High quality echocardiography labs should closely follow the guidelines and standards and adhere to the recommendations of the consensus statements. Note is made that these documents are regularly updated and it expected that high quality echocardiography laboratories will train staff to the newest version of the document whenever an update occurs.

Minimal standards for the imaging views and types of information acquired (imaging, PW, CW, color Doppler) in order to address the majority of indications for echocardiography are in turn captured through that IAC echo standards [2] http://www.intersocietal.org/echo/seeking/echo_standards.htm. These, in effect, constitute minimal requirements for echocardiographic transthoracic, transesophageal and stress studies with comparable requirements elucidated in the Pediatriac Echocardiography standards document http://www.intersocietal.org/echo/standards/IACPedEchoStandardsJuly2014.pdf and in Tables 28.1, 28.2, and 28.3.

Table 28.1 Standard components of a trans-thoracic echocardiogram (Adapted with permission from the Intersocietal Accreditation Commission Standards and Guidelines for Adult Echocardiography Accreditation)

A complete transthoracic imaging and Doppler echocardiographic examination is one that:
Includes standard views from multiple planes including views of all cardiac structures and selected extracardiac structures. These include, but are not limited to:
(i) Left ventricle;
(ii) Right ventricle;
(iii) Left atrium;
(iv) Right atrium;
(v) Aortic valve;
(vi) Pulmonic valve;
(vii) Mitral valve;
(viii) Tricuspid valve;
(ix) Proximal ascending aorta;
(x) Aortic arch (when indicated);
(xi) Inferior vena cava; and
(xii) Pericardium
Includes spectral Doppler and/or color flow interrogation of all normal and abnormal flows within the heart including the valves, the great vessels and the atrial and ventricular septa
The complete exam must include (except where technically unobtainable), but not be limited to:
The following standard 2-D views:
(i) Parasternal long axis view;
(ii) Parasternal short axis views (at the level of the aortic valve, left ventricle at the basal, mid and apical levels);
(iii) Right ventricular inflow view (from anteriorly directed parasternal long axis view);
(iv) Apical four-chamber view;
(v) Apical two-chamber view;
(vi) Apical five-chamber view;
(vii) Apical long axis view;
(viii) Subcostal four chamber view;
(ix) Subcostal short axis view (when indicated);
(x) Subcostal IVC/hepatic vein view; and
(xi) Suprasternal notch view (when indicated)
The following 2-D or M-Mode measurements of the left heart:
(i) Left ventricular internal dimension at end-diastole;
(ii) Left ventricular internal dimension at end-systole;
(iii) Left ventricular posterobasal free wall thickness at end-diastole;
(iv) Ventricular septal thickness at end-diastole;
(v) Left atrial dimension at end-systole or left atrial volume index; and
(vi) Aortic root dimension at end-diastole

Table 28.1 (continued)

The following standard Doppler flow evaluations:	
(i)	Four cardiac valves – forward flow spectra for each valve, and any regurgitation, shown in at least two imaging planes with color Doppler;
(ii)	Also use of non-imaging Doppler Transducer to assess stenotic valves, valvular regurgitation or whenever indicated;
(iii)	Tricuspid regurgitation spectrum must always be sought with CW Doppler from multiple views for estimation of systolic right ventricular pressure when tricuspid regurgitation is present;
(iv)	Atrial and ventricular septa – color Doppler screening for defects;
(v)	Left ventricular outflow tract velocity;
(vi)	Velocity-time integrals and hepatic and pulmonary vein flow spectra are optional
(vii)	For aortic stenosis, the systolic velocity must be evaluated from multiple transducer positions (e.g., apical, suprasternal and right parasternal). This must include interrogation from multiple views with a dedicated non-imaging continuous wave Doppler transducer (at least one clear envelope must be obtained)
Use of contrast for suboptimal image quality – contrast is indicated for use when two contiguous segments are not visualized in any three of the apical views (poor endocardial border definition) as it provides greater accuracy in determining left ventricular function	

Table 28.2 Standard components of a transesophageal echocardiogram (Adapted with permission from the Intersocietal Accreditation Commission Standards and Guidelines for Adult Echocardiography Accreditation)

A complete transesophageal imaging and Doppler echocardiographic examination is one that:	
Includes the following standard views while allowing for patient tolerance and safety:	
(i)	Gastric short axis and long axis views;
(ii)	Standard 2 and 4 chamber views;
(iii)	Short and long axis views of the aortic valve with appropriate Doppler;
(iv)	Multiple imaging planes of the mitral valve with appropriate Doppler;
(v)	Multiple imaging planes of the tricuspid valve with appropriate Doppler;
(vi)	Longitudinal view of the pulmonic valve with appropriate Doppler;
(vii)	Multiple imaging planes of the right atrium, left atrium and left atrial appendage with appropriate Doppler;
(viii)	In cases of suspected cardiac source of emboli, appropriate use of contrast methods to evaluate for the presence of intracardiac shunting;
(ix)	Multiple imaging planes of the atrial septum and foramen ovale with appropriate Doppler
(x)	Imaging of the pulmonary veins with appropriate Doppler, when mitral regurgitation is present;
(xi)	Short axis views of the ascending, descending and transverse arch of the aorta;
(xii)	Long axis views of the main pulmonary artery and proximal portions of the right and left pulmonary arteries;
(xiii)	Images of the proximal inferior and superior vena cava; and
(xiv)	Imaging of the pericardial space and pericardium

Table 28.3 Standard components of a stress echocardiogram (Adapted with permission from the Intersocietal Accreditation Commission Standards and Guidelines for Adult Echocardiography Accreditation)

Stress echocardiograms must be comprehensive and include the following standard components	
(i)	Treadmill stress echo: images must be obtained at baseline and immediately post exercise. All LV segments need to be visualized and compared side by side (baseline vs. peak exercise). The required views are parasternal long axis view, parasternal short axis view, apical four-chamber view and apical two-chamber view, or apical long axis, apical four-chamber view, apical two-chamber view and apical short-axis view
(ii)	Bicycle stress echo protocols: at a minimum, images must be obtained at baseline and immediately post exercise. All LV segments need to be visualized and compared side by side. The required views are parasternal long axis view, parasternal short axis view, apical four-chamber view and apical two-chamber view or apical long axis, apical four-chamber view, apical two-chamber view and apical short-axis view
(iii)	Pharmacologic stress echo: images must be obtained at baseline and three other phases. Common protocols include digitizing rest, low-dose, pre-peak and peak, or rest, low-dose, peak and recovery. All LV segments need to be visualized and compared side by side. The required views are parasternal long axis view, parasternal short axis view, apical four-chamber view and apical two-chamber view, or apical long axis, apical four-chamber view, apical two-chamber view and apical short-axis view
(iv)	Contrast stress echo: facilities using contrast must have a written protocol for use of contrast agents for stress echocardiography
(v)	A Doppler stress echocardiogram includes interrogations of flow velocities (from the same site) before, during and/or immediately following stress. Doppler stress echocardiography may be utilized to document gradient changes that occur with stress, or to evaluate diastolic filling pattern changes that occur with stress

Contrast Echocardiography

The American Society of Echocardiography has recommended the use of echocardiographic contrast agents when endocardial delineation of two or more of the 17 left ventricular myocardial segments is inadequate. The derived quality measure is the percent of studies deemed inadequate by this definition in which contrast is used. It is estimated that 10–20 % of TTEs should include contrast administration. The number is arguably higher for stress echocardiograms in which it is critical to acquire diagnostic images within 60 s of the conclusion of treadmill stress during which time patients are typically tachypneic and unable to perform the breath-holding that may be necessary for adequate images. However with it being estimated that contrast is used in only 5 % of studies, frequency of appropriate contrast utilization is a quality measure that is frequently not met. The major obstacles to contrast utilization are related to the availability of personnel for establishing intravenous access that is not otherwise required for resting TTE or exercise stress testing and the availability of those whose scope of practice includes the ability to inject contrast agents. While some states permit sonographers to acquire these skills, others limit these to nurses, nurse practitioners or physicians. Laboratory accreditation recommends but does not mandate the ASE recommendation for contrast use is met.

Image Review and Analysis

The standard for image review and analysis is one in which digitally stored images can be rapidly retrieved with a system that allows the checking and correcting, if needed, of measurements that have been made by the sonographer at the time the study is recorded. Additionally, the ability to retrieve and simultaneously display images from prior studies is essential for the side-by-side comparisons that may be required to detect subtle but clinically important changes e.g. worsening of a wall motion abnormality in a patient with coronary disease, or growth of a vegetation in a patient with infective endocarditis. Highly desirable is the ability to capture images of new measurements embedding them into the original study. These capabilities are not universally available in commercially available systems. Remote secure web-based access, ideally with the full functionality of the on-site system is also an important feature that makes it easier for physicians to review studies in a timely fashion.

State-of- the- art systems also include the ability to review and perform reconstructions of three dimensional volume sets as well as to provide an analysis of strain, strain-rate, rotation and torsion.

Reporting

Quality in echocardiographic reporting incorporates elements of the report, structure/format of the report, timeliness of the report, report communication, and, of course, the quality of the interpretation. The ASE and IAC provide recommendations as to the core elements of echocardiographic reports, which emphasize a systematic and comprehensive commentary of cardiac structure and function that includes statements indicating where certain views were attempted but inadequate for interpretation. Equally important is the use of a standard structured report i.e. all reports for a given lab should be formatted in the same way, use standard language to communicate common findings, and present elements of the report in the same sequence. Although this can be achieved with dictated reports, it is facilitated by the use of a computer based reporting system, ideally interfaced with the image archive and analysis system and linked to report communication vehicles including fax machines and direct feed to electronic medical records. Reports must provide key patient demographics that would permit the accurate identification of each individual patient and facilitate the identification of prior studies that should be compared with the current study. Additionally, they must include heart rate (and rhythm where possible) and blood pressure as important conditions that are assessed with echocardiography, notably many forms of valve disease, may vary in severity or hemodynamic impact depending on heart rate and/or blood pressure. A method for locking reports once signed and an audit trail that highlights any changes to the original signed report are also desirable. There are a number of commercially available echocardiography reporting systems as well as excellent systems that have been home grown, typically at large academic medical centers. Some systems possess the ability to archive images from and generate reports for other imaging modalities which can greatly facilitate quality assurance activities that involve comparing the echocardiographic findings with those from an independent reference standard.

Minimum standards for the time from study conclusion to report generation are included in the ASE quality and IAC reporting documents with high quality labs meeting the higher standard of report completion on the same day that the study is performed. The ASE and IAC documents provide an additional time window from the time the report is generated to the time that it is signed and finalized but for computer generated reports, this is a non-issue since reports are electronically signed at the time the report is generated. The simultaneity of report generation and signature provides another strong argument for computer-based report generation.

Reporting is a physician responsibility and although competent sonographers should recognize key findings and may include them on a worksheet for the reading physician's reference, sonographers should not communicate results either verbally or in writing to anyone other than the interpreting physician. Very rare exceptions can be made for critically ill and unstable patients in whom life-threatening conditions are unequivocally diagnosed with an echocardiogram and when there is no interpreting physician immediately available. However, under such circumstances, the interpreting physician must be contacted immediately so that he/she can confirm the observed findings and complete the report. Image archival and reporting systems that allow remote web-based access greatly facilitate rapid review of emergency studies highlighting the desirability of this feature in an archival/reviewing and reporting system.

While physician credentialing may provide one indirect measure of the quality of the study interpretation, peer review and correlation of echocardiographic interpretations with the results of other studies is important (e.g. stress echocardiography and coronary angiography, transthoracic echocardiography and cardiac MRI). Where these processes identify deficiencies in a reader's abilities, there must be a mechanism in place for remediation and either restricting that physician's ability to read echoes or having his/her studies over-read by a qualified reader until such time as it is determined that the reader is able to read independently. For hospital based laboratories, the ongoing physician professional evaluation (OPPE) and focused physician professional evaluation (FPPE) processes may be involved. In some instances, where remediation, typically focused on education in the form of live, CD/DVD or web-based education, fails, it may be necessary for the physician to stop reading echocardiograms.

Each echocardiography laboratory must have a policy concerning communication of critical findings where simply generating a written report in a timely fashion will be inadequate, even if the report is immediately uploaded to an electronic record. Key elements of such a policy are: identification of the most common scenarios for which such communication would be required e.g. aortic dissection, pericardial effusion with tamponade physiology; identification of the person to whom the results should be communicated, typically an attending physician; and a method for documenting that the communication has taken place. The recommendations for study reporting are summarized in Table 28.4.

Table 28.4 IAC and ASE recommendations for reporting Trans thoracic Echocardiograms

Timeliness:
STAT echo – result available immediately
Inpatient echo – 24 h
Outpatient echo – by the end of the following business day
Final signed report – within 48 h
Report:
Demographics:
Date and time[a] of the study
Name and/or identifier of the facility
Name/or identifier of the patient
Date of birth and/or age of the patient
Indication for the study
Name or initials of the performing sonographer
Name of the ordering physician and/or identifier
Height
Weight
Blood pressure
Study quality[a]
Patient location[a]
2D and/or M-mode measurements:
Left ventricular end-diastolic dimension
Left ventricular end-systolic dimension
Basal anteroseptal end-diastolic wall thickness
Basal inferolateral end-diastolic wall thickness
Left atrial dimension at end-diastole or indexed LA volume
Aortic root dimension at end-diastole or ascending aorta
Doppler assessment:
Evaluation of peak and mean gradients (if senosis is present)
Valve are (if senosis is present)
Degree of regurgitation
Right ventricular systolic pressure
LV diastolic function[a]
Report must include comments on:
Left ventricular size, ejection fraction and regional dysfunction
Right ventricular size and function
Right atrium
Left atrium
Mitral valve
Aortic valve
Tricuspid valve
Pulmonic valve
Pericardium
Aorta

[a]Recommended by ASE only

References

1. Picard MH, Adams D, Bierig SM, Dent JM, Douglas PS, Gillam LD, et al. American Society of Echocardiography recommendations for quality echocardiography laboratory operations. J Am Soc Echocardiogr. 2011;24(1):1–10.
2. Intersocietal Commission Standards for the Accreditation of Echocardiography Laboratories. [Internet] http://www.intersocietal.org/echo/seeking/echo_standards.htm. 2015. Available from: URL: http://www.intersocietal.org/echo/seeking/echo_standards.htm
3. Lang RM, Badano LP, Mor-Avi V, Afilalo J, Armstrong A, Ernande L, et al. Recommendations for cardiac chamber quantification by echocardiography in adults: an update from the American Society of Echocardiography and the European Association of Cardiovascular Imaging. J Am Soc Echocardiogr. 2015;28(1):1–39.
4. Nagueh SF, Appleton CP, Gillebert TC, Marino PN, Oh JK, Smiseth OA, et al. Recommendations for the evaluation of left ventricular diastolic function by echocardiography. J Am Soc Echocardiogr. 2009;22(2):107–33.
5. Rudski LG, Lai WW, Afilalo J, Hua L, Handschumacher MD, Chandrasekaran K, et al. Guidelines for the echocardiographic assessment of the right heart in adults: a report from the American Society of Echocardiography: endorsed by the European Association of Echocardiography, a registered branch of the European Society of Cardiology, and the Canadian Society of Echocardiography. J Am Soc Echocardiogr. 2010;23(7):685–713.
6. Zoghbi WA, Enriquez-Sarano M, Foster E, Grayburn PA, Kraft CD, Levine RA, et al. Recommendations for evaluation of the severity of native valvular regurgitation with two-dimensional and Doppler echocardiography. J Am Soc Echocardiogr. 2003;16(7):777–802.
7. Baumgartner H, Hung J, Bermejo J, Chambers JB, Evangelista A, Griffin BP, et al. Echocardiographic assessment of valve stenosis: EAE/ASE recommendations for clinical practice. J Am Soc Echocardiogr: Off Publ Am Soc Echocardiogr. 2009;22(1):1–23. Ref Type: Abstract.
8. Lopez L, Colan SD, Frommelt PC, Ensing GJ, Kendall K, Younoszai AK, et al. Recommendations for quantification methods during the performance of a pediatric echocardiogram: a report from the pediatric measurements writing group of the American Society of Echocardiography Pediatric and Congenital Heart Disease Council. J Am Soc Echocardiogr. 2010;23(5):465–95.

Chapter 29
Quality Control: Laboratory Accreditation

Linda D. Gillam and Sofia Shames

Abstract The accreditation process plays an important role in the quality assessment and improvement of echocardiography laboratories. The accreditation process will be reviewed along with criticism and changes to the process over time. Many measures of the individual steps in the accreditation process as well as more global measures of quality are included in the standards required for laboratory accreditation through the Intersocietal Commission. This section also provides links to additional sources of information concerning each of these measures.

Keywords Echocardiography • Quality • Laboratory accreditation • Intersocietal commission

Accreditation for echocardiography laboratories is provided through the Intersocietal Accreditation Commission for Echocardiography (IAC Echo) formerly known as the Intersocietal Commission for the Accreditation of Echocardiography Laboratories (ICAEL). The IAC standards for accreditation for adult and pediatric echocardiography labs http://www.intersocietal.org/echo/seeking/echo_standards.htm incorporate a number of structure and process measures but, to date, no outcomes measures. They should be considered to set the minimum standard for an echocardiography laboratory whether ambulatory or inpatient.

Specifically the standards include requirements/recommendations for organization of the laboratory, examinations and procedures, and quality improvement. The requirements for the organization of the laboratory include those related to: the training and ongoing continuing medical education of the medical and technical staff as well as the designation of medical and technical directors for whom higher

L.D. Gillam, MD, MPH (✉)
Department of Cardiovascular Medicine, Morristown Medical Center, 100 Madison Avenue, Morristown, NJ 07962, USA
e-mail: linda.gillam@atlantichealth.org

S. Shames, MD
Department of Cardiology, Columbia University Medical Center, PH 3-342, 622 West 168th street, New York, NY 10032, USA
e-mail: ss3972@cumc.columbia.edu

P.L. Tilkemeier et al. (eds.), *Quality Evaluation in Non-Invasive Cardiovascular Imaging*, DOI 10.1007/978-3-319-28011-0_29

training standards are set; physical layout and safety of the echocardiography laboratory; maintenance of the equipment; components and structure of the echocardiographic report as well as requirements for timely report completion and communication and a policy for critical findings; and administrative requirements including those related to patient confidentiality, complaints and primary source verification. Standards related to examinations and procedures cover the scheduling and allocation of adequate time for testing, equipment capabilities and required elements of the echocardiographic examination, minimum procedural numbers for the laboratory as a whole, sonographers and physicians. Quality improvement requirements included implementation of a quality improvement program that includes independent review of studies and correlation of echocardiographic findings with those obtained with other modalities, Implementation of the appropriate use criteria, with meetings and documentation is required as well as quality assurance processes. Accreditation may be granted for transthoracic echocardiography, stress echocardiography and transesophageal echocardiography and there is a mechanism for accrediting laboratories with multiple sites. Once granted, accreditation must be renewed every 3 years.

Responding to criticisms that the process is largely based on an honor system as well as an internal decision to provide laboratory performance assessment more often than 3 year intervals, the Intersocietal Accreditation Commission (IAC) has implemented a process of mid-cycle audits to ensure that the reported adherence to standards actually occurs. With an overall philosophy of helping laboratories that do not initially meet the standards make improvements that will allow them to do so, laboratory accreditation can be viewed to be not only as a quality measure but also a quality improvement tool.

Endorsement of Laboratory Accreditation

As professional societies that supported the creation of the Intersocietal Accreditation Commission and its accreditation of echocardiography laboratories, the American College of Cardiology and American Society of Echocardiography have also endorsed the link between laboratory accreditation and payment. These societies have proposed that payment should be limited to testing performed in accredited labs or, short of this concept that payments for tests performed in non-accredited labs be discounted. However, it has been frustratingly difficult to achieve buy-in from payers particularly commercial ones that this link should occur. While a standard argument against mandating lab accreditation is that access to services would be limited by such a policy, there are well-over 3,000 accredited laboratories at well over 5,000 sites (some laboratories have multiple sites), suggesting that this argument would not hold true in most regions. While it may be that payer decision making is governed by drivers other than quality, it can also be argued that the provider community and its professional societies as well as accrediting/credentialing organizations need to provide more data as to the value of accreditation as well as sonographer and physician credentialing.

Achieving and Maintaining Accreditation and Credentialing

For laboratories seeking accreditation, there are commercial consultants that can help with the creation of required policies and procedures and give guidance as to how to structure peer – review and other quality improvement processes. Additionally, as part of the accreditation process, feedback is given regarding areas of deficiency, reinforcing the concept that accreditation is viewed as having an inclusionary rather than an exclusionary policy.

For echocardiographic accreditation or re-accreditation, both interpreting physicians as well as sonographers are required to have completed continuing medical education. There area number of opportunities for meeting the physician and sonographer continuing education requirements for lab accreditation and physician/sonographer credentialing. For example, the American Society of Echocardiography provides a number of educational opportunities for sonographers and physicians including live programming, such as an annual scientific session and several multi-day courses, webinars, DVD's and a textbook. ASE also cosponsors many programs developed by other CME providers and supports regional CME activities provided by local groups. A calendar of activities is available at http://asecho.org/. Other professional organizations such as the American College of Cardiology and academic medical centers also offer a variety of educational options. Thus, achieving the continuing education requirements should not pose a problem.

The peer review process may pose challenges in some environments particularly if deficiencies in the quality of interpretations cannot be remediated and the laboratory may need to eliminate one or more of the physician readers. In this difficult situation, external peer review may be helpful. The American Medical Foundation, a not-for-profit peer review and quality improvement organization, has the ability to assist with issues related to quality in echocardiography. http://www.medicalfoundation.org/.

Chapter 30
Exploring the Dimensions of Quality and Future Directions

Linda D. Gillam and Sofia Shames

Abstract Echocardiography as with other imaging techniques has many outcomes measures that are related to structure and process. True outcome measures, that is, how an echocardiogram result directly affects a patient outcome, are very difficult to develop at the present. Many efforts are underway to develop outcome measures for imaging and those will be explored as well as future directions for quality initiatives in echocardiography and the societies and boards involved in quality assessment.

Keywords Echocardiography • Quality • Outcome measures • Laboratory accreditation • Intersocietal accreditation commission • National board of echocardiography

The American College of Cardiology has hosted two think tanks directed toward expanding the understanding of the dimensions of quality in imaging (including but not limited to echocardiography) and developing strategies for quality improvement. These have included multiple stakeholders including payers, equipment manufacturers, representatives of credentialing and accreditation bodies, as well as imaging societies including the American Society of Echocardiography, The summaries of these sessions have been reported [1, 2] and have provided dimensions of care framework for evaluating quality in imaging starting with patient selection, including image acquisition, image interpretation, results communication and concluding with an impact on patient management and/or outcomes. This framework highlights the fact that the literature linking imaging quality to outcomes remains

L.D. Gillam, MD, MPH (✉)
Department of Cardiovascular Medicine, Morristown Medical Center, 100 Madison Avenue, Morristown, NJ 07962, USA
e-mail: linda.gillam@atlantichealth.org

S. Shames, MD
Department of Cardiology, Columbia University Medical Center, PH 3-342, 622 West 168th street, New York, NY 10032, USA
e-mail: ss3972@cumc.columbia.edu

P.L. Tilkemeier et al. (eds.), *Quality Evaluation in Non-Invasive Cardiovascular Imaging*, DOI 10.1007/978-3-319-28011-0_30

underdeveloped. Indeed, the quality metrics that have been discussed here are largely structure and process measures with few if any outcomes measures.

Developing outcomes measures for testing is challenging because clinical outcomes are typically influenced by many variables other than the imaging test (e.g. patient characteristics, treatments) and links between the imaging test and a clinical outcome may be indirect and identifiable after only an extended period of observation. However, such studies will be necessary to validate the approaches taken to date and to establish a value proposition for imaging quality. The American Society of Echocardiography Foundation funds a small number of research grants and welcomes submission related to quality in imaging. Additionally, the Intersocietal Accreditation Commission (IAC) offers research grants for studies to explore the link between laboratory accreditation and other dimensions of quality. Interested investigators can submit letters of intent early in the year with a subset of studies selected to submit more detailed proposals in late spring. Additional information is available on the IAC website http://www.intersocietal.org/. Finally, the National Board of Echocardiography is also exploring means of funding research to explore the link between physician credentialing (Board Certification) and other dimensions of quality.

References

1. Douglas P, Iskandrian AE, Krumholz HM, Gillam L, Hendel R, Jollis J, et al. Achieving quality in cardiovascular imaging: proceedings from the American College of Cardiology-Duke University Medical Center Think Tank on Quality in Cardiovascular Imaging. J Am Coll Cardiol. 2006;48(10):2141–51.
2. Douglas PS, Chen J, Gillam L, Hendel R, Hundley WG, Masoudi F, et al. Achieving quality in cardiovascular imaging II: proceedings from the second American College of Cardiology-Duke University Medical Center Think Tank on Quality in Cardiovascular Imaging. J Am Coll Cardiol Img. 2009;2(2):231–40.

Part VII
Laboratory Perspectives

Chapter 31
Developing a Quality Improvement Program

Peter Tilkemeier

Abstract Developing a quality improvement program is a multifaceted process that requires the identification and empowerment of a diverse team to identify and implement change in an existing process. The quality improvement process is initiated by targeting those areas which are important for the organization to improve. This can be done through a number of internal processes, comparison to external standards or external analyses. Data needs to be collected in a meaningful and reproducible way for analysis regarding current processes. Once the data collection has been completed and analyzed, the team can develop solutions for change that are then implemented on an organizational wide basis. After the recommended changes have been implemented, it is important to monitor results to ensure that the changes have resulted in improvement and that this is maintained over time. Quality improvement plans will play an important role in the future of imaging as we move from volume based to value based payment methodologies.

Keywords Quality improvement • Quality management team • Quality improvement process • Data collection • Data analysis • Quality improvement monitoring • Root cause analysis

Developing a Quality Improvement Program

Quality improvement programs are a necessary component of every facility's function. A process that addresses quality performance within the facility is a necessary component of regulatory organizations, insurers, patient and referring healthcare provider expectations and because it is the right thing to do. There are numerous regulatory organizations including The Joint Commission, the American College of Radiology, the Inter-societal Accreditation Commission, American Board of Medical Specialties and all of its member organizations, governmental organizations and the insurers. At

P. Tilkemeier, MD, MMM
Department of Medicine, Greenville Health System,
701 Grove Road, Support Tower 5, Greenville, SC 29605, USA
e-mail: ptilkemeier@gmail.com

P.L. Tilkemeier et al. (eds.), *Quality Evaluation in Non-Invasive Cardiovascular Imaging*, DOI 10.1007/978-3-319-28011-0_31

the present time, the efforts of these organizations are focused on utilizing reimbursement or lack thereof as a mechanism for enforcing compliance with quality improvement initiatives. It is important that we understand the components of a program to address quality performance within an organization if we are to be successful. These include: (1) quality control, processes for monitoring and improving technical performance; (2) quality assurance, a comprehensive process used to monitor and evaluate the quality and appropriateness of patient care and the clinical performance of practitioners; (3) quality improvement, proactive activities aimed at improving the processes and enhance the quality of care and services; (4) performance improvement, improving output, efficiency or effectiveness based on performance data; (5) total quality management, a large program encompassing all of the efforts of quality performance programs; (6) patient's safety programs, mechanisms to identify and mitigate potential problems that would affect patient's; and (7) risk management programs, programmatic efforts to help prevent accidents, injuries and mitigate risk across a health system [1, 2]. Additionally, for a facility to implement successful quality management a number of items must be in place. These include institutional leadership and support, lack of a blaming culture, mechanisms for managing customers and engaging physicians, the ability to capture, analyze and report quality on a systematic basis, safety improvement programs and educational programs [1]. Additionally, a quality improvement team must be assembled with individuals that are empowered to analyze data and make recommendations for change as well as work with leadership to implement change. The system must make this participation a reward rather than a burden [3].

Components of a Quality and Safety Program

Quality and safety programs can be focused around five major areas including patient safety, customer relations, and technical performance including physician performance, education and process improvement. These areas can be approached from multiple perspectives including administrative measures, clinical measures (including technical parameters of image acquisition and physician interpretation) and system measures such as cost effectiveness and business analytics. A robust methodology for gathering data that is perceived as representative of clinical practice along with methods for analyzing the data that is meaningful to those who will utilize it and mechanisms for communication of the results and plan for change are foundational.

The Quality Management Team

For a quality management team to be effective it must have the right membership, support from institutional leadership and be supported by the culture of the organization. Members need to be familiar with the processes that are going to be

Table 31.1 Quality improvement team members and their roles

Member	Role
Executive sponsor	Senior management leadership, institutional alignment, access to resources
Nursing	Clinical input
Technologist	Clinical input
Physician	Clinical input
Information technology	Clinical input, data harvesting and analysis, development of monitoring processes
Business planning	Data harvesting, analysis and ongoing monitoring
Marketing	Survey data results, ongoing survey generation, celebrating success
Development	Placing projects in strategic planning process, aligning with institutional goals
Patient	Provide patient perspective and input

evaluated by the team; furthermore the team must be diverse to allow a broad system based approach to solving problems. This will include nursing, information technology, business planning, technical and physician operations and marketing and development. The most effective teams now include patient representatives as well (Table 31.1). Each member of the team must be fully engaged in the process and not feel as if this is just another assignment in their day. Many times this results in significant team effort being spent on understanding the importance of the problem and its impact on the patient and the healthcare system [3].

The team must function to engage the staff in the quality process in a continuous manner. This will ensure alignment of goals and minimize "sabotage" to the quality improvement process. For this engagement to occur several elements are required including: (1) identifying a common purpose; (2) reframing values and beliefs; (3) using and gauging improvement methods; (4) providing back up to the staff and; (5) adopting an engaging style [4].

The Quality Improvement Process

The first step in any quality improvement project is to identify areas which are opportunities for improvement. This identification process is crucial for the success of the program. Initial projects should be those which will be readily achievable and will have visible impact to the organization. This will allow some early "wins" for the quality improvement committee and process and will make the more difficult improvement processes more readily achievable as the committee addresses them. It is important when identifying opportunities for quality improvement that the opportunity be recognized by many, have the potential to impact processes widely with minimal intervention and current practice, have measurable data both initially and upon implementation of the change process to ensure adequate feedback change has occurred and that the new process is sustainable from an institutional perspective including financial and business models.

Table 31.2 Features of a quality improvement process

Phase of process	Action items
Discovery	Identify opportunity
	Identify needs to attain opportunity
	Identify team members
	Collect baseline data
Analysis	Analyze data
	Insure baseline process in control
	Identify opportunities for change
	Identify appropriate comparative data
Action	Develop plan for change
	Implement changes
	Analyze effectiveness of change
	Develop monitoring plan
	Celebrate accomplishment

Following identification of projects for improvement, data must be collected and analyzed in a meaningful way. This should include the ability to identify contributing and root causes to a process in need of improvement. The third step should be to generate potential solutions and develop mechanisms for implementing change. The fourth step would be to ensure that there are mechanisms in place to monitor the results of the change and reengage the committee as necessary to ensure sustained improvement [5]. Each of these will be examined in depth (Table 31.2 and Fig. 31.1).

Identifying Areas for Improvement

There are many ways to identify opportunities for improvement within an organization as outlined in Table 31.3. These can include results from participation in quality improvement projects on a national basis where the opportunity is identified as an organization with a significant shortfall relative to a benchmark, customer surveys including staff feedback in either an anonymous or identified manner, issues identified through patient safety reporting, direct observation of management and in discussion with staff, identifying the" pain" points in the system, peer review and reporting, assessment of compliance with current local and national guidelines and standards, and in-depth internal analyses.

Examples in these areas can include patient satisfaction, referring physician satisfaction, scheduling, patient throughput, report turnaround time, appropriateness of referral, image quality, patient preparation, adequacy of testing, intra and/or inter-observer variability of image interpretation, peer review image interpretation, comparison of image interpretation with other modalities, appropriateness of care, deficits in education identified through testing or participation in continuous maintenance of certification cost effectiveness or other business analytics and those

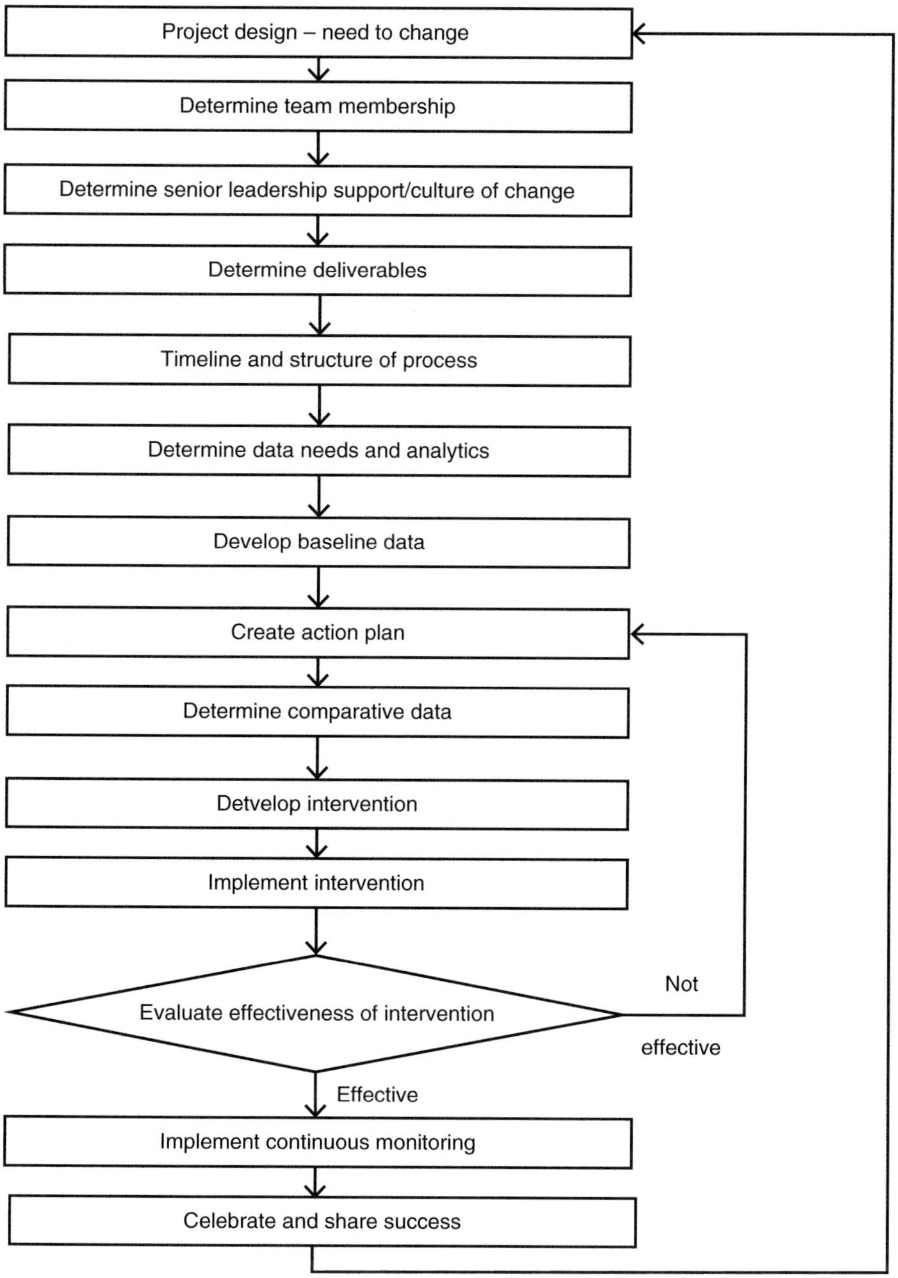

Fig. 31.1 Flow chart of a successful quality improvement process [25]

Table 31.3 Identifying areas for improvement

Opportunity	Example
National benchmark comparison	Appropriate use criteria
Customer surveys (including staff)	Patient and referring provider satisfaction surveys
Patient safety reporting	Untoward event reporting and tracking
Direct observation	Focused professional practice evaluations, staff performance reviews
Barrier identification	Group interviews and surveys
Peer review	Image interpretation review
Internal analyses	Report turnaround time, delays in scheduling

Table 31.4 Data collection and analysis

Data source	Data collection mechanism	Analytic tools
Local studies	1. Surveys	1. Flow charts
	2. Data collection tools	2. Cause and effect diagrams
	3. Practice specific data harvesting	3. Process control charts
		4. Histograms
		5. Scatter diagrams
		6. Radar charts
Large scale studies	1. Registries	1. Group comparisons
	2. Claims data	2. Statistical modeling
	3. Data mining	3. Mortality and outcomes data
	4. Outcomes data	
Financial and business analytics	1. Claims data	Cost effectiveness analysis
	2. Outcomes data	
	3. Alternatives to care	

items identified through brainstorming or team analysis of potential areas for improvement [3, 5–7]. As many of these processes have variable definitions for their indicators that do not necessarily cross institutions, it would be exceptionally helpful if societies were to develop a set of definitions for quality improvement programs that could be uniformly adopted [8].

Data Collection and Analysis

Depending upon the metric that is being evaluated, the source, mechanism of collection and analysis can vary widely as shown in Table 31.4. For some local processes a small survey can be adequate, however, for larger outcomes studies, national or international registries will need to be developed and participated in by a large number of facilities in order to have meaningful data for analysis. The data collection process, whether it is for a small local study or participation in a large registry project, needs to have internal and external validity to ensure effective use of the data to implement change. Given the scientific nature of the physicians usually involved in the quality improvement process or affected by the quality improvement process, the same degree of scientific analysis applied in large studies should be applied to local quality initiatives.

Analysis of the data can occur with a variety of tools. These can include flow charts, cause-and-effect diagrams, Radar diagrams, control charts, histograms and scatter diagrams [5, 9]. Many of these analytic tools will not be familiar to the staff, technical or physician, and will require additional education regarding how they are utilized in a meaningful way that can be derived from the analysis. These are discussed in greater detail in the chapter entitled reporting quality and national/international benchmarks. Other methods include the use of the root cause analysis which allows a more systematic approach to a problem. The root cause analysis establishes a sequence of events that elucidates the relationship between contributing factors in the temporal manner. Through this mechanism, the root cause of the event can usually be identified. Additionally, decision prioritization matrices and relationship diagrams can be utilized as mechanisms to assist in identifying major contributing root causes [10, 11].

When data are collected on larger scales and compiled in large databases, such as registries, the analytic tool is referred to as "data mining". Utilizing "big data" is most useful when evaluating and developing changes to practice and guidelines. This practice, allows the identification of physician specific practice patterns, appropriateness of referrals for imaging studies, appropriateness of care following imaging studies, and the development of evidence-based decision support to impact the guideline development process [8].

From a financial and business analytics perspective, one of the most effective tools has been the utilization of cost-effectiveness analysis. This tool has been utilized in imaging for more than 25 years with increasing frequency more recently. It is a method of economic evaluation in which costs and outcomes of a program and at least one method of alternative care are compared over time [12, 13]. Unfortunately, in a study published in 2008 over the 25 years evaluated there was no significant improvement in the quality of these studies [14].

Generating Solutions and Implementing Change

Once opportunities for improvement have been identified through the mechanisms noted previously and analyzed with regards to the institutional data, the process of generating solutions and implementing change begins and are summarized in Table 31.5. Although the prior steps in a quality improvement project seem difficult, generating solutions and implementing change is probably the most challenging to achieve within an organization. It is clear that few like change and one of the greatest fears can be that the alterations implemented will result in processes that are potentially worse than the initial condition. It is important to bear this in mind throughout the solution generation phase.

Table 31.5 Generating solutions

Potential mechanism for generating solutions
1. Brainstorming
2. Survey tools
3. Root cause analysis
4. Maintenance of certification/licensure
5. Decision support tool data harvesting
6. Laboratory accreditation application
7. National benchmarking

Generating solutions can occur in many ways. Those involved in the process can assist with brainstorming to develop a new preferred state, customer survey tools can help to identify the new preferred state, and comparison to other programs can help identify the ideal future state. Just as a root cause analysis has been utilized to help identify those processes needing improvement, it can be utilized on the preferred future state to identify those changes that will have the potential largest impact on achieving the preferred state. This ensures the "largest bang for the buck" when change is being implemented. There are trade-offs to this approach. Often times to get the largest impact the most change must occur. For many organizations this can be difficult, if not impossible, to achieve either in reality or that which is perceived. Sometimes, it is necessary for an organization to have "small wins" that can affect change and improve processes to a minimal extent. This approach provides the opportunity for the organization to understand that change is possible and that it can positively affect quality measures. Once these small wins are in place, the larger change processes can be initiated as the organization now realizes the true potential of the quality improvement process.

Utilizing the mechanisms afforded through the Part IV maintenance of certification (MOC) projects of the American Board of Medical Specialties focused on physician and facility based quality improvement projects, healthcare facilities have engaged physician populations who will need to be active participants in the quality improvement process including solution generation and implementation. With regard to potential topics in Part IV MOC regarding the imaging community there are a number of challenges including: practice settings, administrative versus actively practicing physicians, the broad spectrum of disease encompassed by the specialists, the effect of specialist versus generalists performing imaging, and national healthcare priorities [15]. Additional sources of potential quality improvement solutions can be generated from decision support implementation. The results from composite evaluation of the utilization of decision support software either on a voluntary or mandatory basis and its effect on changing physician behavior can have a significant impact on informing the organization regarding potential solutions for change. These can range from substitution of one test for another due to time of day or day of week, perceived versus real risk, prior test results bias or many other factors [8]. As important as the quality team is for implementing change, it is essential for the team's success to have effective team building, assessment of team morale and events to improve this if necessary, and finally, celebrations of success throughout the organization to reward all for implementing change.

Monitoring Results and Maintaining Improvement

Following the implementation of a change to improve a quality process, it is important to monitor and reassess whether or not the change was effective and if it continues to maintain its effectiveness. Multiple tools are in place to assist in this process. The most frequently used tools are process control charts. Control charts follow a process over time to allow identification of whether a change in the process is related to usual variation or special cause and effect. Usual variation is felt secondary to random effect while special cause variation is that which is due to outside effects on the process. The methodology requires statistical analysis to develop upper and lower limits for a process associated with a mean. Depending upon the pattern of the data, one of eight potential patterns can identify special cause variation. These were identified by Shewhart and will be discussed in depth in Chap. 33 [16, 17]. The response to special cause variation depends upon the type of variation that is present. It is important to study a process prior to implementing change to ensure that it is under control and that the lack of control following implementation is not incorrectly attributed to the change itself. Once a steady-state has been established, change can be implemented. The effect of this change can then be followed on the control chart to ensure the change has been successful. Continued monitoring via the flow chart will ensure that the improvement has been maintained. If special cause variation results from the change, further intervention may be necessary [17]. Upon completion of the initial change cycle and reestablishment of a control state, further opportunities for process improvement can be undertaken as the quality cycle repeats itself.

Image Interpretation and Reporting as an Example

One of the steps common to all of the imaging modalities considered in this text is accurate image interpretation and reporting of results. An important method to ensure accurate image interpretation is utilization of peer review. In order for this to be effective, it will be important that there be education regarding the best practices for performing image review, how to use the review in an impactful manner in a practice to change physician behavior, classification of the peer review process and utilization of the peer review process on an enterprise wide basis. The principals of a comprehensive peer review program including appropriate feedback to the interpreting physician, reporting all of the areas to the organization as a whole so that everyone can learn from the mistakes of others in a non-punitive manner, and use of continuous quality control measures to ensure that the organization as a whole is improving with ongoing peer-reviewed processes. The first step is to ensure adequate education regarding the process of peer review. It is important in this process to identify the balance between true and important errors and those which are more a matter of individual style. This requires everyone's participation and the development of a process to adjudicate differences in opinion [18].

Classifying the errors into major categories can help to identify those practices which are suitable to the greatest degree of emphasis and potential change. Working collaboratively, Duke and Emory Universities developed a classification schema including five major categories. These are failure to detect a finding, wrongly interpreted a finding as abnormal, recognize an abnormality but minimize this as normal or artifact, recognize an abnormality but assign incorrect etiology to it, or failure to recognize limitations of imaging techniques and recommendations regarding next diagnostic or treatment steps [19]. As an example of a potential mechanism to improve interpretation, computer aided abnormality detection software has been developed. The use of computer aided detection of imaging abnormalities has been shown to provide a "second opinion" of image interpretation. This can lead to an increase in false positive findings however usually increase the accuracy of the interpretation [20, 21]. Following accurate interpretation of the study, reporting templates have been utilized to promote guideline based interpretation of images. This is necessary secondary to the large number of deficits noted in reporting in a clinical setting [22]. The development of templates allows for implementation of practice guidelines and documentation of the imaging study according to those guidelines [23]. This may include the necessary information required to meet national reporting measures. Use of a structured document through using coded information such as that identified by the American College of Radiology and the American College of Cardiology allows future evaluation of the adequacy of the report as well as incorporation of the data into quality measures, databases and registries [23, 24].

This example demonstrates the process of improvement starting with identification of a process needing improvement by using data comparing to national results, development of mechanisms to evaluate and develop new processes at a local level, implementation of those measures and the potential mechanisms for evaluating the effect of the change in the future.

The Future of Quality Improvement Plans for Imaging

The role of quality improvement in all of the imaging modalities will be increasingly important as we move forward to a value based as opposed to a volume based reimbursement methodology. The development and implementation followed by ongoing monitoring with a well-established quality improvement plan will be necessary for the success of all imaging modalities [6]. It will be imperative for organizations to develop an active quality control, quality assessment and quality improvement program for all imaging modalities that has full engagement of the organization from its highest leadership to the technologist and staff performing the studies including the physician partners in the process. These programs will need to address every aspect of imaging including appropriate ordering, timely delivery, appropriate care, timely and accurate reporting and understanding of the need to exceed the expectations of all parties involved in the process.

References

1. Kruskal JB, Anderson S, Yam CS, Sosna J. Quality initiatives: strategies for establishing a comprehensive quality and performance improvement program in a radiology department. RadioGraphics. 2009;29(2):315–29.
2. Erturk SM, Ondategui-Parra S, Ros PR. Quality management in radiology: historical aspects and basic definitions. J Am Coll Radiol. 2005;2(12):985–91.
3. Kanne JP. Quality management in cardiopulmonary imaging. J Thorac Imaging. 2011;26(1): 10–7.
4. Reinertsen JL, Gosfield AG, Rupp W, Whittington JW. Engaging physicians in a shared quality agenda. IHI Innovation Series white paper. Cambridge, MA: Institute for Healthcare Improvement. [Internet]. 2007 [cited 2014 Nov 30]. Available from: http://www.ihi.org/resources/Pages/IHIWhitePapers/EngagingPhysiciansWhitePaper.aspx.
5. Kruskal JB, Eisenberg R, Sosna J, Yam CS, Kruskal JD, Boiselle PM. Quality initiatives: quality improvement in radiology: basic principles and tools requires to achieve success. RadioGraphics. 2011;31(6):1499–509.
6. Intersocietal Accreditation Commission. XXX nuclear facility quality improvement plan. [Internet]. 2012 [cited 2014 Nov 30]. Available from: www.intersocietal.org/nuclear/forms/Sample_QI_Plan.doc.
7. MacFarlane CR. ACR accreditation of nuclear medicine and PET imaging departments. J Nucl Med Technol. 2006;34(1):18–24.
8. Rubin DL. Informatics in radiology: measuring and improving quality in radiology: meeting the challenge with informatics. RadioGraphics. 2011;31(6):1499–509.
9. Tague NR. The quality toolbox. American Society for Quality. Milwaukee: Quality Press; 2005.
10. van Wagtendonk I, Smits M, Merten H, Heetveld MJ, Wagner C. Nature, causes and consequences of unintended events in surgical units. Br J Surg. 2010;97(11):1730–40.
11. van Noord I, Eikens MP, Hamersma AM, de Bruijne MC. Application of root cause analysis on malpractice claim files related to diagnostic failures. Qual Saf Health Care. 2010;19(6), e21. doi:10.1136/qshc.2008.029801. Epub 2010 Jul 14.
12. Neumann PJ, Rosen AB, Weinstein MC. Medicare and cost-effectiveness analysis. N Engl J Med. 2005;353(14):1516–22.
13. Glassman PA, Model KE, Kahan JP, Jacobson PD, Peabody JW. The role of medical necessity and cost-effectiveness in making medical decisions. Ann Intern Med. 1997;126(2):152–6.
14. Otero HJ, Rybicki FJ, Greenberg D, Neumann PJ. Twenty years of cost-effectiveness analysis in medical imaging: are we improving? Radiology. 2008;249(3):917–25.
15. Strife JL, Kun LE, Becker GJ, Dunnick NR, Bosma J, Hattery RR. The American board of radiology perspective on maintenance of certification: part IV – practice quality improvement in diagnostic radiology. AJR. 2007;188:1–4.
16. Pujar S, Calvert S, Cortina-Borja M, Chin RF, Smith RA, Cross JH, Das K, Pitt M, Scott RC. Statistical process control (SPC) – a simple objective method for monitoring seizure frequency and evaluating effectiveness of drug interventions in refractory childhood epilepsy. Epilepsy Res. 2010;91(2-3):205–13.
17. Cheung YY, Jung B, Sohn JH, Ogrinc G. Quality initiatives: statistical control charts: simplifying the analysis of data for quality improvement. RadioGraphics. 2012;32(7):2113–26.
18. Butler GJ, Forghani R. The next level of radiology peer review: enterprise-wide education and improvement. J Am Coll Radiol. 2013;10(5):349–53.
19. Provenzale JM, Kranz PG. Understanding errors in diagnostic radiology: proposal of a classification scheme and application to emergency radiology. Emerg Radiol. 2011;18(5):403–8.
20. Doi K. Computer-aided diagnosis in medical imaging: historical review, current status and future potential. Comput Med Imaging Graph. 2007;31(4-5):198–211.
21. Yoshida H, Näppi J. CAD in CT colonography without and with oral contrast agents: progress and challenges. Comput Med Imaging Graph. 2007;31(4-5):267–84.

22. Tilkemeier PL, Serber ER, Farrell MB. The nuclear cardiology report: problems, predictors, and improvement. A report from the ICANL database. J Nucl Cardiol. 2011;18((5):858–68.
23. Kahn CE, Heilbrun ME, Applegate KE. From guidelines to practice: how reporting templates promote the use of radiology practice guidelines. J Am Coll Radiol. 2013;10(4):268–73.
24. Hendel RC, Budoff MJ, Cardella JF, Chambers CE, Dent JM, Fitzgerald DM, Hodgson JM, Klodas E, Kramer CM, Stillman AE, Tilkemeier PL, Ward RP, Weingold WG, White RD, Woodward PK, ACC/AHA/ACR/ASE/ASNC/HRS/NASCI/RSNA/SAIP/SCAI/SCCT/SCMR/SIR. Key data elements and definitions for cardiac imaging: a report of the American College of Cardiology/American Heart Association task force on clinical data standards (writing committee to develop clinical data standards for cardiac imaging). Circulation. 2009;119(1):154–86.
25. Steele JR, Schomer DF. Continuous quality improvement programs provide new opportunities to drive value innovation initiatives in hospital-based radiology practices. J Am Coll Radiol. 2009;6(7):491–9.

Chapter 32
Preparation for Accreditation or Reaccreditation

Peter Tilkemeier

Abstract The process of accreditation or reaccreditation of a facility is one which insures high-quality throughout the entire imaging chain. The major accrediting bodies include The Joint Commission, the American College of Radiology, and the Inter-societal Accreditation Commission in the United States and the European Society of Cardiology in Europe. These organizations have developed a set of criteria necessary for a facility to be accredited. These include: the standards, staff training, clinical protocols, results communication, and quality improvement programs. The process is one of developing a gap analysis for the laboratory relative to the standards and addressing those gaps. This process should be one of continuous quality improvement ensuring that the facility is in a constant state of readiness with regard to the most recent standards.

Keywords Accreditation • Reaccreditation • Accrediting bodies • Continuous quality improvement • Gap analysis

Preparation for Accreditation or Reaccreditation

There are a number of steps that an organization can take to optimize their readiness for submission of an initial accreditation or reaccreditation application. There are also some steps that apply only to the reaccreditation process. The steps for success are similar among all accreditation processes independent of the accrediting body. The first step to accreditation is to decide which accrediting body best fits your clinical setting. It is important to recognize the differences among the three major accreditation organizations for advanced diagnostic imaging in the United States as those are the ones that are certified to meet the requirements for reimbursement for Medicare. The situation is somewhat different in Europe as accreditation is not a

P. Tilkemeier, MD, MMM
Department of Medicine, Greenville Health System,
701 Grove Road, Support Tower 5, Greenville, SC 29605, USA
e-mail: ptilkemeier@gmail.com

P.L. Tilkemeier et al. (eds.), *Quality Evaluation in Non-Invasive Cardiovascular Imaging*, DOI 10.1007/978-3-319-28011-0_32

Table 32.1 Comparison of accreditation and reaccreditation requirements by organization

Organization	ACR	TJC	IAC	EACVI
Modalities supported	CT, MRI, nuclear, PET	CT, MRI, nuclear, PET	CT, Echo, MRI, nuclear, PET, vascular	Echo
Initial accreditation				
Application	Yes	No	Yes	Yes
Image submission	Yes	No	Yes	Yes
Site visit	No	Yes	No	No
Reaccreditation				
Application	Yes	Online prep tool	Yes	Yes
Image submission	Yes	No	Yes	Yes
Site visit	No	Yes	No	No
Interim audit				
Audit	Yes	Yes	Yes[a]	No
Site visit	No	Yes	Yes[a]	No

CT computed tomography, *Echo* echocardiography, *MRI* magnetic resonance imaging, *Nuclear* nuclear medicine, *PET* positron emission tomography, *Vascular* non-invasive vascular imaging
[a]Randomly selected for audit or site visit

current requirement for payment. Major differences among these three organizations are reflective of the type of facility they principally serve. For example, The Joint Commission (TJC) is most commonly seen as an accrediting body for hospitals and ambulatory care centers performing advanced diagnostic imaging as the accreditation visit can be part of the usual Joint Commission patient visit [1]. Similarly, the American College of Radiology (ACR) accreditation pathway is most often seen in settings where multiple imaging modalities are present. For example, freestanding imaging centers and hospitals are prevalent in this pathway as they can accredit multiple modalities through a single source [2]. The Intersocietal Accreditation Commission (IAC) has had a greater focus in the accreditation of facilities performing cardiac and vascular imaging [3]. As a result of this their principal constituency is the private office setting. To assist the facility in making the right choice for accreditation, it is important to get a copy of the standards from each accrediting organization and review them to assess which accreditation organization is going to offer the most beneficial pathway for the facility. Details of the differences among all the organizations offering accreditation as shown in Table 32.1.

When reviewing the accreditation standards of each organization important things to additionally note are the deadlines and timelines for submission and expiration dates. It will be important to ensure that these coordinate with the timelines for other projects that may be occurring in the imaging facility. Additionally, consideration should be given for a facility which desires to harmonize reaccreditation in existing modalities with a new modality accreditation. Having selected the appropriate accreditation organization, the next step would be an in-depth review of the requirements of the application process as some may require significant lead time in order to meet them prior to submission. Many facilities have found it helpful to "reverse engineer" the application process from the deadline backward to establish important milestones in the submission process. Examples include ensuring appropriate board certification, licensure or continuing education requirements that are required prior to submission that all can require significant lead time to accomplish. If reimbursement is tied to accreditation, allowing an opportunity to respond to requests for additional information prior to the deadline in case accreditation is not granted on first application is also an important consideration. The review process once the application is completed varies between the organizations dependent upon their philosophy. TJC does not require an application and bases their decision upon the site visit with subsequent final notification of results in approximately 4–6 weeks. The ACR and IAC approach requires submission of materials, review of those materials by staff followed by peer review and then recommendation to the governing body for final determination of accreditation status.

All of the accreditation organizations, whether in the United States or Europe, have provided access to their standards to afford the facility the ability to create a checklist for submission [4–13]. Many facilities find it extremely helpful to appoint an individual to lead the accreditation and or reaccreditation process, someone with excellent organizational skills and an ability to motivate everyone in the facility towards completion of their individual requirements. Working from a copy of the application requirements and knowledge of the facility applying for accreditation, it is helpful to create a gap analysis to establish those areas where documentation, training or processes may not be meeting the standard. An improvement plan to close the gap(s) can then be put in place to ensure success when the application is submitted.

There are five major areas common to all of the accreditation organizations that contribute to the delays in achieving accreditation. The first of these is non adherence to standards. The standards include requirements for staff training, protocols for testing, imaging equipment performance or the contents of the reports. It is necessary to understand the standards of the accreditation organization that has been selected implicitly. Language such as must or required imply full compliance with the standard is necessary for accreditation to be granted, should, may or suggested implies that there is some degree of variability allowed in the response. Attention to this level of detail will help ensure success in the application process.

The second area of concern is staff training. Whether it be documentation of initial training including board certification and licensure to more frequently, lack of adequate documentation regarding continuing education that is relevant to the field for either the physician or technologist. For example, CME credit for attending an interventional cardiology conference is most likely not relevant to the accreditation of a nuclear cardiology facility. Efforts are underway to facilitate the use of continuing education credits for multiple purposes simultaneously such as maintenance of licensure, maintenance of certification and accreditation. This should help ease the burden of continuing education credits required for accreditation.

Ensuring compliance with clinical protocols is a third major area of concern. As most accreditation standards are based on published guidelines and expert opinion, it is imperative to ensure that these are implemented in the facility. Whether it be the number of required images or method of acquisition of those images for a vascular study, appropriate radiation dosimetry for a study utilizing ionizing radiation, or attention to appropriate selection of patients for the study, attention to protocols and ensuring they are up to date and specific to the facility is an important marker of quality within the facility.

The inability to communicate results in a timely, uniform and succinct fashion compliant with the standards can be a major source of delay in the accreditation process. Utilizing different templates for every physician can certainly raise concern from the review perspective. Given that the reports are critical to so many functions; documenting what was performed, the source of billing information, and conveying the clinical results of the study, significant attention should be placed on the report format and content by the facility. Reporting errors were a major source of delaying accreditation in a recent study [14].

The fifth and final area of concern is the facility's quality improvement program. A robust quality improvement program is essential to ensuring initial and ongoing accreditation of a facility. A high performing quality improvement process demonstrates that a facility is focused on continual improvement and ensuring compliance with evolving guidelines and standards. Numerous chapters in this book are dedicated to the quality improvement process with specific emphasis in each modality. From an overall viewpoint it is helpful to consider the perspectives of those using the facility-the patient, the referring physician and the staff. Numerous examples of potential quality improvement programs are available electronically [15].

Reaccreditation of facilities is focused on ensuring the facility remains up-to-date regarding implementation of guidelines and standards for the entire imaging process. This includes the same five major areas of interest noted earlier in this chapter. Additionally, special emphasis should be placed on commentary and feedback from the prior accreditation visit. Independent of the accreditation organization, this is a uniform area of focus at the time of reaccreditation. Other areas of interest are the updates to standards that have occurred since the prior accreditation date. Knowledge of and adherence to these updates demonstrates the facility's ongoing commitment to quality imaging. A helpful tool for the facility can be to retain a copy of the standards that were in place at the time of the prior accreditation evaluation as a baseline for comparison against updates to the standards as they occur. Ongoing adherence to standards must be a continuous process, not one of updating all the facility's policies and procedures every 3 years to be compliant with current standards when accreditation is due [16]. This process of continuous quality improvement is actually much easier to achieve and ensures ongoing highest-quality patient care as opposed to the every 3 year major overhaul approach to ensuring a facility's ongoing accreditation.

As part of the philosophy that accreditation should be a continuous process, all of the accreditation organizations have moved towards implementation of an intra-cycle assessment of compliance with the accreditation standards. This can be performed either through an audit of these laboratories processes electronically or via an on-site visit. The usual cycle for accreditation is 3 years with the intra-cycle visit occurring somewhere between 12 and 24 months. It is therefore essential for the facility to be performing continuous quality improvement to ensure ongoing compliance with the most current set of guidelines and standards of practice.

The accreditation and reaccreditation process is an in-depth one, however, it is designed with this degree of depth and breadth to ensure that the patient and referring physician get the highest quality imaging to assess and answer the clinical question. Structured constant contact with the accrediting organization will ensure that the facility has access to the most recent standards. The accrediting organizations are committed to an open communication process with the facilities in all steps of either the initial accreditation or ongoing accreditation of the facility.

References

1. Accreditation handbook for diagnostic imaging centers. Oak Brook: Joint Commission Resources; 2011. Feb [cited 26 Jul 2014]. Available from: http://www.jointcommission.org/assets/1/18/2011_IMG__Hdbk.pdf.
2. MacFarlane CR. ACR accreditation of nuclear medicine and PET imaging department. J Nucl Med Technol. 2006;34(1):18–24.
3. Intersocietal Accreditation Commission. Getting started with IAC accreditation. [Internet]. 2014. [Cited 26 Jul 2014]. Available from: http://www.intersocietal.org/iac/accreditation/gettingstarted.htm.
4. Standards for diagnostic imaging services. Oak Brook: Joint Commission Resources; 2014.
5. American College of Radiology. CT Accreditation program requirements. [Internet]. 2013. [Cited 26 Jul 2014]. Available from: http://www.acr.org/~/media/ACR/Documents/Accreditation/CT/Requirements.pdf.
6. American College of Radiology. MRI Accreditation program requirements. [Internet]. 2013. [Cited 26 Jul 2014]. Available from: http://www.acr.org/~/media/ACR/Documents/Accreditation/MRI/Requirements.pdf.
7. American College of Radiology. Nuclear medicine accreditation program requirements. [Internet]. 2014. [Cited 26 Jul 2014]. Available from: http://www.acr.org/~/media/ACR/Documents/Accreditation/NuclearMedicinePET/Requirements.pdf.
8. American College of Radiology. PET Accreditation program requirements. [Internet]. 2014. [Cited 18 Oct 2014]. Available from: http://www.acr.org/~/media/ACR/Documents/Accreditation/NuclearMedicinePET/PETRequirements.pdf.
9. Intersocietal Accreditation Commission. IAC standards and guidelines for vascular testing accreditation. [Internet]. 2013. [Cited 26 Jul 2014]. Available from: http://www.intersocietal.org/vascular/main/vascular_standards.htm.
10. Intersocietal Accreditation Commission. IAC standards and guidelines for nuclear/PET accreditation. [Internet]. 2012. [Cited 26 Jul 2014]. Available from: http://www.intersocietal.org/nuclear/main/nuclear_standards.htm.
11. Intersocietal Accreditation Commission. IAC Standards and guidelines for adult echocardiography accreditation and the IAC Standards and guidelines for pediatric echocardiography accreditation. [Internet]. 2014. [Cited 26 Jul 2014]. Available from: http://www.intersocietal.org/echo/main/echo_standards.htm.
12. Intersocietal Accreditation Commission. IAC standards and guidelines for MRI accreditation. [Internet]. 2014. [Cited 26 Jul 2014]. Available from: http://www.intersocietal.org/mri/main/mri_standards.htm.
13. European Society of Cardiology. Accreditation of echocardiographic laboratories in transthoracic, transesophageal and stress echocardiography. [Internet]. 2014. [Cited 26 Jul 2014]. Available from: http://www.escardio.org/communities/EACVI/accreditation/echocardiography/lab/Pages/welcome.aspx.

14. Tilkemeier PL, Serber ER, Farrell MB. The nuclear cardiology report: problems, predictors, and improvement. A report from the ICANL database. J Nucl Cardiol. 2011;18(5):858–68.
15. Intersocietal Accreditation Commission. IAC Nuclear/PET: reaccreditation simplified [Internet]. 2013. [Cited 26 Jul 2014]. Available from: http://www.intersocietal.org/nuclear/ondemand/IACNuclear_ReaccreditationWebinar.pdf.
16. Cohen M. Maintenance of certification and accreditation: a call for daily deeds rather than periodic paper pushing. J Nucl Cardiol. 2010;17(2):342–3.

Chapter 33
Reporting Quality and Determining Benchmarks

Peter Tilkemeier

Abstract The reporting of data regarding a facility's quality measures is a complex one requiring excellent and effective communications to everyone involved. The methodology chosen to present and display the data can have significant impact on its interpretation and application in the clinical setting. There are a number of types of displays available including: tables, bar graphs, scatter diagrams, Pareto charts, radar charts and statistical process control charts. Each of these chart types will be explored in depth. Choosing comparators or data for bench marking is an important choice within an organization depending upon its philosophy regarding process improvement. A number of sources are available for gathering these data. The reporting of a facility's quality of care and comparison to bench marking data will be ever more important as medicine progresses towards a system that is more focused on quality rather than quantity.

Keywords Data reporting • Graphical display • Process control charts • Comparators • Benchmarks

Reporting Quality and Determining Benchmarks

The steps that are necessary for developing a quality improvement program have been previously outlined. As it was noted, specific outcome measures were selected for their importance to the processes in the facility. A component that is essential for the plan's success is the ability to communicate the results in an effective manner to all parties involved. This includes physician and technical staff, quality oversight committees within the facility, patients and payers. The mechanisms for reporting the outcomes will vary depending upon the type of measure being evaluated and the desired effect. These measures are important because it is probable that

---

P. Tilkemeier, MD, MMM
Department of Medicine, Greenville Health System,
701 Grove Road, Support Tower 5, Greenville, SC 29605, USA
e-mail: ptilkemeier@gmail.com

P.L. Tilkemeier et al. (eds.), *Quality Evaluation in Non-Invasive Cardiovascular Imaging*, DOI 10.1007/978-3-319-28011-0_33

other organizations are evaluating a facility's quality data and will be utilizing that to assist in paying for performance to ensure the highest value for the healthcare dollar [1].

Data can be reported utilizing absolute numbers, percentages, averages or ratios. Each of these measurement types affords a different look at the data. For example, if one were examining appropriate use criteria implementation in the facility, the impression from the data would vary depending upon the measurement type. Different conclusions are drawn when data are presented as: there are ten rarely appropriate studies, 10 % of xxx (number) studies were rarely appropriate, an average of rarely appropriate studies over a month was 10 %, or the ratio of rarely appropriate to appropriate studies was one in ten. The absolute number gives the reviewer no relative sense as to the severity of the problem as there is no evaluation of the total volume in which these ten studies occurred. In the example just given, the percentage analysis allows a better sense of the effect of rarely appropriate studies in the facility as the percentage allows evaluation of both the numerator and denominator. It is important in this case to ensure that the denominator matches the evaluative criteria established to determine the numerator. The average of 10 % rarely appropriate studies allows a different evaluation of the data in that it will allow determination of outliers. If the system average was 10 % and one site was 15 % and another 5 %, this would be a very different data set with a resultant change in the action plan. The use of ratios is helpful if there is a comparison to be drawn between two facilities. Similar ratios would suggest similar outcomes from process improvements [2].

The display of the data will need to vary depending upon the data being analyzed, the complexity of the analysis, and the timeframe for which the data are being measured. Tabular reports or bar graphs are most helpful for examining single or multiple points in time. Bar graphs allow a visual representation of multiple variables at similar or multiple points in time. Scatter diagrams allow presentation of all of the data points along with developing the concept of a correlation of the two variables in the data set. This correlation can be in either a positive, negative or random pattern. The Pareto chart is a display that allows an analysis of the cumulative effect of processes, focusing the organization on those which are going to most likely have the greatest impact on improving performance. When evaluating complex interrelated systems results, radar charts can be most useful. For example the relationship between staff compensation, patient satisfaction and follow-up visit "no show" rates across a multi-site practice would best be examined using a radar chart as it allows analysis of relative strengths and weaknesses and the interdependency of each variable to the others [3].

Once a particular quality parameter has been defined as well as the expected performance measure, the use of statistical process control charts can be very helpful in analyzing variance and performance over time. Process control charts display the performance on a single variable over time. If enough data are available such that a normal distribution results this allows calculation of standard deviations, which can then be utilized to calculate upper and lower control limits. The usual display of these data is the utilization of the mean as a central line with either two or three standard deviations being used as the upper and lower confidence limits above and below the central line. Significant trends are those for which at least seven of the data points exhibit a pattern, such as all seven greater than the mean (process improving), less than the mean (process declining), a single data point above or below the upper or lower confidence limits. This would suggest that the process is out of control most likely due to special cause variation, usually resulting from a change in process. Variation within the upper and lower confidence limits results from common cause variation which occurs in all processes over time [4, 5].

A single example that is common to all imaging, appropriate use criteria, will be used to explore each of these graphical displays in greater depth. As many are familiar, appropriate use criteria were developed in response to the perception that overutilization of technology has resulted in an increase in healthcare delivery costs and inappropriate studies being performed [6]. As of 2014, the three AUC categories that have been agreed upon are: Appropriate; Usually appropriate; and rarely appropriate. For all of the following data and examples, a hypothetical data set will be utilized. An example of a bar graph or data table for demonstration of AUC results would be an interdepartmental comparison of the number of rarely appropriate studies within a single timeframe. Multiple vertical bars could easily represent different time frames. An example bar graph with its corresponding tabular data is demonstrated in Fig. 33.1. Figure 33.1a demonstrates this data without a national benchmark displayed and Fig. 33.1b includes national benchmark data. The resulting interpretation can be significantly different. In panel A, it is clear that the all departments are doing quite well, however when the data is evaluated in panel B, it is clear there is significant room for improvement in the Family Medicine department.

A scatter plot demonstrating the rate of rarely appropriate studies in a region by facility volume is shown in Fig. 33.2. A scatter plot allows visualization of the degree of variability of rarely appropriate studies in a facility based on volume. Additionally, it allows analysis of the data in such a way to determine if there is a positive or negative trend associated with appropriateness and increasing facility volume. The hypothetical data demonstrates a positive trend for this relationship.

The use of the Pareto chart to evaluate the most common diagnoses associated with rarely appropriate studies is demonstrated in Fig. 33.3. From a single facility's appropriate use data, the clinical indications associated with rarely appropriate studies were compiled. These are displayed in decreasing frequency from left to right on the x-axis. A summation of the percentages comprises the data displayed by the line. This type of graphical analysis allows a facility to evaluate those clinical indications which led to ordering of 80 % of the rarely appropriate studies. This would allow focused education regarding ordering of these studies within this facility.

A radar chart could be useful to evaluate multiple cause-and-effect relationships that could be associated with rarely appropriate studies. An example is demonstrated in Fig. 33.4. If a system wants to evaluate the interdependence of multiple variables, such as facility where the study was performed, specialty of the ordering physician, if the study was performed for preoperative evaluation, patient age less than 30 and history of prior coronary events on the rate of rarely appropriate studies the radar

a

	Q1	Q2	Q3	Q4
Medicine	4.3	2.4	2	1.6
Surgery	2.5	4.4	2	3
Anesthesia	3.5	1.8	3	3.2
Family med	4.5	2.8	5	4.4

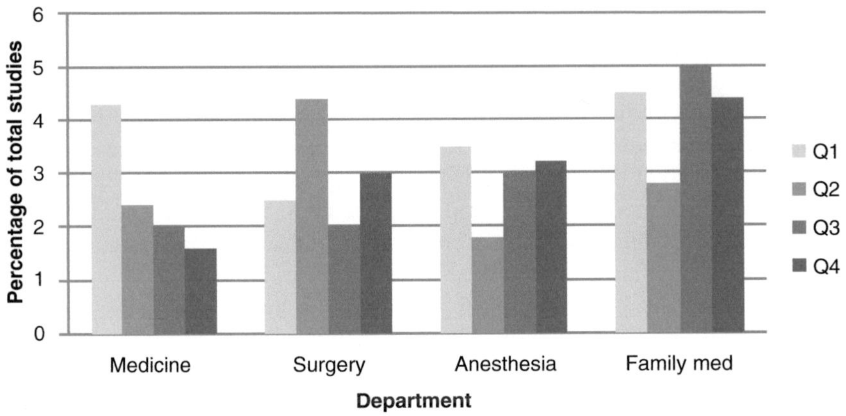

b

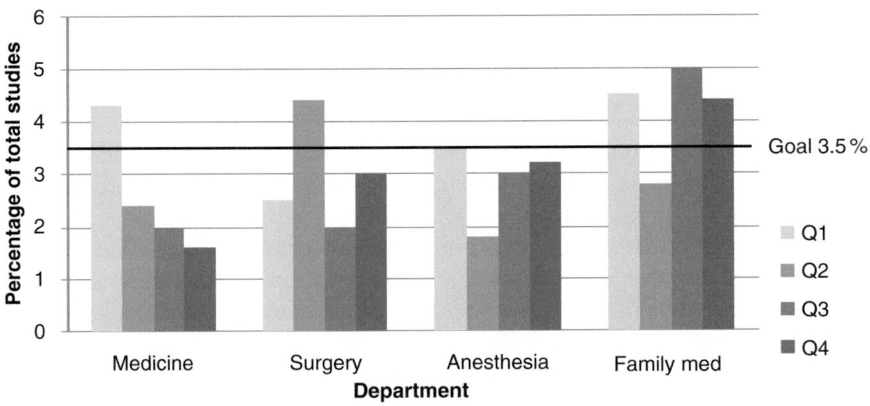

Fig. 33.1 (**a**) Bar graph with tabular data demonstrating the percentage of the total number of studies that were rarely appropriate over a four quarter time frame (**b**) The same bar graph shown in (**a**) with a line defining national benchmark data for comparison of performance

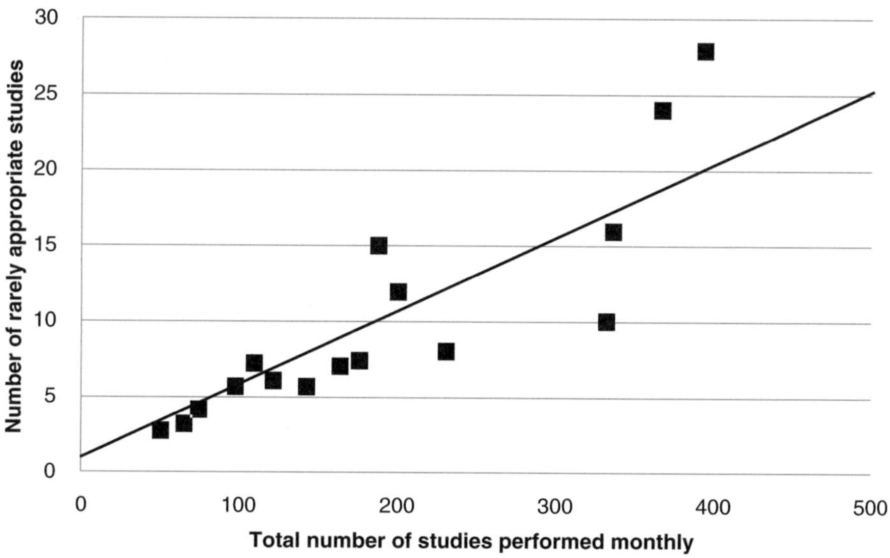

Fig. 33.2 Scatter plot format with a regression line evaluating the number of rarely appropriate studies relative to monthly volume

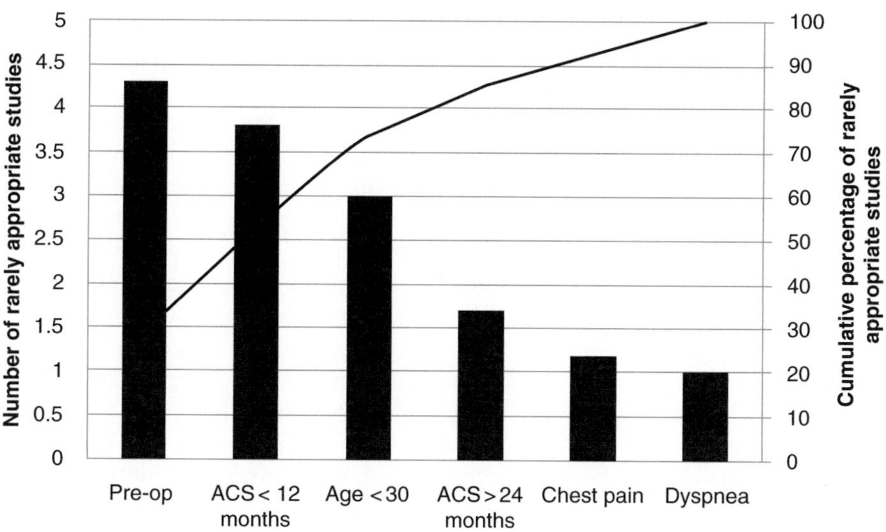

Fig. 33.3 Pareto chart showing the relationships among the number of rarely appropriate studies, reason for study and the contribution to the cumulative percentage of rarely appropriate studies

plot in Fig. 33.4 could be a potential result. The hypothetical data displayed here should focus the system's attention on patient age less than 30 and preoperative evaluation as major areas for improvement. This example is the same data set that was displayed in the Pareto chart that has now been expanded to include factors beyond common diagnoses and indications.

Statistical process control charts for the rate of rarely appropriate studies for a single facility are shown in Fig. 33.5. The average rate for the facility is displayed as the centerline with the upper and lower confidence intervals set at two standard deviations. The data displayed here shows that the process is in control with common cause variation occurring. The data displayed in Fig. 33.6 is from a lab with a decreasing trend in rarely appropriate studies over time. This is the case as the last seven data points all show a decline in the percentage of rarely appropriate studies. Figure 33.7 demonstrates that the percentage of rarely appropriate studies has had significant special variation due to one of the data points being above the upper confidence limit. Investigation as to why this occurred would be indicated.

In the context of understanding the different methods for reporting quality data, if one is to determine if a quality improvement program is necessary, comparison or benchmarking data for these quality indicators needs to be part of the analysis. In order for comparison or benchmarking data to be relevant, the facility utilizing the data must have evaluated the data source to ensure its comparability to the facility's own data. For example, it would not be recommended to utilize comparison or benchmark data from a large academic health system to evaluate a small private practice performing cardiovascular imaging. There would be inherent differences in referral patterns, utilization rates, use of decision-support algorithms and multiple other variables. At the same time, however, this may be the only data available to use as a comparable site or benchmark for comparison. Many of the current registries and databases that are available for assessing quality measures in cardiovascular imaging have wide enough participation that they are able to perform this level of matching when generating an individual facility report. For example, the National Cardiovascular Data Registry sponsored by the American College of Cardiology, divides their reports into similar sized hospitals and major hospital types such as university affiliated or non-affiliated. This allows some degree of certainty that the report compares your data to similar organizations with regard to overall performance. Hypothetically, this type of comparison allows the facility to understand how it ranks relative to other facility's performance. The use of comparative data allows a facility to compare their results to that of similar facilities while use of a benchmark is a comparison to the data of the best performing facility available in the data set to which all should be striving. Either can be used as long as there is clear understanding by the organization using the data and the intent of that use, driving to improvement within the group or to become the highest performing facility, the decision as to whether to use comparison or benchmark data can be made. The choice as to whether to use comparison or benchmark data will also be driven by the organization's philosophy regarding process improvement and if there is value in achieving best in class as opposed to best in a particular area or region.

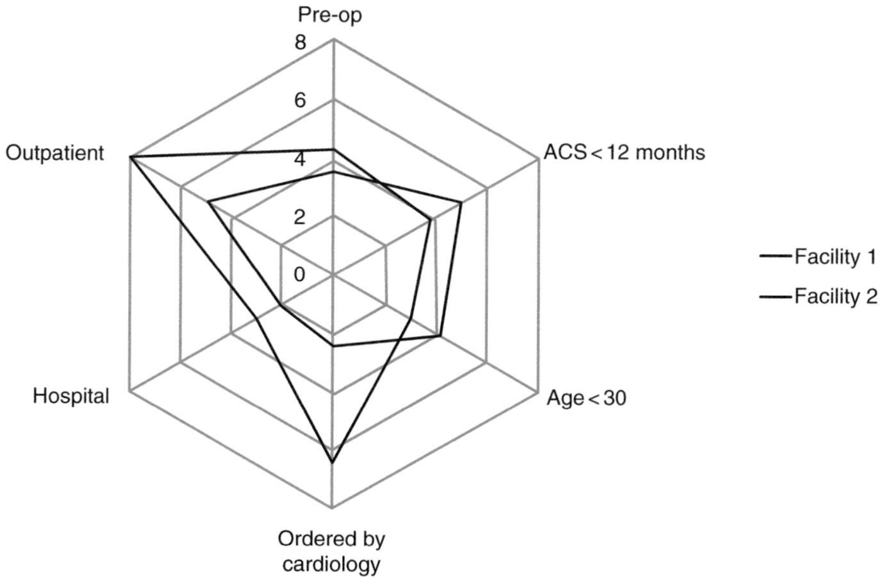

Fig. 33.4 Radar chart evaluating the differences in cause and effect on the percentage of rarely appropriate studies between two facilities

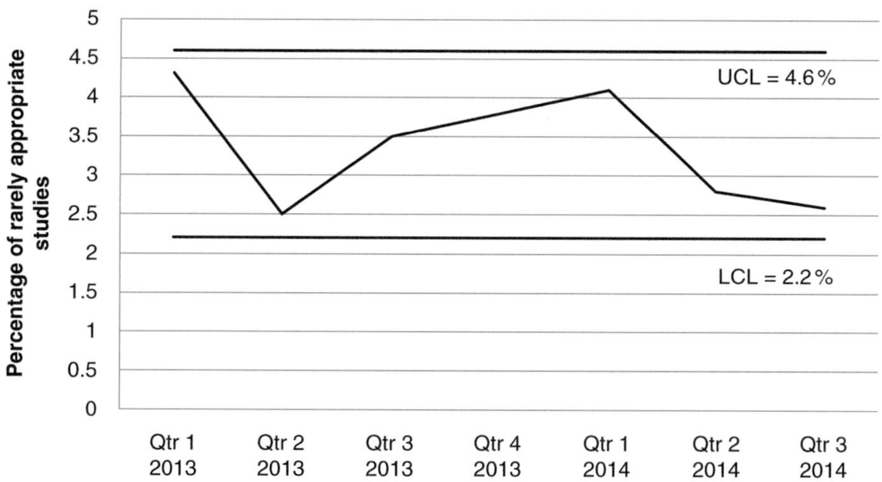

Fig. 33.5 Statistical process control chart for a single facility's percentage of rarely appropriate studies over time. The graph displays a process in control

There are multiple sources for comparison or benchmarking data. These include governmental such as the Center for Medicare Services, societal, as demonstrated by the National Cardiovascular Data Registry of the American College of Cardiology, public domain in the case of The Commonwealth Fund and its website www.whynotthebest.org, and private organizations such as the Medical Group

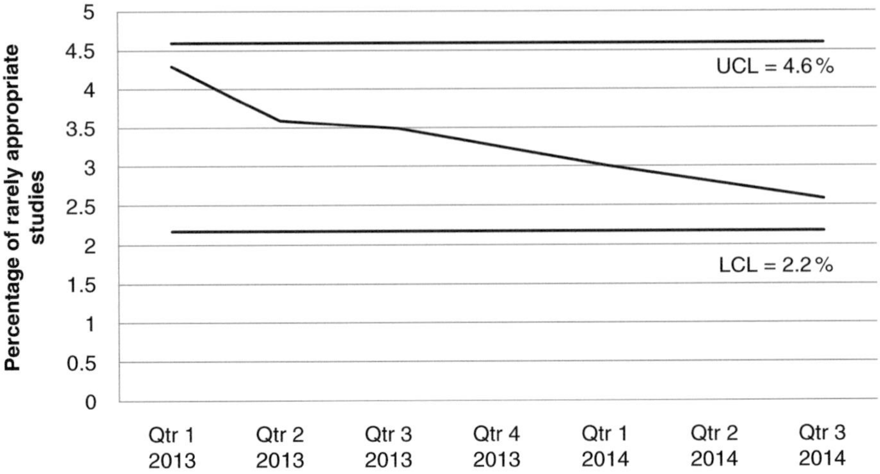

Fig. 33.6 Statistical process control chart for a single facility's percentage of rarely appropriate studies over time. The graph displays a process improving over time with a decreasing percentage

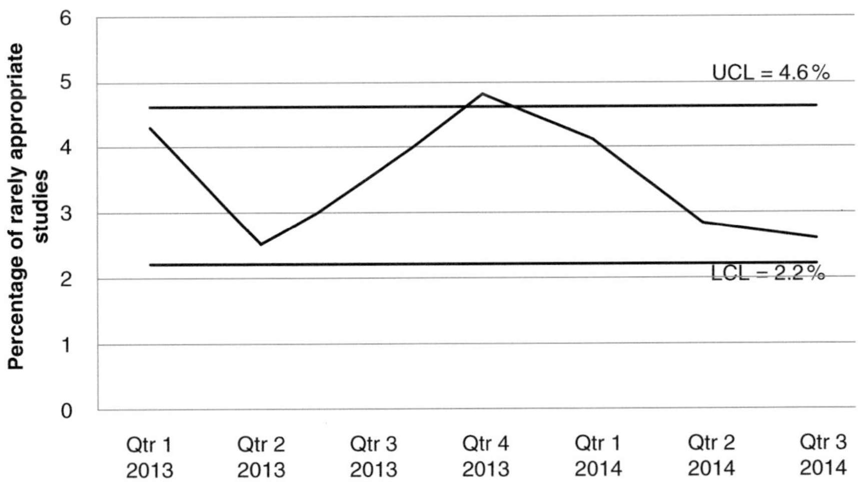

Fig. 33.7 Statistical process control chart for a single facility's percentage of rarely appropriate studies over time. The graph displays a process with significant variation warranting further investigation

Management Association or The Joint Commission [7–11]. Similar benchmarks are available from the European Society of Cardiology for the quality indicators considered important to their leadership [12]. As was mentioned previously, it is important when using these benchmarks to understand the demographics of the participating facilities. Additionally, as was noted previously it is important to understand the characteristics of the denominator for the cases included in the benchmark for the indicator the facility has chosen to evaluate.

In summary, numerous methodologies for reporting quality data have been evaluated and demonstrated. Some of the potential areas for error in applying this data have been explored. Mechanisms to best identify sources for benchmarking or comparing with a particular facility and its quality data to determine if a quality improvement program is truly necessary or if ongoing quality monitoring is sufficient have been discussed. It is clear that everyone will be evaluating the facility's quality of care delivery particularly in regard to high expense items such as cardiovascular imaging. In the evolving world of healthcare delivery today, quality becomes an ever increasing component of payment for services [13–15]. It behooves every facility, not only for those in the United States but also globally, to have extensive knowledge regarding their perceived quality and to implement quality improvement programs where the data indicate this is necessary [16].

References

1. Seidel RL, Nash DB. Paying for performance in diagnostic imaging: current challenges and future prospects. J Am Coll Radiol. 2004;1:952–6.
2. Spath PL. Introduction to healthcare quality management. 2nd ed. Chicago: Health Administration Press; 2013. p. 74–109. Chapter 4, Evaluation performance.
3. Johnson SP, McLaughlin CP. Measurement and statistical analysis in CQI. In: Mclaughlin CP, Kaluzny AD, editors. Continuous quality improvement in healthcare. Gaithersburg: Aspen Publishers; 1999.
4. Schmaltz S, Loeb JM, Hanold LS, Koss RG. Statistical tools for quality improvement. In: Ransom ER, Joshi MS, Nash DB, Ransom SB, editors. The healthcare quality book. 2nd ed. Chicago: Health Administration Press; 2011.
5. Provost LP, Murray SK. The health care data guide: learning from data for improvement. San Francisco: Jossey-Bass; 2011.
6. Hendel RC. Utilization management of cardiovascular imaging, pre-certification and appropriateness. JACC Cardiovasc Imaging. 2008;1(2):241–8.
7. American College of Cardiology Foundation. National cardiovascular data registry. [Internet]. 2014. [Cited 26 Jul 2014]. Available from: https://www.ncdr.com/webncdr/.
8. Centers for Medicare and Medicaid Services. Quality measures and performance standards. [Internet]. 2014. [Cited 26 Jul 2014]. Available from: http://www.cms.gov/Medicare/Medicare-Fee-for-Service-Payment/sharedsavingsprogram/Quality_Measures_Standards.html.
9. The Commonwealth Fund. Why not the best? [Internet]. 2014. [Cited 26 Jul 2014]. Available from: http://www.whynotthebest.org.
10. Medical Group Management Association. Benchmarking resources. [Internet]. 2014. [Cited 26 Jul 2014]. Available from: http://www.mgma.com/industry-data/all-data-resources/benchmarking-tools-from-mgma-surveys.
11. Joint Commission Resources. 2014 Core measure sets. [Internet]. 2014. [Cited 26 Jul 2014]. Available from: http://www.jointcommission.org/core_measure_sets.aspx.
12. Executive Agency for Health and Consumers. The EURHOBOP project [internet]. 2013. [Updated 3 Sep 2013; cited 26 Jul 2014]. Available from: http://www.eurhobop.eu.

13. Tynan A, Berenson RA, Christianson JB. Health plans target advanced imaging services: cost, quality and safety concerns prompt renewed oversight. Issue Brief Cent Stud Health Syst Chang. 2008;118:1–4.
14. Goldsmith J. The future of radiology in the new health care paradigm: the Moreton lecture. J Am Coll Radiol. 2011;8(3):159–63.
15. Krishnaraj A, Weinreb JC, Ellenbogen PH, Patti JA, Hillman BJ. Radiology in 2022: challenges and opportunities in the coming decade – proceedings of the 12th annual ACR forum. J Am Coll Radiol. 2013;10(1):15–20.
16. Unger F. Health is wealth: considerations to European healthcare. Contrib Sec Biol Med Sci. 2012;33(1):9–14.

Chapter 34
Additional Quality Activities and the Future

Peter Tilkemeier

Abstract As medicine and particularly cardiovascular procedures move into the future of value based strategies, cardiovascular imaging will need to provide documented value. For this to occur, robust quality will become an important aspect to reduce unnecessary downstream testing and provide the best diagnostic accuracy. Future mechanisms to demonstrate and improve quality are constantly evolving. These include the use of behavioral theory and feedback, team based quality improvement initiatives, utilization of online learning communities, public reporting mechanisms and the development of registries for cardiac imaging data. These initiatives will require further refinement and implementation as part of electronic health records to improve their accuracy and efficiency. Utilization of the data from these tools will play important roles as we develop clinical decision support systems that can be implemented at the point of care. This will ensure the highest value imaging based upon individual patient characteristics as part of population analysis.

Keywords Quality improvement • Value • Behavioral feedback • Learning communities • Public reporting • Data registries

As society moves from volume based to value based reimbursement models for the delivery of medical care and as a result of this change in the current paradigm, cardiac imaging will no longer be a "profit" center for a facility. Cardiovascular imaging will now become part of the cost of care delivery for a patient and a patient population. The change in care model delivery is coming quickly through government mandated changes as noted by the Department of Health and Human Services initiatives detailed in Fig. 34.1. The Department of Health and Human Services is particularly encouraging the expansion of these initiatives into the broader insurance marketplace through its creation of a Healthcare Payment Learning and Action Network [1]. In order to effectively respond to these types of initiatives, it will be important that cardiovascular imaging develop new tools that

P. Tilkemeier, MD, MMM
Department of Medicine, Greenville Health System,
701 Grove Road Support Tower 5, Greenville, SC 29605, USA
e-mail: ptilkemeier@gmail.com

P.L. Tilkemeier et al. (eds.), *Quality Evaluation in Non-Invasive Cardiovascular Imaging*, DOI 10.1007/978-3-319-28011-0_34

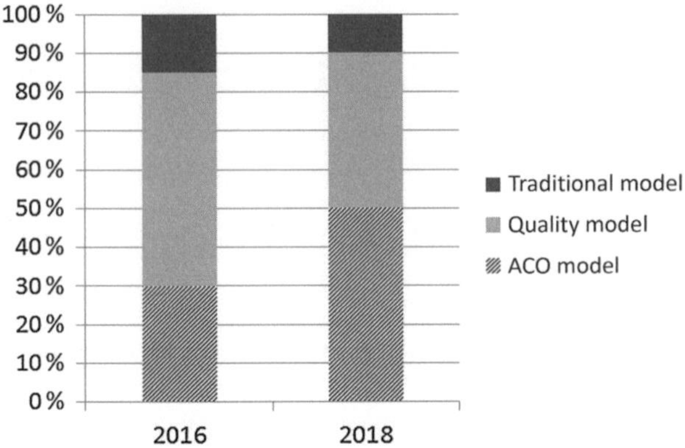

Fig. 34.1 The rapid progression of Centers for Medicare Services changes in payment methodology to move from volume to value [1]

allow us to assess quality and value of imaging in a real or close to real time network. Additionally, a recent Institute of Medicine report defined a "learning healthcare system" that would provide real time data and feedback to physicians and other healthcare providers allowing continuous quality improvement at the point of care [2]. Furthermore, those involved in the process understand that this is the beginning and there is a long journey before we begin reaching goals. We must begin to implement tools that put our guidelines into practice. The existence of published evidence-based guidelines does not guarantee their implementation in clinical practice. It is only through ongoing processes and continual feedback to the healthcare team providing a service that quality improvement can be successful [3, 4].

As guidelines are developed and placed into practice, it is important to recognize the level of evidence of the documents utilized in their development. It is also important to acknowledge that gaps in guidelines may be present due to a lack of sufficient data to allow the writing committees to develop consensus. Development of a mechanism to ensure that guidelines and measures can be meaningfully created for those technologies that are not supported by class I, level A evidence will be necessary, as this degree of supporting evidence exists for only a small portion of today's guidelines. The American College of Cardiology Foundation and the American Heart Association have published a methodology for the development of quality measures for cardiovascular technology. This includes a proposed framework for the development of quality measures for therapeutic procedures as well as measures for cardiovascular technology. With regard to therapeutic procedures the four steps have been developed and include: preprocedural evaluation of patient characteristics, determination of short-term (technical) and long-term (clinical) success, communication of results including outcomes, and outcomes associated with the procedure both positive and negative. For cardiovascular technology, appropriate use measures and structure and safety measures can be developed through use of the existing evidence, review of the current appropriate use criteria documents and ensuring concordance of multiple documents that may address similar technological

Table 34.1 New directions in quality improvement tools

Methods	Tools needed to implement
Team based quality improvement	Quality management tools, team involvement in process
Focused continuous quality improvement initiatives	Quality management tools, infrastructure to identify areas for improvement
Public reporting and benchmarking	Validated performance measures, standardized data submission, data attribution, cost analysis and risk adjustment models
Implementation of behavioral theory with immediate benchmark feedback	Behavioral interventions to change behavior, data collection tools consistent with benchmark data
Use of immediate benchmark feedback for individual practitioners	Integration of EHR data with national databases
Development of learning communities	Infrastructure for learning community to acquire, analyze and share data and methods
Registries with centralization of data and collaboration	Structured data, data reporting standards, registry structure

implementations followed by review and publication. Each of the performance measures should be developed in response to a defined gap in care or quality issue and should be developed in a number of practice settings to ensure widespread applicability [5].

There are a number of projects that allow a glimpse into the future of quality improvement in practice. These include team based quality improvement, focused continuous quality improvement initiatives, public reporting and bench marking, the implementation of behavioral theory with immediate benchmark feedback, use of immediate benchmark feedback for individual practitioners, the development of learning communities, and the utility and value of registries with centralization of data and collaboration across sites and specialties as a mechanism to improve quality. Each of these will be examined separately and are summarized in Table 34.1.

Team-Based Quality Improvement

It is becoming clear that quality improvement is a team sport. Everyone involved in a particular process must be identified and participating in any efforts for improvement. Utilizing techniques outlined earlier such as Lean and Six Sigma, the team based approach can be highly successful in implementing change in all aspects of clinical care. Kanne outlines the important members of the team and utilization of data to drive quality improvement. Potential projects he identified ranged from radiation safety, image interpretation, reporting of results and communication of critical results. He additionally includes the importance of the adoption of a culture of quality and safety in a non-blaming organization [6].

Focused Continuous Quality Improvement Initiatives

Utilization of focused continuous quality improvement initiatives will be an important mechanism to continue to improve quality in an ongoing manner as we move forward. Baseline information is utilized to develop the scope of an initiative for quality improvement. Multiple studies have demonstrated the success of a multistep intervention with ongoing feedback to promote continued quality improvement. Following identification of the need for quality improvement, the first step involves ensuring the entire team understands and agrees with the need for improvement. Second, process change needs to be implemented in a stepwise manner to ensure the ability to assess the effect of each of the interventions. Following the implementation of a new process, follow-up with feedback to the group is necessary to ensure that significant change has occurred. One of the potential positive outcomes from this process includes greater staff autonomy and increased potential for the staff to be functioning at their highest level of training and qualification. Ongoing reevaluation of the effectiveness of the intervention is necessary until it becomes part of the routine clinical practice within a facility or healthcare system [4, 7].

Public Reporting and Bench Marking

The use of public reporting of outcomes can be a powerful tool in quality improvement, and its use is increasing across medicine. The methodology can, however, have unintended consequences. Regarding any measures that are publicly reported it is important to note a number of characteristics to ensure their success. Public reporting programs should be designed to promote quality improvement, utilize performance measures that are scientifically validated, utilize reporting measures that are developed in partnership with practicing physicians, understand the importance of covariates which may affect performance and that are audited frequently, utilize a standardized submission process for all participating sites, correctly attribute and report the data at a meaningful level of accountability, understand the potential impact of unintended consequences, integrate quality and cost, use similar and valid cost measurement analysis methods, and finally provide no incentive for poor quality care. As has been found in public reporting efforts, the potential for avoiding high-risk cases when data is not adjusted can be significant and a potential down-side to such a program and patient care [8]. Implementation of public reporting programs should address this potential effect prior to implementation. Additionally to assist in putting the data into perspective, the development of national and regional databases and registries will be essential to the success of public reporting mechanisms going forward. Public reporting can certainly be a double-edged sword that when used in an appropriate manner can be very impactful on changing behaviors and quality outcomes [9].

Implementation of Behavioral Theory with Immediate Benchmark Feedback

The use of behavioral theory and immediate benchmark feedback has been shown to be quite effective in at least two programs aimed at reducing radiation exposure. It has been noted that the use of education alone is not sufficient stimulus to ensure behavioral change. There was some effect when the feedback was performed on an annual basis [10]. As part of the behavioral mechanism approach, interventions have included mandatory education and participation in the initiative, continuous education and feedback to the participants and emphasis on the importance of the change that was being addressed. The inclusion of comparative benchmark data and potential patient risk was identified as having significant impact on the overall outcome of the intervention. Education was further stratified based upon the quartile of individuals participating in the trial. Greater improvement was noted in the groups which have the greatest potential for improvement. There was some improvement in all quartiles which was potentially secondary to the Hawthorne effect (knowing you are being observed) [11, 12]. Additional benefit of a behavioral approach was noted with regard to radiation dose reduction in terms of patient and algorithm selection as well as the need for implementation of new technologies to limit radiation exposure over time. Again, required participation was necessary in all phases of this trial for success [13].

Use of Immediate Benchmark Feedback for Individual Practitioners

The use of real-time feedback compared to benchmark data may well become the norm in the future as we are able to acquire more data electronically at the time of the procedure. The Department of Veterans Affairs has utilized their clinical assessment reporting and tracking program to capture clinical information at the point of care and compare it to national data in a real-time manner such that as the clinician finishes a procedure they are provided with their data. This technology also allows centralization of outliers for review of major adverse events and unexpected complications. This simultaneous data acquisition reduces the potential for data entry errors and misinterpretation should this data need to be acquired following the procedure. As we move towards greater integration of our electronic health records and ability to share electronic data through health information exchanges the potential for real time quality improvement initiatives will increase. This will certainly be an important contributor to the ability to deliver value to the patient and system [14].

Development of Learning Communities

Another progressive methodology that could have potential impact in the future is the development of learning communities to promote improvement and widespread dissemination of quality improvement mechanisms. The American College of Cardiology through its Formation of Optimal Cardiovascular Utilization Strategies (FOCUS) program has shown the ability of such a learning community to have significant impact on appropriate use criteria and reduction of inappropriate or rarely appropriate studies. The program was developed in three parts: Part 1 involved entering patient cases to establish a baseline; Part 2 was to evaluate the data and develop and implement an action plan with quality improvement activities included; and Part 3 was reevaluation of patient cases to identify the effect of the intervention. As part of their participation in the program the physicians were required to share their findings as part of an online community. The action items that were utilized most frequently included increasing education, physician feedback, physician review meetings, education of referring physicians and the use of standardized tools to assess appropriateness. This effort continues today and has participants from across the United States in a wide range of practice demographics. Use of similar learning communities in other areas of noninvasive imaging could have significant potential impact in the future [15].

Utility and Value of Registries with Centralization of Data and Collaboration Across Sites and Specialties

As we begin to report data regarding our patients in a standardized manner the ability to centralize this data in registries becomes possible. The use of large data registries that will allow us to compare patient outcomes across regions, populations and modalities for specific indications will lead to even greater opportunities for quality improvement initiatives. The development of the ImageGuide™ registry for nuclear cardiology is an example [16, 17]. The expansion of imaging registries to multiple modalities will be important going forward. These goals were outlined as part of the American College of Cardiology-Duke University Medical Center Second Think Tank on quality in cardiovascular imaging. They specifically identified the need for creation of a multicenter imaging registry that allows for multimodality and multi-specialty participation and investigates mechanisms to incent participation at the physician and facility level. The development of such a registry will allow us to collect data necessary for prospective registry based trials, understand the gaps in knowledge and the trials necessary to fill the gaps as well as the potential for new technology to fill the gaps and truly understand the value of cardiac imaging in a new value based paradigm [18].

Summary

There are many new methods in development and the potential for greater implementation of those methods in clinical practice for quality and value improvement in noninvasive cardiac imaging. The implementation of many of these methodologies requires greater utilization of electronic data and standardized and structured data formats as part of the reporting process. Incorporation of the quality improvement process into the daily workflow has been shown to be most impactful. This process reduces the cost of data gathering, increases the data accuracy, has the greatest potential impact on modifying physician performance and as a result of these three, should support the value equation for noninvasive cardiac imaging. The potential for utilizing this data to drive decision support tools that can be utilized throughout the continuum of patient practice will have even greater impact. The degree of impact will need to be further evaluated as these tools are developed and utilized clinically.

References

1. U.S. Department of Health & Human Services. Better, smarter, healthier: in historic announcement, HHS sets clear goals and timeline for shifting Medicare reimbursements from volume to value. [Internet]. 2015 [cited 2015 Feb 22]. Available from: http://www.hhs.gov/news/press/2015pres/01/20150126a.html.
2. Committee on the Learning Health Care System in America. Smith M, Saunders R, Stuckhardt L, McGinnis JM, editors. Best care at lower cost: the path to continuous learning health care in America. Washington, DC: The National Academies Press. [Internet]. 2012 [cited 2015 Feb 25]. Available from: http://books.nap.edu/openbook.php?record_id=13444.
3. Martin RP. Quality is job one, and our patients and our profession deserve it. J Am Soc Echocardiogr. 2011;24(11):1180–2.
4. Johnson TV, Rose GA, Fenner DJ, Rozario NL. Improving appropriate Use of echocardiography and single-proton emission computed tomographic myocardial perfusion imaging: a continuous quality improvement initiative. J Am Soc Echocardiogr. 2014;27(7):749–57.
5. Bonow RO, Douglas PS, Buxton AE, Cohen DJ, Curtis JP, Delong E, Drozda Jr JP, Ferguson Jr TB, Heidenreich PA, Hendel RC, Masoudi FA, Peterson ED, Taylor AJ, American College of Cardiology Foundation; American Heart Association Task Force on Performance Measures. ACCF/AHA methodology for the development of quality measures for cardiovascular technology: a report of the American College of Cardiology Foundation/American Heart Association Task Force on Performance Measures. Circulation. 2011;124(13):1483–502.
6. Kanne JP. Quality management in cardiopulmonary imaging. J Thorac Imaging. 2011;26(1):10–7.
7. Greaves C, Gilmore J, Bernhardt L, Ross L. Reducing imaging waiting times: enhanced roles and service-redesign. Int J Health Care Qual Assur. 2013;26(3):195–202.
8. Resnic FS, Welt FGP. The public health hazards of risk avoidance associated with public reporting of risk adjusted outcomes in coronary intervention. J Am Coll Cardiol. 2009;53(10):825–30.
9. Klein LW, Ho KK, Singh M, Anderson HV, Hillegass WB, Uretsky BF, Chambers C, Rao SV, Reilly J, Weiner BH, Kern M, Bailey S, Society of Cardiovascular Angiography and

Interventions. Quality assessment and improvement in interventional cardiology: a position statement of the Society of Cardiovascular Angiography and Interventions, part II: public reporting and risk adjustment. Catheter Cardiovasc Interv. 2011;78(4):493–502.

10. Smith IR, Foster KA, Brighouse RD, Cameron J, Rivers JT. The role of quantitative feedback in coronary angiography radiation reduction. Int J Qual Health Care. 2011;23(3):342–8.
11. Adair JG. The Hawthorne effect: a reconsideration of the methodological artifact. J Appl Psychol. 1984;69(2):334–45.
12. Smith IR, Cameron J, Brighouse RD, Ryan CM, Foster KA, Rivers JT. Impact of quantitative feedback and benchmark selection on radiation use by cardiologists performing cardiac angiography. Radiat Prot Dosimetry. 2013;155(1):32–41.
13. Chinnaiyan KM, Boura JA, DePetris A, Gentry R, Abidov A, Share DA, Raff GL, Advanced Cardiovascular Imaging Consortium Coinvestigators. Progressive radiation dose reduction from coronary computed tomography angiography in a statewide collaborative quality improvement program: results from the Advanced Cardiovascular Imaging Consortium. Circ Cardiovasc Imaging. 2013;6(5):646–54.
14. Maddox TM, Plomondon ME, Petrich M, Tsai TT, Gethoffer H, Noonan G, Gillespie B, Box T, Fihn SD, Jesse RL, Rumsfeld JS. A national clinical quality program for Veterans Affairs catheterization laboratories (from the Veterans Affairs clinical assessment, reporting, and tracking program). Am J Cardiol. 2014;114(11):1750–7.
15. Saifi S, Taylor AJ, Allen J, Hendel R. The use of a learning community and online evaluation of utilization for SPECT myocardial perfusion imaging. JACC Cardiovasc Imaging. 2013;6(7):823–9.
16. Shaw LJ, Wang TY, Mahmarian JJ, Tilkemeier PL, Douglas PS, Arrighi JA, Denton EA, Flood KB. Registry. J Nucl Cardiol. 2013;20(4):655–6.
17. Tilkemeier PL, Wang TY, Lytle BL, Denton EA. Milestones: ASNC ImageGuide™: cardiovascular imaging data registry. J Nucl Cardiol. 2013;20(6):1186–7.
18. Douglas PS, Chen J, Gillam L, Hendel R, Hundley WG, Masoudi F, Patel MR, Peterson E. Achieving quality in cardiovascular imaging II: proceedings from the Second American College of Cardiology – Duke University Medical Center Think Tank on Quality in Cardiovascular Imaging. JACC Cardiovasc Imaging. 2009;2(2):231–40.

Index

P.L. Tilkemeier et al. (eds.), *Quality Evaluation in Non-Invasive Cardiovascular Imaging*, DOI 10.1007/978-3-319-28011-0

Q

R

S

T

V

MIX
Papier aus verantwortungsvollen Quellen
Paper from responsible sources
FSC® C105338

If you have any concerns about our products,
you can contact us on
ProductSafety@springernature.com

In case Publisher is established outside the EU,
the EU authorized representative is:
Springer Nature Customer Service Center GmbH
Europaplatz 3, 69115 Heidelberg, Germany

Printed by Libri Plureos GmbH
in Hamburg, Germany